SMALL

ANIMAL

ANESTHESIA

by
WILLIAM V. LUMB,
D.V.M., M.S., Ph.D.

*Professor of Veterinary Medicine, Colorado
State University, Fort Collins, Colorado*

125 Illustrations, one in color

Lea & Febiger

Philadelphia   1963

Library of Congress Catalog Card Number 63:16704

Printed in the United States of America

To my father,
J. W. Lumb, D. V. M.

PREFACE

In the past twenty years veterinary anesthesiology has made great strides. New equipment, new drugs, and new techniques have developed with amazing rapidity. While teaching small animal anesthesiology it became apparent to me that although much information on this subject has been published, most of it is quite inaccessible to the student or practitioner. Thus a need existed for a comprehensive text which contained material from widely diverse sources and which integrated this information. It is believed that this text will introduce the veterinary student to anesthetic principles and serve as a reference for those already familiar with common techniques. It will also prove useful to persons other than veterinarians who have reason to anesthetize animals.

No attempt has been made to make the contents strictly "practical"; rather, emphasis has been placed on basic principles and broad coverage of the subject matter. References are furnished for those desiring to investigate specific topics more thoroughly. The pharmacology of many drugs is outlined, since this knowledge is essential for proper use; similarly, instructions for operating many types of anesthetic equipment are also included.

Appendix A has been added so the reader can obtain any drug or equipment described. Appendix B contains standard values and conversion tables, while Appendix C is a formula for euthanasia solution.

As with all texts, some controversial material is included. I have used most of the techniques described in the Small Animal Clinic of the Colorado State University College of Veterinary Medicine. In instances where a procedure is considered definitely undesirable, attention is directed to this fact and the reasons stated. Accounts of experiences with various anesthetic techniques and constructive criticism of the text from readers will be appreciated.

So many persons have contributed to preparation of this book that it is impossible to acknowledge the assistance of each. Though they remain nameless their help was invaluable.

The author is deeply indebted to Dr. Lee R. Phillips of Denver, Colorado and Dr. N. H. Booth of Fort Collins, Colorado who critically reviewed the manuscript and made many suggestions for its improvement. Drs. R. W. Davis, W. A. Wolff, and A. B. Dodge gave valuable information concerning deer, elk, and falcons respectively. Art work and line drawings were done by Mrs. Pat Dietemann who also designed the cover. Mrs. Phyllis Davis, Mrs. Ann Thomason, Mrs. Mary Carroll and Mrs. Rosemary Peake typed most of the manuscript.

Thanks are due my colleagues who have shown remarkable forebearance in assuming part of my clinical duties during the past three years.

My wife, Lilly, has contributed materially through encouragement, suggestions, typing, and proofreading during the entire period of preparation.

WILLIAM V. LUMB

FORT COLLINS, COLORADO

CONTENTS

AN OUTLINE OF SMALL ANIMAL ANESTHESIA

Chapter 1

Introduction

Anesthesia is one of the great miracles of medicine. It has reduced pain in both man and animals and has enabled surgeons to save untold numbers of lives. The never-ending search for better anesthetic agents and techniques has been mutually beneficial to both veterinary and human patients. As veterinary medicine matures, safe efficient small animal anesthetic techniques are becoming a reality.

Definitions

The word anesthesia comes from the Greek word *anaisthesia*, meaning "insensibility or not feeling." Anesthesia is produced by agents which depress the activity of nervous tissue either locally or generally. A number of terms are used in describing depression of nervous tissue:

1. *Analgesia* refers to relief from pain.

2. *Tranquilization* is a state of behavioral change in which the patient is relaxed and unconcerned by his surroundings. In this state he is often indifferent to minor pain.

3. *Sedation* is a mild degree of central depression in which the patient is awake but calm.

4. *Narcosis* in man is defined as a drug-produced state of deep sleep accompanied by analgesia. In veterinary medicine the narcotized patient is seldom asleep but is sedated and oblivious to pain.

5. *Hypnosis* is a condition of artificially induced sleep, or a trance resembling sleep, resulting from moderate depression of the central nervous system.

(9)

6. *Local anesthesia* is loss of sensation in a limited body area.

7. *Regional anesthesia* is insensibility in a larger though limited body area.

8. *Basal anesthesia* is a light level of general anesthesia usually produced by preanesthetic agents. It serves as a basis for deeper anesthesia on administration of other agents.

9. *General anesthesia* is complete unconsciousness.

10. *Surgical anesthesia* is unconsciousness, accompanied by muscular relaxation to such a degree that surgery can be performed painlessly and without struggling on the part of the patient.

History of Small Animal Anesthesia

The high standards and achievements of modern surgery have resulted to a great extent from the application of two discoveries, anesthesia and aseptic technique. Prior to the introduction of general anesthesia, surgery was a horribly painful experience for the patient and was often accompanied by fatal shock. To reduce the agony, surgeons attempted to operate as fast as possible; consequently, hemostasis was poor and delicate or meticulous operations were impossible. Those patients which survived the operation and immediate postoperative period often died from sepsis during convalesence.

The ancients used narcotics, alcohol, and even asphyxia to alleviate pain during surgical procedures. About 1540, Paracelsus produced ether and noted its soporific effect on fowls. Joseph Priestly laid the foundation for anesthesia through his discovery of carbon dioxide (date unknown), oxygen (1771), and nitrous oxide (1772). Sir Humphrey Davy published a book in 1800 on "Researches, Chemical and Philosophical; Chiefly Concerning Nitrous Oxide . . ." which suggested the possible anesthetic qualities of this gas. In 1824 H. H. Hickman, an English surgeon, conducted several experiments in administration of carbon dioxide to animals on which he then operated. Hickman is credited with first proving by animal experimentation that the pain of a surgical operation could be abolished by inhalation of a gas.

Dr. C. W. Long of Jefferson, Georgia was first to perform an actual surgical operation on a person under ether anesthesia in 1842. His discovery was not widely published and its use, therefore, did not become general until others, working independently, made the same discovery. In 1844 Dr. Horace Wells, a dentist of Hartford, Connecticut, discovered the general anesthetic properties of nitrous oxide. Although he failed to convince medical science of its value, he is credited with publicizing the possibility of its use in surgery. The first major surgical operation performed on a person under ether anesthesia was done in the year 1846 at the Massachusetts General Hospital in Boston. Dr. W. T. G. Morton, a dentist who administered the anesthetic, is said to have previously practiced the technique on a puppy.

Dr. C. T. Jackson, a Boston physician, was perhaps the first to use ether to any extent on animals. Writing in 1853 he stated,

> "In 1846 . . . I also indicated its use in preventing all sensation in domestic animals upon which surgical operations were to be performed. . . . The means is easy, safe and efficient and any intelligent person can administer the ether. . . ."

In January of 1847, Edward Mayhew, an English veterinarian, reported experiments on dogs and cats in which the head of the animal was introduced into a bladder connected to an ether-filled flask (Smithcors, 1957). He claimed that cats were anesthetized in as little as 10 seconds and dogs in 15 to 45 seconds!

Chloroform was discovered by von Liebig in 1831. It was used for general anesthesia in animals by Flourens, a French physiologist, in 1847 and, in the same year, in man by Dr. J. Y. Simpson of Edinburgh, Scotland. In 1848 Thomas Nunneley, an English surgeon, introduced "A.C.E. mixture" containing 1 part alcohol, 2 parts chloroform, and 3 parts ether, and described its use on cats (Clark, 1938).

At least one American physician turned veterinarian was quick to appreciate the possibilities of these new discoveries; G. H. Dadd, in the 1850's, was routinely using general anesthesia. Dadd's book, *The Modern Horse Doctor* (1854), was the first in America to advocate humane treatment of animals and the application of scientific principles in veterinary practice.

In 1806 Friedrich W. Sertürner, a German chemist, discovered morphine. However, efficient use was not made of this drug until development in 1853 of the hollow needle by Wood and the hypodermic syringe by Pravaz. The latter discoveries also laid the foundation for use of cocaine which was isolated by Albert Niemann of Germany in 1860. In 1878 von Anrep suggested the possibility of using cocaine for local anesthesia after injecting himself in the arm with a weak solution (Keys, 1942). In 1884 Karl Koller introduced cocaine for local anesthesia of the eye, and Halstead described nerve block anesthesia a year later. Sir Fredrick Hobday, an English veterinarian, popularized its use for veterinary surgery. J. L. Corning, using cocaine, is credited with inducing spinal anesthesia in a dog in 1885. However, from his description it would appear that he probably produced epidural anesthesia. In 1898 August Bier of Germany produced true spinal anesthesia in animals and then in himself and an assistant (Keys, 1942). Meanwhile, the use of morphine and chloral hydrate intraperitoneally for anesthesia in the dog was reported from France (———, 1892).

Perhaps due to unfavorable sequelae, general anesthesia was not readily adopted by the veterinary profession. Until well into the 20th century a heavy hand, without anesthesia, was the stock in trade of the average veterinarian. In a paper describing "ovariotomy", presented to Cornell University in 1900 for the degree of Doctor of Veterinary Medicine, Jewell stated,

> "The securing of the smaller animals is simple. Place the animal outstretched upon an inclined surface with the side upward on which the incision is to be made, the mouth being previously muzzled if a dog or cat. The legs should be secured with small ropes and fully extended. An assistant should hold the animal firmly."

While practices such as these were being condoned and even taught in veterinary schools, others, fortunately, were taking a more progressive stand. In 1900 Dr. R. W. Ellis, a practitioner, reported the successful correction of a ventral hernia in a cat under ether anesthesia. Explaining his reasons for reporting the case, he stated,

> ". . . another reason is, to encourage the use of ether in all operative procedures with cats, whether it be simply the extraction of a tooth, castrating a developed male (not necessary with very young kittens), or the more important and intricate operations that may present themselves. The administration of ether to cats is reasonably safe—the more you use it the more confident you will grow on that point; but if you wait for major operations, you will be long in becoming familiar with its use."

Veterinary anesthesiology has made tremendous strides since 1900. New groups of drugs, such as the barbiturates and tranquilizers, have been introduced and special equipment has been developed specifically for small animals. The fact that today veterinarians have a wide choice of anesthetic agents and techniques is due to the foresight, imagination, and perseverance of these early pioneers.

Theories of Anesthesia

Substances producing general anesthesia cause a descending paralysis of the central nervous system beginning in the cortex, progressing to the spinal cord and finally affecting the vital centers of the medulla. Anesthetic agents differ greatly in structure since they include hydrocarbons, alcohols, ethers, urethanes, sulfones, and amides. It is impossible, except in a homologous series of substances, to show any relationship between anesthetic action and chemical constitution. Therefore, many of the theories of narcosis have been based on physical properties of the anesthetics. The Meyer-Overton theory is an example. (Sollmann, 1948) It states that there is a relationship between anesthetic activity and the distribution of certain drugs in a lipoid-water system. It has also been shown that there is an alteration in the permeability of the cell membrane. These observations, however, simply give an indication of how the drug may gain access to the cells or cell surfaces. They do not explain how function of the cell is influenced.

The cerebral cortex can easily be depressed by altering its blood supply. Also, there is a definite relationship between the physiological activity of the brain and its utilization of oxygen and glucose. It is this relationship which appears to be affected by anesthetics. When the cerebral circulation of the dog is perfused with pentobarbital sodium at a constant rate, the oxygen uptake of the brain and utilization of glucose is reduced approximately 30% (Handley et al., 1941). Working with brain slices in vitro, Quastel and coworkers (Jowett, 1937a, b; Michaelis, 1941) demonstrated that such drugs as ether, chloretone, and barbiturates inhibit the respiration of brain tissue in concentrations which cause deep narcosis in vivo. The effect is rapid and reversible and brain tissue has been shown to be much more sensitive to this effect than kidney, liver, spleen, and testes. Michaelis and Quastel (1941) stated,

> "The fact that glucose oxidation is quantitatively the most important respiratory process in brain in vivo makes it likely that in vivo as well as in vitro, narcotics exert inhibitory effects on glucose oxidation by the brain."

Based on statements by Michaelis and Quastel, Greig (1946) drew the following chart showing the narcotic sensitive region in the oxidation process and possible sites of narcotic block (Fig. 1–1).

She further showed that pentobarbital caused blocking at position II where flavoprotein is oxidized by the cytochrome system. In vitamin C deficient guinea pigs, pentobarbital anesthesia is prolonged but will be reduced if these animals are given ascorbic acid. Greig (1947) found that when ascorbic acid is added to brain suspensions containing pentobarbital, glucose metabolism is increased despite the presence of pentobarbital. She suggested that ascorbic acid offers an alternative route for the oxidation of carbohydrate by providing a bypass between flavoprotein and cytochrome c (Fig. 1–2).

According to Wilson (1949), ether and chloroform affect acetylcholine metabolism of the central nervous system more directly than

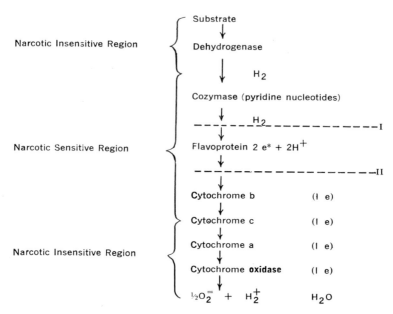

FIGURE 1–1. Possible sites of narcotic action in the oxidation process are indicated at I and II (*e = electron). (Greig, M. E.: The Site of Action of Narcotics on Brain Metabolism. J. Pharm. & Exper. Therap., *87*, 185, 1946.)

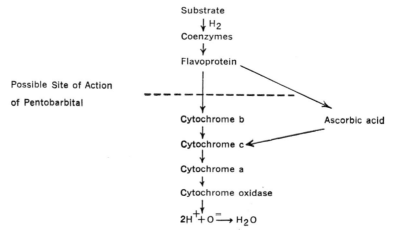

FIGURE 1–2. Bypass for carbohydrate oxidation provided by ascorbic acid. (Greig, M. E.: The Effect of Ascorbic Acid in Reducing the Inhibition of Brain Metabolism Produced by Pentobarbital *in Vitro*. J. Pharm. & Exper. Therap., *91*, 317, 1947.)

do barbiturates. Since different areas of the brain vary greatly in
ability to synthesize acetylcholine and in cholinesterase content, it
is possible that the different effects of volatile anesthetics and barbiturates may be due to variation in sites of action.

Both the volatile anesthetics and barbiturates have one point in
common; the synthesis of acetylcholine is dependent on carbohydrate metabolism. It may be that this synthesis is affected by the
various agents at different stages.

Reasons for Administration of Anesthetics

Because anesthesia was first developed to alleviate pain and
provide relaxation for surgery, its use for other purposes is sometimes overlooked. It is employed in small animals for a wide variety
of procedures most of which are listed below:

A. RESTRAINT
    1. Splinting.
    2. Wound dressing.
    3. Grooming fractious or matted animals.
    4. Radiotherapy.
    5. Cleaning ears.
    6. Prevention of wound irritation by licking, chewing, scratching.

B. EXAMINATION
    1. Eye.
    2. Ear.
    3. Nose.
    4. Throat.
    5. Palpation of abdomen (relaxation of abdominal musculature).
    6. Skeletal system.
    7. Endoscopic examination.
        a. bronchoscopy.
        b. esophagoscopy.
        c. gastroscopy.
        d. proctoscopy.
        e. vaginoscopy.
    8. Radiography.

C. MANIPULATION
    1. Closed reduction of fractures, luxations.
    2. Breakdown of rectal impactions.
    3. Catheterization.

D. SURGERY OF ALL KINDS

E. CONTROL OF CONVULSIVE SEIZURES
    1. Poisoning.
    2. Encephalitis.
    3. Epilepsy.

F. EUTHANASIA
    1. Generally accomplished by an overdose of an anesthetic.

Types of Anesthesia

Because of the diversity of uses for which anesthetic agents are employed, no agent administered by a single route can effectively perform all these tasks efficiently. For this reason many agents, which may be administered by a variety of methods, are utilized. Anesthesia has been divided into types according to the route of administration and drug employed:

A. INHALATION
Anesthesia is produced by inhalation of gases or vapors of volatile liquids.

B. INTRAVASCULAR
A solution of the anesthetic is injected into the blood stream by one of the following routes:
1. Intravenous
2. Intra-arterial
3. Intracardial
4. Intramedullary (marrow puncture)

C. INTRAPERITONEAL
A solution of the anesthetic is injected into the peritoneal cavity from which it is absorbed into the systemic circulation.

D. INTRATHORACIC
A solution of the anesthetic is injected into the thoracic cavity following which it is absorbed into the general circulation.

E. SUBCUTANEOUS OR INTRAMUSCULAR
Aqueous or oily solutions of soluble drugs are injected into subcutaneous or muscle tissue.

F. ORAL
Solid or liquid drugs are given *per os* and are absorbed from the upper gastrointestinal tract.

G. RECTAL
An enema of an aqueous or oily solution is given and is absorbed into the systemic circulation.

H. TOPICAL
An agent is applied on the surface of a tissue to block the nerve endings.

I. INFILTRATION
Anesthesia is accomplished by injecting the anesthetic into the tissues to be cut, blocking the nerve endings that will actually be disturbed by the surgeon.

J. FIELD BLOCK
Anesthetic solution is injected around the periphery of the surgical area.

K. CONDUCTION (NERVE BLOCK OR REGIONAL)
Anesthesia is induced by blocking nerves at a site distant from the operation. This can be subdivided into:
1. Nerve block
The agent is deposited around a nerve trunk.

2. Epidural (extradural, peridural, caudal)

The anesthetic is deposited in the epidural space so that it contacts the spinal nerves where they emerge from the dura and before they leave the spinal canal.

3. Spinal

The drug is injected into the subarachnoid space so that it contacts the anterior and posterior (dorsal and ventral) roots and the sympathetic fibers of the nerve as it passes from the spinal cord.

L. ELECTRONARCOSIS

An electrical current is passed through the cerebrum.

M. HYPNOSIS

Anesthesia is induced by placing the patient in a trance-like state.

N. HYPOTHERMIA

The body temperature is lowered, either locally or generally, to the point where anesthesia is produced.

References

CLARK, A. J.: Aspects of the History of Anaesthetics. Brit. Med. J., *2*, 1029, 1938.

DADD, G. H.: *The Modern Horse Doctor.* J. P. Jewett and Company, Boston, 1854.

ELLIS, R. W.: Hernia in a Cat—Surgical Interference—Recovery. Am. Vet. Rev., *24*, 427, 1900.

GREIG, M. E.: The Site of Action of Narcotics on Brain Metabolism. J. Pharm. & Exper. Therap., *87*, 185, 1946.

GREIG, M. E.: The Effect of Ascorbic Acid in Reducing the Inhibition of Brain Metabolism Produced by Pentobarbital *in Vitro.* J. Pharm. & Exper. Therap., *91*, 317, 1947.

HANDLEY, C. A., SWEENEY, H. M., and BROOKMAN, B. T.: Metabolism in Perfused Dog's Head during Sodium Pentobarbital Depression and Metrazol Stimulation. Proc. Soc. Exper. Biol. & Med., *48*, 670, 1941.

JACKSON, C. T.: *Etherization of Animals.* Report of the Commissioner of Patents for the Year 1853. Beverly Tucker, Senate Printer, Washington, D. C. p. 59, 1853.

JEWELL, C. H.: Ovariotomy in the Domestic Animals. Am. Vet. Rev., *24*, 353, 1900.

JOWETT, M. and QUASTEL, J. H.: LXXIX. The Effects of Narcotics on Tissue Oxidations. Biochem. J., *31*, 565, 1937.

JOWETT, M. and QUASTEL, J. H.: CXLVI. The Effects of Ether on Brain Oxidations. Biochem. J., *31*, 1101, 1937.

KEYS, T. E.: The Development of Anesthesia. Anesthesiology, *3*, 11, 1942.

MICHAELIS, M. and QUASTEL, J. H.: 53. The Site of Action of Narcotics in Respiratory Processes. Biochem. J., *35*, 518, 1941.

SMITHCORS, J. F.: The Early Use of Anaesthesia in Veterinary Practice. Brit. Vet. J., *113*, 284, 1957.

SOLLMANN, T.: *A Manual of Pharmacology.* 7th ed., W. B. Saunders Co., Philadelphia, p. 604, 1948.

WILSON, A.: The Pharmacological Basis of Modern Anaesthesia, Proc. Roy. Soc. Med., *42*, 522, 1949.

————————: De l'anesthesie par l'injection intra-peritoneale d'une solution de chloral seul ou associé a la morphine. Ann. med. Vet., *41*, 345, 1892.

GENERAL
CONSIDERATIONS

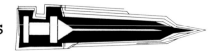

Chapter 2

Factors Altering Anesthesia

Anesthesia is of necessity a reversible process. Knowledge of the factors underlying production of anesthesia, and those which may modify it, is essential to success of the procedure. It should be remembered that the dose of an anesthetic and the technique for its administration are based on the *average* animal. However, because of the many phenomena which modify the effect of an anesthetic agent, it is unlikely that any given animal will be exactly "average."

Marked variations in response to a standard dose of anesthetic result from the interplay of many factors. Since detoxification of anesthetics depends on the metabolic processes of the animal, conditions affecting the metabolic rate exert a marked influence on anesthetic effect. Among these are the following:

1. *Relative Size.* Small animals have a higher basal metabolic rate per unit of body weight than large animals; therefore, the smaller the animal the larger the dose per unit of body weight necessary for anesthesia (Fig. 2–1). The larger breeds of dogs, which require relatively small amounts of pentobarbital compared to toy breeds, are an example of this.

2. *Physical Condition.* Animals with large quantities of fat, which is a relatively inactive non-metabolizing tissue, will have a lower basal metabolic rate per unit of body weight and will require less anesthetic than lean muscular animals in good condition. Greyhounds, an example of the latter, are notorious for their tendency toward hyperesthesia on induction and recovery (Knight, 1949).

Animals in poor condition also require less anesthetic. De Boer (1947) found that dogs kept on a low food intake resulting in weight losses of 10 to 20% showed a marked increase in duration of anesthesia following a single injection.

3. *Age.* In the newborn, the basal metabolic rate is low. It grad-

(18)

ually increases to its highest point at the time of puberty through early adulthood and then gradually declines (Fig. 2–2).

De Boer (1947) has shown that there is a variation in sleeping time caused by a standard dose of anesthetic in dogs of various ages. Very young animals and older adult animals were found most sensitive; whereas, dogs in the age range from 3 to 12 months were anesthetized the shortest period of time. The total amount of thiopental necessary to inhibit respiration was greater in dogs 3 to

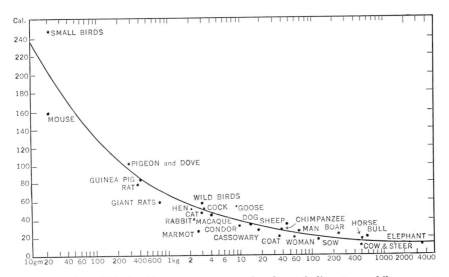

FIGURE 2–1. Relationship between average basal metabolic rate per kilogram per day of different species (vertical axis) and average body weight (abscissa). The weight range is from 20 gm. to 4000 kg. Semilogarithmic chart. (From Benedict, Vital Energetics: A Study in Comparative Basal Metabolism. Carnegie Institution of Washington Publ. No. 503, 1938.)

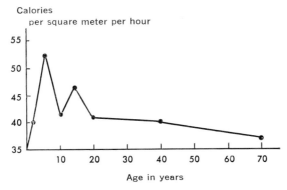

FIGURE 2–2. Graph of basal metabolism, expressed in calories per square meter of body surface area per hour, as related to age in man. (From Collins, V. J.: *Principles and Practice of Anesthesiology.* Lea & Febiger, 1952.)

12 months old than in older and younger dogs. In addition, when multiple injections were given every 15 minutes until death occurred, animals in the 3 to 12 month group survived the longest.

4. *Sex.* The basal metabolic rate of males is approximately 7% higher than females. In the female a rise occurs during pregnancy due to the metabolic activity of the fetuses. Conflicting evidence concerning sex differences in susceptibility to anesthetics has been presented. The anesthetic used may be the determining factor.

Nicholas and Barron (1932) showed that definite sex variance existed in the susceptibility of rats to sodium amytal anesthesia. Pregnant females were most susceptible, nonpregnant females less, and male rats least susceptible. Pregnant females required an average dose of only 10 mg./100 gm., whereas, males required 20 mg./100 gm. On the other hand, Kennedy (1934) could find no sex variance in mice to hexobarbital anesthesia. Cameron (1938) has shown that normal females are less susceptible to pentobarbital sodium than spayed females, as evidenced in the latter by longer duration of anesthesia and increased mortality. Sex hormones may also cause differences in response to an anesthetic agent other than those resulting from the change in metabolic rate (See page 22).

5. *Recent Feeding.* According to Dukes (1947) a large meal of meat may increase the metabolic rate of dogs as much as 90% above the basal level (specific dynamic effect). Carbohydrate and fat also produce this elevation, though to a lesser extent. It is usually 12 to 18 hours after the last meal before the basal metabolic rate is attained in carnivorous animals.

6. *Activity.* The metabolic rate increases with activity; hence, very active animals require relatively large doses of anesthetic agents.

7. *Preanesthetic Medication.* Morphine lowers the metabolic rate; atropine causes a slight rise. When administered in combination, however, the metabolic rate is decreased. Tranquilizers usually lower the metabolic rate.

8. *Fear and Excitement.* It is a well known fact that animals showing a period of excitement on induction of anesthesia always require more anesthetic. This causes a tendency toward overdosing with its attendant dangers. For this reason preanesthetic sedation is recommended.

9. *Concurrent Disease.* The effect of disease on the metabolic rate usually varies with its duration. In the early febrile stage the rate may be increased; however, as the disease progresses toxemia may reduce it to very low levels. Fever increases the metabolic rate in accordance with van't Hoff's law, which states that for each degree Fahrenheit the temperature rises, the metabolic rate is increased 7%. When animals suffer from toxemia or liver disease, the functions

of this organ are impaired and the ability of the animal to detoxify short-acting barbiturates is depressed. Under these circumstances the dose of pentobarbital may be reduced to one-tenth of that usually required. Shock lowers the metabolic rate and, because of circulatory inefficiency, decreases absorption and distribution of anesthetic agents; therefore, their full effect may not be manifest in the normal time.

Guinea pigs with vitamin C deficiency have been shown to be more susceptible to anesthesia as evidenced by earlier induction, deeper anesthesia, and slower recovery (Beyer et al., 1944). Vitamin C deficient guinea pigs recover slowly, if at all, from anesthesia which has little apparent after-effect on animals injected daily with ascorbic acid.

Hyperthyroidism is accompanied by an elevated metabolic rate, whereas hypothyroidism is accompanied by lowering of the metabolic rate. Totally thyroidectomized dogs require very small doses of anesthetic.

Leukemia in some forms increases the metabolic rate as does severe pain (Adriani, 1958).

Apart from things which alter the metabolic rate, and hence the activity of a given dose of anesthetic agent, other factors may modify its action:

1. *Concentration and Rate of Administration of the Anesthetic Agent.* With short-acting barbiturates particularly, concentration and rate of injection of a given dose will affect anesthetic action. The more dilute the agent or the slower the injection, the less effect produced.

2. *Tolerance.* Green and Koppanyi (1944) demonstrated that on repeated daily injection of hexobarbital, thiopental, and propallylonal, dogs develop a marked tolerance to these drugs as evidenced by a significant reduction in sleeping time. A cross-tolerance to the other two barbiturates and also to barbital was shown to occur. The tolerance is short-lasting and disappears in less than 2 weeks. Hubbard and Goldbaum (1949) observed the same phenomenon in mice injected with thiopental, sleeping time being reduced 50% after 5 or 6 daily injections. They believed the tolerance mechanism was one of adaptation to higher thiopental tissue levels rather than increased excretion or destruction of drug.

3. *Concurrent Administration of Other Drugs.* It has been shown that sulfonamides cause an increased susceptibility to pentobarbital, ether, and chloroform anesthesia (Butler et al., 1941). This increased susceptibility is great enough to be considered when one large predetermined dose of an anesthetic is administered.

Polymixin B, streptomycin, and neomycin produce partial neuromuscular block. Neomycin produces a far greater block in the presence of ether than by itself. Deaths in humans undergoing anesthesia have been attributed to the combination, death being due to prolonged respiratory paralysis (Sabawala and Dillon, 1959).

4. *Hemorrhage.* Removal of 2% of the body weight in blood tremendously prolongs the recovery time from thiopental anesthesia in dogs (De Boer, 1947). It may be concluded that hemorrhage, such as might accompany a surgical procedure, will significantly increase sleeping time.

5. *Recent Feeding.* In addition to altering the metabolic rate, feeding increases chylomicrons in the blood stream. It has been shown that thiobarbiturates will localize in these and the duration of anesthesia will be shortened (Anderson and Magee, 1956).

6. *Sex.* Selye (1941) demonstrated that steroid hormones injected intravenously or intramuscularly in massive doses are capable of producing general anesthesia in experimental animals. This action is limited to steroids with hormonal action. Females are more susceptible than males to this type of anesthesia. Spayed females show no alteration in susceptibility, but castrated males are as susceptible as females. The administration of androgens lessens the susceptibility of females and castrated males to the point that it equals that of intact males. Partial hepatectomy increases the anesthetic action of the steroids in both sexes. Cameron (1949) has theorized that testosterone is in some way connected with hepatic detoxification mechanisms.

Physical Examination

"For every mistake that is made for not knowing, a hundred are made for not looking."
—Anonymous

A thorough preoperative physical examination of the patient is essential to successful anesthesia and surgery. It will often save the veterinarian later embarrassment. The following should be included:

1. Inspection of the skin and hair coat.
2. Examination of the conjunctiva, mouth and throat, and other body orifices.
3. Palpation of the superficial lymph nodes.
4. Palpation of the abdominal viscera.
5. Auscultation of the heart and lungs.
6. Determination of body temperature.

Ancillary examinations which may be indicated include:

1. Red, white, and differential blood counts.
2. Hemoglobin and/or hematocrit determinations.
3. Urinalysis.
4. Fecal examination.
5. Determination of blood urea nitrogen.
6. Clotting time.
7. Examination for filaria.
8. X-ray or fluoroscopic examination.

Following examination the physical status of the patient should be classified and recorded if accurate records are kept (Table 2–1). Whether recorded or not, this mental exercise forces the anesthetist to evaluate the patient's condition and proves valuable in proper selection of the agent to be used. Classification of physical status is an essential part of any anesthetic record system (Chapter 19).

Table 2–1.—Classification of Physical Status

Category	Physical Status	Possible Examples of This Category
I	Healthy. No discernible disease.	Animals entered for ovariohysterectomy, ear trim, caudectomy.
II	Pre-existing disease. No discernible systemic symptoms.	Skin tumor, fracture without shock, uncomplicated hernia, localized infection, compensated cardiac disease.
III	Pre-existing disease. Mild systemic symptoms.	Low fever, slight dehydration, slight anemia, slight cachexia.
IV	Pre-existing disease. Severe systemic symptoms.	Uremia, toxemia, severe shock, severe dehydration, anemia, cardiac decompensation, emaciation, high fever. Includes all moribund animals.

The preliminary physical examination should be done in the owner's presence, if possible, so that a prognosis can be given personally. This allows the client to ask questions and enables the veterinarian to allay any fears concerning management of the patient. An experienced veterinarian is always careful to "lay the cards on the table." In response to such a leading question as, "Is there a possibility he may die?" it should be carefully explained that, while there is a possibility that the animal may die, the reason for administration of anesthesia more than justifies the slight risk entailed.

Selection of the Anesthetic Agent

The ideal anesthetic agent is one which:

1. Does not depend on detoxifying mechanisms within the body for its destruction and elimination.

2. Permits rapid induction, quick alteration in depth of anesthesia, and rapid recovery.
3. Does not depress respiratory and cardiac centers.
4. Is not irritant to any tissue.
5. Is inexpensive, stable, noninflammable, and nonexplosive.
6. Requires no special equipment for administration.

No agent available today possesses all these qualities. Therefore, selection of an agent is a compromise based on appraisal of the situation at hand. Factors to be considered include:

1. The patient's species, breed, and age.
2. Physical status of the patient.
3. The time required for the surgical (or other) procedure, its type and severity, and the surgeon's skill.
4. Familiarity with the proposed anesthetic technique.
5. Equipment and personnel available.

Table 2-2 indicates the relationship of some of these factors to anesthetic agents commonly employed.

In general the veterinarian will have greatest success with agents he has used most frequently and with which he is most familiar. The art of administration is developed only with experience, therefore change from a familiar agent to a new one is usually accompanied by a temporary increase in the mortality rate. Clark (1938) speaking of anesthesia in man stated,

> "The outstanding fact is that thorough familiarity with a technique is equivalent at least to a 30 per cent difference in efficiency. If a person has mastered a technique, it is not worth his while changing to a new and unfamiliar one unless the change promises some big advantage."

Often the length of time required to perform a surgical procedure and the amount of help available during this period dictate the anesthetic which is used. Generally, very short procedures are done with short-lasting agents, such as thiobarbiturates, and long procedures with longer-lasting agents, such as pentobarbital. On the other hand, where help is ample, long periods of anesthesia may be maintained by intermittent injections of thiobarbiturates, or by inhalation anesthesia.

Certain agents, such as anesthetic gases, cannot be administered without considerable equipment. Hence, lack of adequate facilities and help for administration automatically rules out certain anesthetics.

Species differences may prevent the use of some drugs. For example, procaine is lethal for parakeets and morphine is excitatory for cats. On the other hand, most agents can be used interchangeably among species at approximately the same dose level per unit of body weight.

Anesthesia in the very young is attended with increased risk. This is due to size limitations, lower metabolic rate and, perhaps, immature detoxification mechanisms. For this reason the use of pentobarbital in the very young is contraindicated.

Aged animals are often poor anesthetic risks due to decreased stamina and the possibility of chronic heart, liver, or kidney disease which may be inapparent on casual examination. These animals, therefore, should not be given agents which are irritant to these body tissues or which require good liver and kidney function for their detoxification or elimination. The same is true of patients in a poor physical state due to febrile disease, since the liver and kidneys usually are somewhat affected, regardless of the location of the disease within the body.

General anesthesia is to be avoided, if at all possible, in animals with an elevated blood urea nitrogen. Local, regional, or epidural anesthesia should be used where possible. If general anesthesia must be used the thiobarbiturates and inhalant anesthetics are preferred; pentobarbital should never be employed under these circumstances.

A cardiac murmur *per se* is not a contraindication for general anesthesia since surprisingly few animals with murmurs die from anesthesia *provided* they are compensated. However, they have less cardiac reserve and require more careful supervision during anesthesia. Dogs with heartworm infestation and congenital lesions of the heart and great vessels also fall in this category. Use of a thiobarbiturate or a thiobarbiturate in combination with an inhalant anesthetic is indicated.

Brachycephalic dogs, because of their pendulous soft palate and restricted respiratory passages, have difficulty in breathing even when awake. Under anesthesia this difficulty is compounded and many of these animals die because a patent airway is not maintained. Therefore, it is wise to use agents which are short-lasting, and with which the depth of anesthesia can be easily controlled so that a prolonged recovery period is avoided. Many small animal facilities are now air-conditioned and year-round surgery can be undertaken without considering the weather. During the summer months, in hospitals which are not air-conditioned, anesthesia may present a problem. This is particularly true of brachycephalic breeds. In hot, humid weather it is sometimes better to delay surgery on these animals than chance losing them through anesthesia and attendant struggling during the recovery period.

Table 2-2.—Indications and Contraindications for Some Common Anesthetic Agents

Physical Condition or Reason for Anesthesia	Agent or Technique									
	Pentobarbital	Thiamylal	Thiopental	Halothane	Methoxyflurane	Ether	Morphine-Apomorphine	Infiltration, field, or nerve block	Epidural	Tranquilizer
Animals Under 6 Weeks of Age	No	X (2%)	X (3.2%)		With caution	X	No	X	No	With caution
Aged Animals	With caution	X	X	X	X	X	X	X	X	X
Brachycephalic Dogs	Only if necessary	X	X	X	X	X	X	X	X	X
Cesarean Section	No	Not advisable		X	X	X	X	+ Tranquilizer	X	+ Another agent
Febrile Animals	Only if necessary	X	X	X	X	If necessary	X	X	X	X

Condition									
Shock	No	With extreme caution				No	X	No	With extreme caution
Uremia	No	Use only when absolutely necessary				No	X	X	With caution
Cardiac Disease — Compensated	Only if necessary	Use only when absolutely necessary	X	X	X	X	X	X	X
Cardiac Disease — Uncompensated	No		X	X	X	No	X	No	When absolutely necessary. Reduce dose
Respiratory Disease	No	X	Suitable in conditions where lung irritation is not important			No	X	X	
Hepatic Disease	No	No	Use only when absolutely necessary			No	X	X	When necessary. Reduce dose

X = Generally suitable for use.

In animals with diaphragmatic hernia, pentobarbital is not as safe as intermittent doses of thiobarbiturate or thiobarbiturate plus an inhalation anesthetic.

As a group the barbiturates are contraindicated for cesarean section because of the respiratory depression which is produced in the newborn. Also, there is some indication that pentobarbital should not be used for any reason in pregnant animals if the effect on the fetuses is a consideration. Becker *et al.* (1958) have shown that administration of pentobarbital to pregnant guinea pigs on either the 22nd, 42nd, or 63rd day of gestation resulted in high mortality in the young. In addition, symptoms of neural damage were seen in the survivors. Thiobarbiturates can be used for cesarean section either alone or in combination with an inhalant but a lower survival rate in the young will result. This is particularly true when the operation follows a prolonged labor.

A number of satisfactory anesthetic techniques are available for cesarean section including administration of inhalants, use of narcosis, or tranquilization and injection of local or epidural anesthetics.

Patient Preparation

Too often, operations are undertaken with inadequate preparation of the patient. A little foresight here will pay big dividends. With most types of general anesthesia it is best to have the patient off feed for 12 hours previously. Water, in most instances, can be offered up to the time that preanesthetic agents are given. It should be remembered that many old dogs suffer from nephritis. While these animals remain compensated under ideal conditions, the trauma of hospitalization, water deprivation, and anesthesia, even without surgery, may cause acute decompensation. To withhold water from these animals, even for short periods, may prove fatal.

Systemic administration of antibiotics preoperatively is a helpful prophylactic measure if shock or contamination of the operative site are anticipated. Oral antibiotics have been shown to "sterilize" the bowel very effectively and should be used prior to elective surgery of the gastrointestinal tract. In surgery of the colon, rectum, and anus, preoperative enemas administered a day or two prior to surgery will remove fecal material and facilitate manipulation. On the other hand, an enema just prior to surgery may complicate the situation, since feces will be very fluid and the operative site may easily become contaminated because of this.

Dehydrated animals should be treated with fluids and vitamins *prior* to surgery. The delay occasioned by administration of fluids will be more than compensated by the animal's increased ability to withstand the shock of anesthesia and surgical trauma. An attempt should be made to correlate the patient's electrolyte balance with the type of fluid which is administered. In those hospitals where electrolyte balance studies are performed, exacting replacement therapy can be administered. Anemia, as determined clinically and with hematocrit and hemoglobin determinations, should be corrected by administration of whole blood. Crowell *et al.* (1959) have shown experimentally that from the standpoint of shock prevention a hematocrit of 42 is optimum for the dog at elevations close to sea level. Patients in shock without blood loss or in a state of nutritional deficiency will be benefited by administration of plasma. Corticosteroids are indicated in aged or debilitated patients and those undergoing extensive surgery. Again, preanesthetic administration is more valuable than during surgery.

A number of conditions may alter normal intrathoracic pressure. Among these are pneumothorax, hemothorax, pyothorax, chylothorax, and diaphragmatic hernia. Affected animals are often in a precarious state of respiratory exchange and any undue struggling on induction of anesthesia may cause them to die. Intrapleural air or fluid should be removed by aspiration prior to induction, since the effective lung volume may be greatly reduced and severe respiratory embarrassment otherwise result. While no attempt should be made to insert an endotracheal catheter in these patients prior to anesthesia, *this must be done immediately following induction.* Many animals have been lost because the anesthetist was not prepared to carry out all phases of induction-intubation-artificial respiration in one continuous operation.

Decompensated heart disease is a contraindication for general anesthesia, since fluid in the lungs reduces respiratory efficiency and the animal may have no cardiac reserve. If these animals must be anesthetized, an attempt at compensation through digitalization and diuresis should be made prior to anesthesia. If ascites is present this fluid should be aspirated to reduce excessive pressure on the diaphragm.

Just prior to induction, it is wise to place the patient on a run for a few minutes to allow defecation and urination. The bladder can be emptied, once the animal is anesthetized, by slow steady compression through the abdominal wall. An empty bladder is an advantage in abdominal surgery, particularly in the male, since urination usually contaminates the operative field.

The patient should be placed on the operating table in a physiological position if possible. Compression of the chest, acute angulation of the neck, and over-extension of limbs can all lead to serious difficulties. Two positions causing trouble are illustrated. Figure 2–3 shows a dog positioned for surgery of the neck region. The legs are pulled posteriorly and the head and neck extended by means of a rope over the upper jaw. An animal so fastened will frequently die of respiratory failure unless an endotracheal catheter is inserted. Figure 2–4 shows a dog in position for surgery of the perineal region. If the stifle joint is held in acute extension for some time, as illustrated, peroneal nerve paralysis may result.

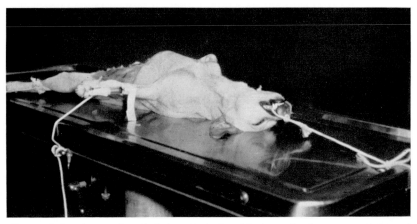

FIGURE 2–3. A sometimes-lethal method of positioning a dog for surgery of the neck. Respiratory arrest frequently occurs.

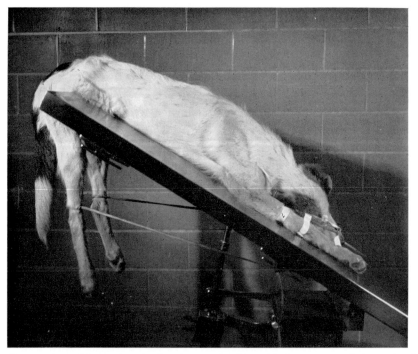

FIGURE 2–4. The patient is placed on a slanting table for surgery of the perineal region. Peroneal nerve paralysis may result.

Kilburn *et al.* (1960) have shown that tilting the patient markedly alters the amount of respiratory gases which can be accommodated in the chest. When pentobarbital-anesthetized dogs were inclined at 30° with the head up, the lung volume* was increased 24% above that in the horizontal position. When the head was declined 30° the volume was decreased by 66%. These figures indicate that tilting the patient head-down should be avoided whenever possible.

References

ADRIANI, J.: Anesthesia for Patients with Uncommon and Unusual Diseases. Anesth. & Analg., *37*, 1, 1958.

ANDERSON, E. G. and MAGEE, D. F.: A Study of the Mechanism of the Effect of Dietary Fat in Decreasing Thiopental Sleeping Time. J. Pharm. & Exper. Therap., *117*, 281, 1956.

BECKER, R. F., FLANNAGAN, E., and KING, J. E.: The Fate of Offspring from Mothers Receiving Sodium Pentobarbital before Delivery. A Study in the Guinea Pig. Neurology, *8*, 776, 1958.

BEYER, K. H., STUTZMAN, J. W., and HAFFORD, B.: The Relation of Vitamin C to Anesthesia. Surg. Gynec. & Obstet., *79*, 49, 1944.

BUTLER, T. C., DICKISON, H. L., GOVIER, W. M., GREER, C. M., and LAMSON, P. D.: The Effect of Sulfanilamide and Some of Its Derivatives on the Reaction of Mice to Anesthetics. J. Pharm. & Exper. Therap., *72*, 298, 1941.

CAMERON, G. R.: The Pharmacological Basis of Modern Anaesthesia. Proc. Roy. Soc. Med., *42*, 522, 1949.

CAMERON, G. R.: Some Recent Work on Barbiturates. Proc. Roy. Soc. Med., *32*, 309, 1938.

CLARK, A. J.: Aspects of the History of Anaesthetics. Brit. Med. J., *2*, 1029, 1938.

CROWELL, J. W., FORD, R. G., and LEWIS, V. M.: Oxygen Transport in Hemorrhagic Shock as a Function of the Hematocrit Ratio. Am. J. Physiol., *196*, 1033, 1959.

DE BOER, B.: Factors Affecting Pentothal Anesthesia in Dogs. Anesthesiology, *8*, 375, 1947.

DUKES, H. H.: *The Physiology of Domestic Animals.* 6th Ed., Comstock Publishing Company, Inc. Ithaca, New York, p. 454, 1947.

GREEN, M. W. and KOPPANYI, T.: Studies on Barbiturates. XXVII. Tolerance and Cross-Tolerance to Barbiturates. Anesthesiology, *5*, 329, 1944.

GREEN, M. W. and MUSULIN, R. R.: Studies on Barbiturates. XXV. The Effect of Vitamin C Level on Barbiturate Depression in Guinea Pigs. J. Am. Pharm. A., *30*, 613, 1941.

HUBBARD, T. F. and GOLDBAUM, L. R.: The Mechanism of Tolerance to Thiopental in Mice. J. Pharm. & Exper. Therap., *97*, 488, 1949.

KENNEDY, W. P.: Sodium Salt of C-C-Cyclohexenylmethyl-N-Methyl Barbituric Acid (Evipan) Anaesthesia in Laboratory Animals. J. Pharm. & Exper. Therap., *50*, 347, 1934.

KILBURN, K. H., McDONALD, J., and PICCINNI, F. P.: Effects of Ventilatory Pattern and Body Position on Lung Volume in Dogs. J. Appl. Physiol., *15*, 801, 1960.

KNIGHT, G. C.: Barbiturate Anaesthesia in Small Animals. Proc. Roy. Soc. Med., *42*, 524, 1949.

NICHOLAS, J. S. and BARRON, D. H.: The Use of Sodium Amytal in the Production of Anesthesia in the Rat. J. Pharm. & Exper. Therap., *46*, 125, 1932.

SABAWALA, T. B. and DILLON, J. B.: The Action of Some Antibiotics on The Human Intercostal Nerve-Muscle Complex. Anesthesiology, *20*, 659, 1959.

SELYE, H.: Studies Concerning the Anesthetic Action of Steroid Hormones. J. Pharm. & Exper. Therap., *73*, 127, 1941.

* As measured by functional residual capacity.

FACILITIES, EQUIPMENT AND PERSONNEL

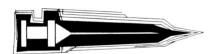

Chapter 3

Facilities and Equipment

Time and thought should be given to preparation of a place in the hospital for anesthetizing animals. All necessary items should be kept in supply and in a state of readiness. When anesthetic emergencies arise, there is no time to hunt equipment which has been mislaid.

The hospital area selected will, in many cases, be the operating room itself. When economically possible, however, it is better to have a separate "prep room" or place for preparing animals. This contributes to cleanliness in the surgery and leaves the operator undistracted. Regardless of the area used, it should be well lighted and equipped with a sink with hot and cold water. A drainboard should be located adjacent to the sink, or a removable metal grate over it, so that animals can be washed and the bladder expressed. When one is working unassisted, a small ring located in the wall over the drainboard or over a small table is advantageous (Fig. 3–1). The patient's collar can be fastened to the ring and the operator can anesthetize animals so restrained without additional help. A convenient method for storing clippers is to attach them to the wall or ceiling overhead using a spring-activated reel.* This arrangement will pay for itself over a period of time since clippers usually break when dropped on the floor. A vacuum cleaner is very useful to remove clipped hair from the patient and surroundings.

Often splint-making and odd jobs requiring tools are performed in the prep room. A workbench with a vise attached can be placed along one wall, and a pegboard fastened on the wall above the table will provide a convenient place to hang the tools. Too frequently the need for storage is overlooked in the operating area. Such things as splint-making materials, sandbags, spare oxygen tanks, and many others are best kept in a storage closet.

* Reelite, see Appendix A, p. 403.

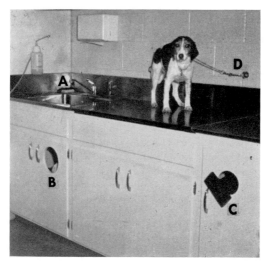

FIGURE 3-1.   A prep area illustrating some useful features: (A) a sink with hot and cold running water, (B) an under-counter waste receptacle, (C) an under-counter vacuum cleaner with flexible hose, and (D) provision for restraining animals by fastening them to the wall.

The following drugs, equipment, and supplies for anesthesia will be found useful in the prep and operating rooms:

Anesthetic agents.
Antiseptics.
Analeptics.
Anesthetic jelly.
Eye ointments.
Electrolyte solutions and infusion equipment.
Plasma expander.
Blood bank and/or disposable blood collection and administration sets.
Nye tourniquet.
Sterile syringes—2, 5, and 10 cc.
1—50 cc. syringe with attached 3-way valve.
1—½ or 1 cc. glass tuberculin syringe graduated in one-hundredths of a cc.
18, 20, 22, and 24 gauge needles.
Clippers.
Scissors.
Rectal thermometer.
Stethoscope.
Endotracheal catheters—various sizes from 12 to 44 French.
Tongue forceps to clamp endotracheal catheter cuff.
Oxygen tank with reduction valve and accessories for connection to endotracheal catheters.
Suction apparatus (Penberthy pump, or other).
Small cart or stretcher on wheels.
Bathroom scale, self-registering.
Balance and weights (metric system) for weighing birds, other small animals.
Infusion stand.
Bath towels.
Nylon or leather thongs.

Sandbags.
Perineal stand.
Trough for table top.
Anesthetist's shield.
Stool for anesthetist.
Cardiac defibrillator.
Cotton, roll.
Gauze, 2 inch rolls.
Adhesive tape, $\frac{1}{2}$, 1, and 2 inch widths.

Most of these items are discussed in this or subsequent chapters.

Ideally, the anesthetized patient is placed in a relaxed comfortable position. An ordinary bath towel put under the patient will help prevent loss of body heat and also absorb any fluids which drain on the operating table.

Conventional small animal operating tables are poorly designed for optimum positioning of the patient. Tables for humans are much

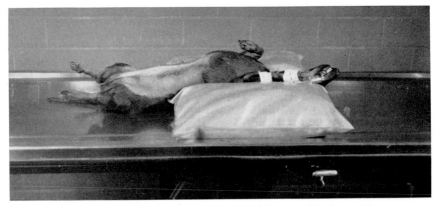

FIGURE 3–2. Plastic-covered sandbags hold the patient in position.

more flexible in that they are jointed and can be adjusted to requirements of the surgeon and comfort of the patient. To overcome the shortcomings of inadequate table design, veterinarians use some additional aids, the least expensive of which is the sandbag. These can be fabricated in several sizes and shapes to fit the needs of various situations. The ordinary canvas-covered sandbag soon becomes blood-stained and unsightly; in addition, it continuously loses a small amount of sand. To correct these deficiencies it can be sealed in a plastic envelope which is water-tight and easily cleaned under the faucet (Fig. 3–2).

In many operations, stretching the patient's legs, by tying them to the operating table with thongs, may complicate the surgical procedure. When a flat-topped operating table is used, it is impossible to tie an anesthetized dog so that it will lie on its back and remain perfectly upright. This is true, despite the fact that this is by

far the most common position used in canine and feline surgery.
Some people have mastered this problem by having operating tables
with trough-shaped tops custom built, while others use portable
troughs of wood or metal placed on conventional tables (Fig. 3–3).

Surgery in the perineal region is often best accomplished by
positioning the patient in ventral recumbency. If the operating
table is horizontal, the surgeon is placed in an awkward position
since the table will be too low. By tilting the table and placing the
patient head-down with rear legs over the high end of the table, the
surgeon will be in a comfortable position with the operating site at
approximately the right height. Care must be taken to see that the

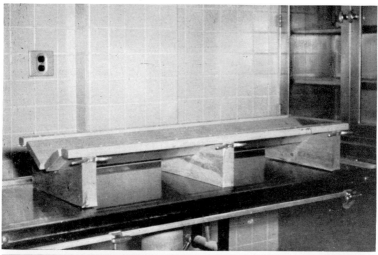

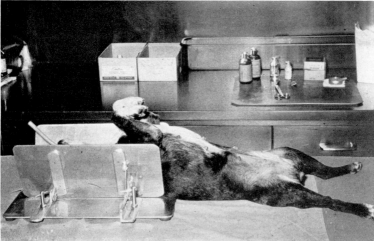

FIGURE 3–3. Wooden and metal troughs for positioning animals on their backs
during surgery. (Lower figure courtesy of Dr. R. L. Leighton, Scarsdale, New York.)

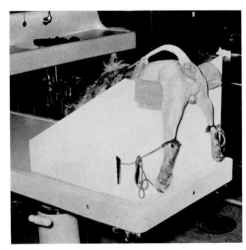

FIGURE 3–4. A perineal stand in use. Note the padding in the inguinal area. Over-extension of the hind limbs with subsequent peroneal nerve paralysis is eliminated when a stand is used.

hind legs are not over-extended at the stifles, since peroneal paralysis may result (Fig. 2–4). A perineal stand will position the patient without the necessity of tilting the table (Fig. 3–4).

Personnel

Well-trained lay personnel can do much to relieve the veterinarian from some of the more routine aspects of patient preparation and anesthesia. The ultimate responsibility for anesthesia rests with the veterinarian, but a lay assistant who does not have a working knowl-edge of these techniques is of little value other than to restrain the animal. For this reason it is essential that the layman be taught the signs of anesthesia and of anesthetic emergencies and be able to initiate steps to cope with the latter. Among the techniques he should know are those of subcutaneous, intramuscular, and intra-venous injection, endotracheal intubation, and oxygen and blood administration. It has been suggested that,

> "... the services of properly trained laymen (to function not only as anesthetists but in a manner analogous to the nurse in the physician's office) should be made available by one or more of our veterinary colleges." (———, 1952).

Considering the financial aspects of practice, a well-trained layman may be worth more to a veterinarian than a second colleague.

References

———: Anesthetic Mortality. N. Amer. Vet., *33*, 6, 1952.

PHYSIOLOGY OF RESPIRATION

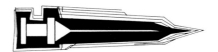

Chapter 4

Definitions

Respiration is the transport of atmospheric oxygen to the body cells and return of carbon dioxide from the cells to the atmosphere. All of the energy utilized by an animal comes from oxidation of complex molecules containing carbon, and one of the end-products of this oxidation is carbon dioxide. A continuous supply of oxygen and constant removal of carbon dioxide are thus essential for animal life.

Pulmonary ventilation is accomplished by expansion and contraction of the lungs. A number of terms are used to describe the various types of breathing which may be observed.

1. *Eupnea* is ordinary quiet breathing.
2. *Dyspnea* is labored breathing.
3. *Hyperpnea* is fast and/or deep respiration, indicating "over respiration".
4. *Polypnea* is a rapid, shallow, panting type of respiration.
5. *Apnea* is transient cessation of breathing.
6. *Hypopnea* is slow and/or shallow breathing, indicating "under respiration".

To describe the events of pulmonary ventilation, air in the lungs has been subdivided into four different *volumes* and four different *capacities* (Fig. 4–1).

1. *Tidal volume*—the volume of air inspired or expired in one respiration.
2. *Inspiratory reserve volume*—the volume of air that can be inspired over and above the normal tidal volume.
3. *Expiratory reserve volume*—the amount of air that can be expired by forceful expiration after a normal tidal expiration.
4. *Residual volume*—the air remaining in the lungs after the most forceful expiration.

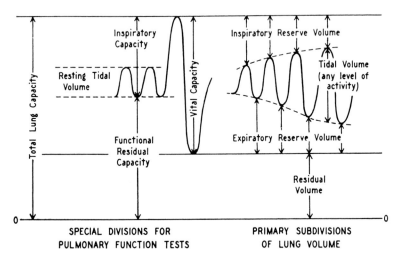

FIGURE 4-1. Lung volumes and capacities. (From ————: Standardization of Definitions and Symbols in Respiratory Physiology. Fed. Proc., *9*, 602, 1950.)

Another term which is frequently used is the *minute respiratory volume* or *minute volume*. This is equal to the tidal volume times the respiratory rate.

Occasionally it is desirable to consider two or more of the above volumes together. Such combinations are termed *pulmonary capacities*.

1. *Inspiratory capacity*—the tidal volume plus the inspiratory reserve volume. This is the amount of air that can be inhaled starting after a normal expiration and distending the lungs to the maximum amount.
2. *Functional residual capacity*—the expiratory reserve volume plus the residual volume. This is the amount of air remaining in the lungs after a normal expiration.
3. *Vital capacity*—the inspiratory reserve volume plus the tidal volume plus the expiratory reserve volume. This is the maxi-

mum amount of air that can be expelled from the lungs after first filling them to their maximum extent.

4. *Total lung capacity*—the inspiratory reserve volume plus the tidal volume plus the expiratory reserve volume plus the residual volume, or the maximum volume to which the lungs can be expanded with the greatest possible inspiratory effort.

The important factor in pulmonary ventilation is the rate at which *alveolar* air is renewed by atmospheric air. This is not equal to the minute respiratory volume because a large portion of inspired air is used to fill the respiratory passages, rather than the alveoli, and no significant gaseous exchange occurs in this air. Air that fills the respiratory passages, the nose, pharynx, trachea, and bronchi, is termed *dead space air*. On inspiration, new air must displace that in the dead space before it reaches the alveoli. The volume of air entering the alveoli with each breath is equal to the tidal volume minus the dead space volume.

Dead space has been further divided into anatomical and physiological divisions. Anatomical dead space is the volume of all spaces of the respiratory system except the alveoli. If alveoli for some reason are nonfunctional, or if pulmonary blood flow to some alveoli is low, then these too may be considered dead space. Thus, physiological dead space includes not only the anatomical dead space, but any alveolar dead space which may be present. In a normal animal the anatomical and physiological dead space are essentially the same, but in pulmonary disease the physiological dead space may be several times larger. Romijn (1943) has described a method for calculating the effective dead space in the dog under normal conditions.

Respiratory Characteristics of Various Species

Data concerning lung ventilation and exchange characteristics of several species are listed in Tables 4–1 and 4–2. The higher metabolic rate of the dog as compared with man is reflected in a relatively high oxygen requirement (Table 4–3).

Anesthesia lowers the metabolic rate and oxygen consumption. Tanaka *et al.* (1961) found that thiopental-anesthetized dogs had a mean oxygen uptake of 10.45 cc./kg./minute. When cooled to 30° C., this was reduced to 6.25 cc./kg./minute.

Farhi *et al.* (1957) made intrapleural pressure measurements in anesthetized dogs and found at the peak of inspiration negative pressure was as much as —14.3 cm. H_2O. At any given point within the pleural cavity, pressures did not vary more than 1 cm.

Table 4-1.—Respiratory Rate, Tidal and Minute Volumes: Vertebrates

Values, unless otherwise specified, are for the resting state.

Animal	Body Weight kg.	Condition	Respiratory Rate breaths/min.	Tidal Volume[1] ml.	Minute Volume L./min.
			Mammals		
Beaver (*Castor canadensis*)	18		16		
Cat (*Felis catus*)	2.45		26	12.4	0.322
Dog (*Canis familiaris*)[2]	30.5 28.6 19.1 16.4		16 (11–18) 17 (11–21) 22 (13–37) 13 (12–16)	432 302 251 296	6.1 (5.1–7.4) 5.3 (4.9–5.4) 5.5 (4.6–6.4) 4.1 (3.3–4.9)
Guinea pig (*Cavia cobaya*)	0.471		90 (69–104)	1.8 (1.0–3.9)	0.16 (0.09–0.38)
Hamster (*Mesocricetus auratus*)	0.091		74 (33–127)	0.8 (0.42–1.2)	0.05 (0.025–0.083)
Manatee, Florida (*Trichechus latirostris*)	250		7 (6–8)	7000 (5000–9000)	45 (35–60)
Marmot (*Marmota marmota*)	2.13	Awake[3] Hibernating[4]	8.0 0.68	22 13 (11.3–14.8)	0.174 0.0089
Monkey (*Macaca rhesus*)	2.68		40 (31–52)	21 (9.8–29)	0.86 (0.31–1.41)
Mouse (*Mus musculus*)	0.0198		163 (84–230)	0.15 (0.09–0.23)	0.023 (0.011–0.036)
Porpoise (*Tursiops truncatus*)[5]	170		1.1 (0.9–1.3)	9000 (8000–10,000)	9.7 (9.0–10.4)
Rabbit (*Lepus cuniculus*)	2.07				0.8 (0.27–1.2)
Rabbit, pigmented White			69 53	21 19	1.45 1.02

Species				
Rat, cotton (*Sigmodon hispidus*)	0.77	94.5 (75–115)	0.35 (0.24–0.70)	0.04 (0.023–0.071)
White (*Rattus norvegicus*)[6]	0.112	85.5 (66–114)	0.86 (0.60–1.25)	0.074 (0.05–0.102)
Seal (*Phoca vitulina*)[6]	27.5 (15–30)	9 (6–12)		3.97
Sloth (*Choloepus hoffmani*)	4.5	13		0.844 (0.78–0.96)
(*Bradypus griseus*)	3.1	6.2 (4.5–8.0)		0.485 (0.33–0.73)
Birds				
Canary		108 (96–120)		
Chicken, ♂		17 (12–21)	45	
♀		28.5 (20–37)		
Duck, ♂		42	36.5 (35–38)[7]	
♀		110		
Goose, ♂		20		
♀		40		
Pigeon		27.5 (25–30)	4.8 (4.5–5.2)[8]	
Turkey		13.4[9]		
Reptile				
Turtle (*Malaclemys centrata*)[10]	0.65–0.72	3.7	14	0.051

[1] Air inspired or expired in one respiration. [2] Measurements made after 30-min. rest in hammock, at 24°C; values corrected to BTPS conditions. [3] Rectal temperature = 37.8°C. [4] Rectal temperature = 5–6°C. [6] Cheyne-Stokes respiration. [7] Standing; supine, 30. [8] Standing; supine, 4.7. [9] Also reported ♂ 28, ♀ 49. [10] Diamond-back terrapin; periodic cycles at 24–29° C. [5] Captive animal. (From N.A.S. *Handbook of Respiration*. W. B. Saunders Co., 1958.)

Table 4–2.—Respiratory Exchange Characteristics: Vertebrates

Volume per cent values are for dry air.

Animal	Inspired Air vol. %		Alveolar Air vol. %		Expired Air vol. %		RQ
	O_2	CO_2	O_2	CO_2	O_2	CO_2	CO_2/O_2
Man (*Homo sapiens*)	20.95	0.03	14.00	5.60	16.30	4.50	0.850
Dog (*Canis familiaris*)			13.66	5.68	16.30	3.46	0.780
Albino rat (*Rattus norvegicus*)							0.894 (0.754–1.072)
Horse (*Equus caballus*)							0.960
Guillemot (*Cepphus grylle*)					15.05	4.83	
Chicken (*Gallus domesticus*)					13.50	6.50	0.764[1] (0.71–0.96)[2]
Turtle (28° C.) (*Malaciemys centrata*)			16.46	4.69			0.71[3]
Frog (20° C.), cutaneous (*Rana esculenta*)							1.92
Frog (20° C.), pulmonary (*Rana esculenta*)							0.32
Puffer fish (20° C.)	0.31		0.31		0.149		

[1] Average for 5 days including day of last feeding.
[2] Range for 1–5 hr. and 4 days after feeding.
[3] Data for painted turtle (*Chrysemys marginata*) included in calculation.
(From Spector, W. S.: *Handbook of Biological Data.* W. B. Saunders Co., 1956.)

Table 4–3.—Comparative Respiratory Exchange

	Oxygen consumed cc./kg./Hour	Carbon dioxide produced cc./kg./Hour
Man	302	257
Dog	847	652

(From Dukes, H. H.: *The Physiology of the Domestic Animals.* 4th ed. Comstock Publishing Co., 1937.)

Control of Respiration

Respiratory movements are regulated to control the rate at which oxygen is added to, and carbon dioxide removed from, the alveolar air of the lungs. Breathing is normally slow and shallow because removal of oxygen from alveolar air and addition of carbon dioxide to it are relatively slow. During exercise both rate and depth of respirations are increased to supply the additional demand for oxygen and to eliminate the increased quantity of carbon dioxide formed in tissue oxidations. Physical and chemical stimuli mediate this response directly or indirectly through the respiratory center.

Increases in carbon dioxide and hydrogen ion concentration (decreased pH) stimulate the neurons of the respiratory center directly. In addition, these neurons produce carbon dioxide through their own metabolic processes. Reduction in blood flow through the medulla is followed by an increase in acidity and carbon dioxide within the respiratory center. As a result, respiration is stimulated.

Decreases in carbon dioxide and hydrogen ion concentration (increased pH) depress the center. If blood flow through the center is increased, a reduction in carbon dioxide and acidity results and respiration is slowed. Blood flow changes, however, are relatively unimportant in their effect on ventilation.

Carotid and aortic bodies are found at the bifurcation of the carotid arteries and in the aorta. These areas each contain two types of receptors, one type (pressoreceptor or baroreceptor) responds to pressure, the other (chemoreceptor) responds to chemical stimulation. Pressoreceptors, which are stimulated by stretching force, are situated in the wall of the carotid sinus and the aortic arch. Stimulation of the pressoreceptors, such as occurs with an abrupt rise in arterial blood pressure, inhibits respiration. In mammals the pressoreceptors do not appear to serve any respiratory function under normal physiologic conditions. They are, however, of great importance in control of circulation.

The chemoreceptors are stimulated by lack of oxygen (oxygen tension in arterial blood of 70 mm. Hg or less). This level can be produced by breathing 18% oxygen or ascending to 4,000 feet. At this altitude the blood is about 92% saturated with oxygen. The chemoreceptors are less sensitive to carbon dioxide and hydrogen ion concentration than the respiratory center, and they normally play little part in control of respiration. Stimuli from chemoreceptors are transmitted to the respiratory center, thence to the respiratory apparatus.

In an emergency the chemoreceptors are of great importance because their chief stimulus is a *decreased oxygen pressure* rather than changes in carbon dioxide and hydrogen ion concentration. Hypoxia is ineffective as a direct stimulus to the respiratory center and produces depression with ultimate failure of the neurons. The chemoreceptor reflex, on the other hand, is quite resistant to hypoxia and stimulates the respiratory center which otherwise is unresponsive to the emergency. The chemoreceptors thus serve as the last line of defense against respiratory failure (Comroe and Schmidt, 1938).

In severe oxygen want, the medullary center can become so depressed that it responds only to chemoreceptor stimulation. When this occurs, administration of oxygen will relieve the hypoxia but will also eliminate the mechanism responsible for stimulation of the respiratory center. Fatal apnea may result (carotid body apnea) if the medullary centers have been sufficiently depressed.

All common anesthetic agents used in veterinary anesthesiology today, except ether, act as respiratory depressants, lowering the sensitivity of the respiratory center and peripheral receptors to various stimuli. During surgery afferent stimuli from the surgical field tend to increase the respiratory rate. These stimuli cease at the close of the operation and respiration at this stage frequently becomes depressed. According to Comben (1950), afferent impulses from the parietal peritoneum act as stimulants to respiration, whereas impulses from certain areas of the visceral peritoneum bring about temporary inhibition of respiration in inspiration. Reflex inhibition of respiration occurs immediately before vomition, during endotracheal intubation, and temporarily with obstruction of the respiratory tree.

In emergencies, advantage has been taken of the fact that certain afferent stimuli tend to produce reflex respiratory movements. Among these stimuli are dilation of the anal sphincter, traction on the tongue, fracture of a long bone, and alternate immersion in hot and cold water. In cats the point of a curved hemostat can be pressed on the hard palate and, with continuing pressure, slid posteriorly onto the soft palate to evoke a reflex respiration. A bilateral respiratory reflex initiated by light pressure on a localized area of the thoracic wall has been described in dogs and rabbits by Whitehead and Draper (1947). The area is approximately $1\frac{1}{2}$ inches in diameter and is located at the point where the scalenus and rectus abdominis muscles and their aponeurotic tendons are in apposition. This is roughly the area on the left chest wall of maximal cardiac impulse and on the right wall is in a corresponding position. Pressure on this area produces smooth normal respirations which are largely diaphragmatic. While the reflex may become fatigued, its sensitivity returns rapidly. It is abolished by severe hypoxia, shock, and deep anesthetic depression. However, compared with anal stretching and tongue traction this is the last reflex to disappear with deepening anesthesia. It has been used effectively as a substitute for artificial respiration following overdoses of barbiturates when depression was not too deep.

Oxygen Transport in the Blood

Under normal conditions oxygen is taken into the lung alveoli and carbon dioxide removed from them at a rate which is sufficient to maintain the composition of alveolar air at a relatively constant concentration. The composition of respiratory gases in man is as follows:

Gas	Inspired Air per cent	Expired Air per cent	Alveolar Air per cent
O_2	20.95	16.1	14.0
CO_2	0.04	4.5	5.6
N_2*	79.0	79.2	80.0

* There is no change in the absolute concentration of N_2. The change in per cent is due to the fact that more oxygen is used than carbon dioxide produced.

At body temperature, alveolar air is saturated with water vapor which has a pressure at 37° C. of 48 mm. Hg. If the pressure in the alveolus is 760 mm. Hg then the pressure due to dry air is 760—48 = 712 mm. Hg. Knowing the composition of alveolar air, the pressure of each gas in the alveolus can be calculated.

Pressure of Respiratory Gases in the Alveolus

$$O_2 = (760–48) \times 0.14 \ \ = 100 \text{ mm. Hg}$$
$$CO_2 = (760–48) \times 0.056 = \ \ 40 \text{ mm. Hg}$$
$$N_2 = (760–48) \times 0.80 \ \ = 570 \text{ mm. Hg}$$

Oxygen pressure in the lungs at sea level is approximately 100 mm. Hg at 38° C. Under these conditions, 100 ml. of plasma will hold 0.31 cc. of oxygen in physical solution. Whole blood, under the same conditions, will hold 20 cc. of oxygen or about 60 times as much as plasma. Carbon dioxide is similarly held by blood. Thus it is apparent that oxygen and carbon dioxide in blood are transported largely in chemical combination, since both are carried by blood in much greater quantities than would occur if simple absorption took place.

Gases always move from high to low pressure areas (Fig. 4–2). If P_1 and P_2 are closed compartments with a small opening between, and the pressure of gas in P_1 is greater than P_2, gas will move from P_1 to P_2 until an equilibrium is reached. The same phenomenon also occurs when gases are dissolved in solutions. In Figure 4–3, P_1 and P_2 are vessels containing a solution. If the solution in P_1 is equilibrated with a high oxygen pressure and P_2 with a low oxygen pressure, oxygen will diffuse from P_1 to P_2 until PO_1 equals PO_2.

In the lung, gas exchange occurs across the alveolar membrane and the capillary membrane. The total distance across which exchange takes place is 1 to 2 microns; therefore, it occurs very rapidly. Equilibrium *almost* develops between blood in the lungs and air in the alveolus, and the P_{O_2} in the blood almost equals the P_{O_2} in the alveolus. At complete saturation, each gram of hemoglobin combines with 1.36 cc. of oxygen. This is the total carrying capacity of hemoglobin, or four oxygen molecules combined with each hemoglobin

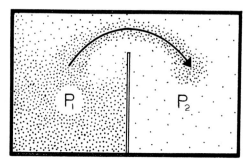

FIGURE 4–2.   If P_1 and P_2 are closed compartments which communicate, and the gas pressure in P_1 exceeds P_2, an equilibrium tends to establish.

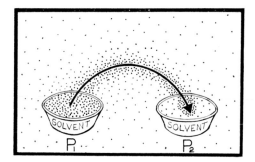

FIGURE 4–3.   If the solvent in P_1 has a high oxygen tension and that in P_2 a low tension, oxygen will diffuse from P_1 to P_2.

molecule. When oxygen is inhaled at a partial pressure of 100 mm. Hg, hemoglobin leaving the lungs is practically saturated. An increase in the partial pressure of alveolar oxygen, therefore, results in only a very small increase in oxygen carried by hemoglobin. Plasma, on the other hand, carries oxygen in an amount directly proportional to the partial pressure of oxygen in the alveoli. At normal atmospheric pressure, breathing air at 38° C., 0.3 cc. of oxygen is carried in solution in 100 ml. of blood.

If pure oxygen is administered, the partial pressure of oxygen in the alveoli is raised from 100 to almost 700 mm. Hg. Plasma oxygen is thus elevated almost seven times, that is from 0.3 to 2.1 cc. of oxygen per 100 ml. of blood. The result is an increase of about 10%

in oxygen carried by the blood. This is of some importance since oxygen transfers from blood to tissues by diffusion, and the process is carried on at a rate proportional to the difference in oxygen tension between plasma and body tissues.

A common misconception is that oxygenation of a patient can be improved by increasing the *pressure* at which oxygen is administered. Actually in clinical practice improved oxygenation of the patient is not obtained by increasing the pressure of the gas mixture, but by increasing the *proportion* of oxygen in the mixture. At a positive pressure exceeding 40 mm. Hg, the capillary circulation in the lungs is inhibited, therefore, it is not practical to administer oxygen at a pressure exceeding this figure.

The partial pressure of oxygen in various body areas is:

Inspired air = 160 mm. Hg
Alveolar air = 100 mm. Hg
Arterial blood = 90–95 mm. Hg
Interstitial fluid = 30 mm. Hg
Intracellular fluid = 10 mm. Hg
Venous blood = 40 mm. Hg

Little oxygen is lost in large blood vessels; a continuous pressure gradient is present from the alveolus to the tissue cell.

Oxygen has a weak covalent link with hemoglobin. Four factors influence oxygen uptake: (1) change in pH due to carbon dioxide, (2) specific effect of carbon dioxide, (3) temperature, and (4) effect of salts.

Decreasing the carbon dioxide tension in blood raises the pH and causes hemoglobin to bind more oxygen. As shown in Figure 4–4, when the carbon dioxide tension increases the curve shifts to the right. Carbon dioxide reacts with hemoglobin to form carbamino-hemoglobin which has much less affinity for oxygen than does hemoglobin; thus it exerts a specific effect also.

Increased temperature favors dissociation of oxyhemoglobin. As metabolic rates increase there is increased heat in the tissues which in turn makes more oxygen available.

The salt or electrolyte concentration of blood has been shown to affect oxygenation though the mechanism of action is obscure. Ordinarily variations in electrolyte concentration of blood have little effect on oxygen transport.

Several factors increase the availability of oxygen in tissues when needed:

1. Increased circulation. Up to three times as much blood may flow through the tissues.
2. Increased respiratory rate. The carbon dioxide tension of the blood regulates the respiratory center.

3. Increased deoxygenation of a given volume of blood. This may be due to: (*a*) lowered oxygen tension in the cells, (*b*) increased temperature with increased dissociation and, (*c*) metabolic products such as carbon dioxide and lactic acid which are acidic.

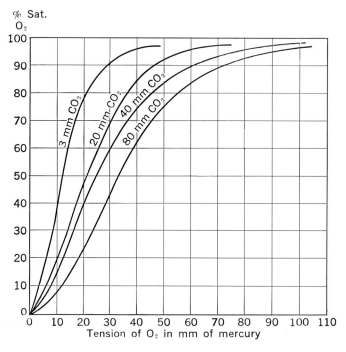

FIGURE 4–4.   Plot of per cent saturation against tension of oxygen in mm. Hg. (From Bock, A. V., Field, H. Jr., and Adair, G. S.: The Oxygen and Carbon Dioxide Dissociation Curves of Human Blood. J. Biol. Chem., *59*, 353, 1924.)

These factors combine to make up to ten times as much oxygen available to tissues as would be available in the resting state. The rate of muscular activity is not limited by oxygen supply since muscle can incur an oxygen deficit.

Oxidation has been defined as any of the following: (1) the addition of oxygen, (2) the removal of hydrogen, or (3) the removal of electrons. In the Krebs' or tricarboxylic acid cycle, oxygen accepts electrons from cytochrome oxidase and combines with hydrogen to form water. Direct addition of oxygen does not take place in living cells though removal of hydrogen or electrons is very common.

Carbon Dioxide Transport and the Chloride Shift

Carbon dioxide is an end product of glucose oxidation. It is pro-

duced by decarboxylation of carboxyl groups according to the reaction:

$$RCOOH \rightarrow RH + CO_2$$

During severe exercise the production of carbon dioxide is increased
enormously. In the tissues carbon dioxide reacts with water to form
carbonic acid.

$$CO_2 + H_2O \underset{\text{Anhydrase}}{\overset{\text{Carbonic}}{\rightleftarrows}} H_2CO_3 \rightleftarrows H^+ + HCO_3^-$$

Because of the blood buffer systems, transport of carbon dioxide
to the lungs for excretion is effected with little change in blood
pH. Under ordinary circumstances the pH of venous blood is only
0.01 to 0.03 lower than that of arterial blood. A carbon dioxide pressure gradient, opposite to that of oxygen, exists from the tissues to
the atmospheric air:

> Tissues = 50 mm. Hg (during exercise may be higher)
> Venous blood = 46 mm. Hg
> Alveolar air = 40 mm. Hg
> Expired air = 32 mm. Hg
> Atmospheric air = 0.3 mm. Hg
> Arterial blood = 40 mm. Hg (equilibrium with alveolar air)

Some carbon dioxide is carried dissolved in the plasma. This is
divided into: (1) H_2CO_3, and (2) carbon dioxide in simple solution.
These are referred to as *carbonic acid*. The amount of carbon dioxide
transported as carbonic acid is about 10% of the total and is found in
the plasma.

The greater portion of carbon dioxide transport is as *bicarbonate*.
This may form: (1) in plasma through buffering action with plasma
protein (this accounts for 5% of carbon dioxide transport), or (2) by
formation in the red blood cell through the chloride shift (this accounts for the largest amount).

As blood passes to the venous side of the vascular system, carbon
dioxide is absorbed and diffuses into the red blood cell (Fig. 4–5).
Here it is converted to carbonic acid. Reduced hemoglobin, a
weaker acid, gives up its alkali, chiefly potassium, to carbonic acid.
As bicarbonate is thus formed and accumulates in the erythrocyte,
the ionic equilibrium between cell and plasma is upset. The corpuscular membrane is impermeable to potassium but bicarbonate
diffuses through into the plasma. Chloride ions in turn shift into the
cell to restore ionic equilibrium and balance the potassium. The
chloride shift enables carbon dioxide to be carried without any
change in blood pH and is the main method of transport.

4

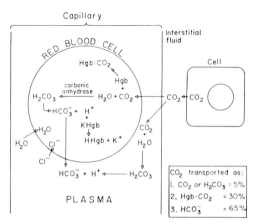

FIGURE 4–5.   Chemical reactions for the transport of carbon dioxide. (From Guyton,
    A. C.: *Textbook of Medical Physiology.* 2nd ed. W. B. Saunders Co., 1961.)

A third method by which carbon dioxide is carried is in the form of
carbamino compound.   Amino acids and aliphatic amines combine
with carbon dioxide to form unstable carbamino compound.   Hemoglobin is the main protein acting in this manner, though many can
do so.

The three mechanisms for carbon dioxide transport are: (1) dissolved carbon dioxide, (2) bicarbonate (HCO_3^-), and (3) carbamino
compound.   With a hematocrit of 40%, carbon dioxide is transported
in the following manner:

Plasma	*Per cent Transport*
Dissolved CO_2	5
HCO_3^-	57*
Cells	
Dissolved CO_2	3
Carbamino Hb	27
HCO_3^-	8

* Due to the chloride shift the plasma carries most of the carbon dioxide.

There are at least three ways that carbon dioxide and oxygen are
integrated in the blood mechanism:

1. The acidity of carbonic acid produced in the tissues favors release of oxygen without a change in oxygen tension.   The release of carbon dioxide in the lungs favors oxygen uptake.
2. Release of oxygen favors carbon dioxide uptake and *vice versa*
   in the carbamino mechanism.
3. The two acid forms of the hemoglobin molecule favor dissociation by shifting from one form to the other.   Oxygen uptake favors carbon dioxide loss and *vice versa*.

Acid-Base Balance

In normal animals the blood pH is 7.4 ± 0.05. If the pH rises above 7.45 the condition is termed *alkalosis*, below 7.35 it is termed *acidosis* (Fig. 4–6). Normal metabolic processes continuously produce acidic substances such as lactic acid, sulfuric acid from protein

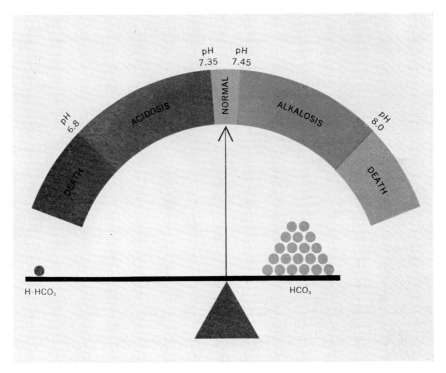

Figure 4–6. "Acid bicarbonate" in a ratio of 1:20 with "base bicarbonate" maintains a normal body pH. (From —————: *Fluid and Electrolytes.* Abbott Laboratories, 1957.)

metabolism, and carbon dioxide. Some alkaline substances are also being added though to a lesser extent. The pH of the blood is kept constant through several mechanisms:

1. Blood buffers
2. Respiration
3. The kidneys

Pathological changes in metabolism almost always result in acidosis. The pH shift during prolonged surgery with poor lung ventilation may result in values below 7. This fact has not been appreciated until lately.

The state of acid-base balance within the body depends primarily upon the relative quantities of carbonic acid and base bicarbonate in the extracellular fluid. Normally these are present in a ratio of 1 to 20 respectively. If this ratio is altered, there is a deviation in pH of the body fluids and a state of acidosis or alkalosis exists. Other buffer systems within the body play only a minor role in regulation of acid-base balance.

Two general types of acid-base imbalances may occur; metabolic disturbances affect *bicarbonate* whereas respiratory disturbances affect *carbonic acid*.

Metabolic Disturbances
    Bicarbonate deficit—acidosis
    Bicarbonate excess—alkalosis

Respiratory Disturbances
    Carbonic acid deficit—alkalosis
    Carbonic acid excess—acidosis

Metabolic acidosis may be caused by such things as diarrhea with loss of sodium bicarbonate in the feces, renal insufficiency with retention of organic acid ions, ketosis with production and accumulation of ketonic acids in the tissues (as occurs with diabetes mellitus or starvation), administration of acidic drugs, or severe infectious disease with production of ketone bodies. The body attempts to compensate for bicarbonate deficit by increased respiratory activity to remove carbon dioxide, and through conservation of bicarbonate ions and excretion of hydrogen ions in the urine.

Metabolic alkalosis may occur as a result of excessive acid loss through vomiting, or through potassium loss such as might occur with overdoses of adrenal corticoids. To correct the imbalance, breathing is slow and shallow. Also, the kidneys excrete bicarbonate ions and retain hydrogen ions.

Respiratory acidosis results from hypoventilation with retention of carbon dioxide. An excess carbon dioxide tension in the blood is termed *hypercapnia* or *hypercarbia*. The kidney compensates by conserving bicarbonate ions and excreting hydrogen ions in the urine.

Respiratory alkalosis occurs with hyperventilation and resultant loss of carbon dioxide. A deficient carbon dioxide tension in the blood is termed *hypocapnia* or *hypocarbia*. The kidneys compensate by excreting bicarbonate ions and retaining hydrogen ions.

Hypoxia

The term *anoxia* literally means without oxygen. Through common usage it has come to mean inability of tissues to receive or utilize an adequate amount of oxygen. Since a literal anoxia seldom

Table 4–4.—Classification of Oxygen Want

Types of Anoxia*	Types of Hypoxia†
1. Anoxic	1. Atmospheric
	2. Tidal
	3. Alveolar
2. Anemic	4. Hemoglobic
3. Stagnant	5. Stagnant
4. Histotoxic	6. Histotoxic
	7. Demand

* Conventional
† Saklad, 1953

Table 4–5.—Blood Values in Various Forms of Hypoxia

Classification of Hypoxia	Arterial Oxygen		Venous Oxygen	
	% Sat.	Vol. %	% Sat.	Vol. %
Atmospheric				
Tidal	75	15	50	10
Alveolar				
Hemoglobic	95	10	35	5
Stagnant	95	19.5	30	5
Histotoxic	95	19.5	85	17
Demand	95	19.5	50	10
Normal	95	19.5	70	14

(From Saklad, M.: *Inhalation Therapy and Resuscitation.* Charles C Thomas, 1953.)

Table 4–6.—Oxygen Capacity, Content, Tension and Arteriovenous Difference in Various Forms of Hypoxia

Hypoxia	Oxygen Capacity	Arterial Oxygen		Venous Oxygen		A-V Difference
		Content	Tension	Content	Tension	
Atmospheric	Normal	Decreased	Decreased	Decreased	Decreased	Decreased
Tidal	Normal	Decreased	Decreased	Decreased	Decreased	Decreased
Alveolar	Normal	Decreased	Decreased	Decreased	Decreased	Decreased
Hemoglobic						
Carbon Monoxide	Decreased	Decreased	Normal	Decreased	Decreased	Decreased
Hemorrhage	Decreased	Decreased	Normal	Decreased	Decreased	Decreased
Stagnant	Normal	Normal	Normal	Decreased	Decreased	Increased
Histotoxic	Normal	Normal	Normal	Increased	Increased	Decreased
Demand	Normal	Normal	Normal	Decreased	Decreased	Increased

(From Saklad, M.: *Inhalation Therapy and Resuscitation.* Charles C Thomas, 1953.)

Table 4-7.—Survival and Revival of Animal Tissues Under Conditions of Hypoxia or Arrested Circulation

Adult tissue, *in situ*, at room temperature, normal body temperature, unless otherwise indicated. N = anoxia produced by cessation of respiration or by administration of nitrogen to animal or to isolated tissue; C = circulation arrested by obstructing or by-passing total afferent blood supply to organ.

Tissue	Animal	Survival Time[1] Minutes	Survival Time[1] Condition	Revival Time[2] Minutes	Revival Time[2] Condition
Brain, cerebral cortex	Cat	$\frac{1}{6}-\frac{1}{4}$	C	<3	C
	Cat			>5–10	C
	Dog			1–8	C
	Dog[3]			12–20	C
	Rabbit	$\frac{1}{3}-2$	N		
	Rat	$1-1\frac{1}{2}$	N		
Brain stem					
Telencephalon and mesencephalon	Rabbit	$\frac{1}{3}-4$	N		
Pupillary centers	Dog	3–4	C[4]		
Medulla	Rabbit	$\frac{1}{2}-8$	N		
Cardioregulatory, vaso-motor, and adrenosecre-tory centers	Dog	4–5	C[4]	15–30	C[4]
	Dog			5–10	C
Respiratory center	Dog, rat	4–5	C[4]	15–30	C
	Dog, rat	$\frac{1}{3}-\frac{1}{2}$	C		
	Rat[3]	20–40	C[5]		
Spinal cord	Cat	$\frac{2}{3}-1$	C	35–45	C
	Cat			90–120	C
	Rabbit	$\frac{2}{3}-2$	C		
Autonomic synapses	Cat	30–40	N, C[6]	120–360+	N[7]
Peripheral nerve	Cat, dog, rabbit	15–45	N[8]		
	Frog	70–360	N[8]		
	Lobster	40–120	N[8]		
Heart	Dog, rabbit, rat	5–20	C		
	Dog, rabbit, rat	4–6	N	8–11	N
	Dog, rabbit, rat[3]	47–111	N		
Lung	Dog			30–45	C[9]
Kidney	Dog			30–60	C[9]
	Dog			>120	C[9]
	Rabbit			60–90	C[9]
	Rat			<120	C[9]
Liver	Dog			20–75	C[9]
	Dog			>60[10]	C[9]
Skeletal muscle	Dog, rabbit, rat	120–360	C	480	C
Smooth muscle, jejunum	Rabbit	1–15	N[8]	>180	N
Small intestine	Dog			120–240+	C[11]
Testis	Rat[12]			10–30	C

[1] Period of anoxia or circulatory arrest during which function persists.

[2] Period of anoxia or circulatory arrest compatible with complete recovery of function, *i.e.*, before irreversible changes occur.

[3] Newborn.

[4] Isolated, perfused head.

[5] Decapitated.

[6] Intact and isolated ganglia.

[7] 25% recovery at 6 hr.

[8] Isolated, *in vitro*.

[9] Criterion: death of animal.

[10] Value for liver at 24°–27° C.

[11] Criteria: electrical reaction and death of animal.

[12] Histological study of spermatogenesis.

(From N.A.S., *Handbook of Respiration*. W. B. Saunders Co., 1958.)

if ever exists, the word *hypoxia*, indicating a state of decreased oxygen availability or diminished utilization of oxygen by tissues, is a preferable term.

Saklad (1953) has classified hypoxia into seven categories in contrast to the four conventional types of anoxia. By so doing, a better etiological designation is achieved (Table 4-4).

Atmospheric hypoxia is due to reduction in available oxygen in the inhaled atmosphere. This could result from high altitude, dilution with inert gases such as anesthetic gases, or confinement in unventilated areas, such as an air-tight box.

Tidal hypoxia is the result of decreased oxygen uptake because of decreased respiratory exchange. Disease, drugs (anesthetic agents are an example), respiratory obstruction, or altered respiratory dynamics (such as convulsions) are causes.

Alveolar hypoxia is produced by a decrease in number or efficiency of the functioning alveoli such as occurs with pneumonia, emphysema, atelectasis, pleural effusion, or intrapulmonary exudates.

Hemoglobic hypoxia is due to reduction in hemoglobin content of the blood, or reduction in available hemoglobin as in carbon monoxide poisoning.

Stagnant hypoxia is the result of poor circulation.

Histotoxic hypoxia results from inability of cells to utilize oxygen properly and may be produced by alcohol, anesthetics, cyanide, or carbon monoxide.

Demand hypoxia is caused by metabolic conditions in which body requirements for oxygen are elevated above normal, such as hyperthyroidism, hyperpyrexia, or blood dyscrasias.

The blood values and characteristics of the various types of hypoxia are shown in Tables 4-5 and 4-6.

There is great variation in dogs' susceptibility to oxygen want (Davis, 1949). Dogs are better able to withstand hypoxia than cats, because of their greater ability to increase ventilatory volume through response to chemoreceptor stimulation (Stacy and Whitehorn, 1947). Resistance to hypoxia is greater in very young animals than in adults. Survival of tissues under hypoxic conditions varies considerably as shown in Table 4-7.

Cardiovascular Effects of Hypoxia

The immediate circulatory response to lack of oxygen is dilation of the coronary and cerebral vessels, elevation of the pulse rate, and increase in cardiac output. The rise in blood pressure is through action of the carotid and aortic bodies, these centers sending afferent impulses to the vasomotor center. In conditions of oxygen deficiency three mechanisms tend to protect the heart: (1) decreased tonicity of the coronary vessels, (2) increased coronary circulation due to greater diversion of the cardiac output, and (3) decrease in cardiac work.

Capillaries are extremely vulnerable to hypoxia, the endothelium being easily injured with resultant relaxation and dilation. They thus become packed with stagnant red blood cells and their walls become progressively permeable to fluid and plasma proteins. This produces a vicious cycle as shown in Figure 4–7.

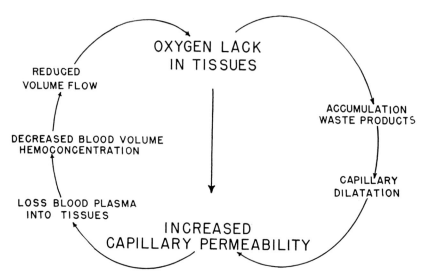

FIGURE 4–7. The vicious cycle of oxygen deprivation and increased capillary permeability. (From Saklad, M.: *Inhalation Therapy and Resuscitation.* Charles C Thomas, 1953.)

Drinker (1925) has pointed out that capillaries in different parts of the body vary in their resistance to hypoxia, and the endothelium of pulmonary capillaries is least resistant to low oxygen tensions. This results in fluid accumulation in the alveolar wall, further obstructing exchange of oxygen and carbon dioxide in the lungs.

The early response to hypoxia is an increased efficiency of the cardiovascular system. Continued lack of oxygen, however, produces a fall in blood pressure, pulse rate, and cardiac output. Fatal hypoxia in dogs almost invariably results in ventricular standstill rather than fibrillation (Harris, 1946).

Effect of Oxygen Deprivation on Liver, Kidney, and Adrenal Gland

The liver parenchyma is quite sensitive to hypoxia, more so than kidney and muscle, and a decrease in hepatic function results. Lack of oxygen caused by ligation of the hepatic artery will produce a lethal bacterial necrosis in dogs. The kidney can tolerate lack of oxygen for approximately 2 hours (Hamilton *et al.*, 1948).

Rats exposed to low oxygen tension for long periods of time have necrosis and hemorrhage in the adrenal glands. Lewis *et al.* (1942) have shown that if adrenalectomized animals are given adrenocortical hormone they withstand oxygen deficit to a greater degree; thus, it appears that the adrenal glands protect against oxygen deprivation to a certain extent.

Blood Changes with Lack of Oxygen

Several chemical changes take place in the blood during hypoxia. Over-ventilation with blow-off of carbon dioxide may cause alkalosis, particularly if the kidneys do not compensate by excretion of bicarbonate. In extreme hypoxia acidosis will result, due to incomplete combustion of carbohydrates resulting in lactic acid formation, and also to decreased respiratory efficiency with carbon dioxide retention (Fig. 4–8).

Lack of oxygen has been shown to produce hyperglycemia with glycosuria. This is probably mediated by the effect of hypoxia on the central nervous system and is associated with increased output of epinephrine.

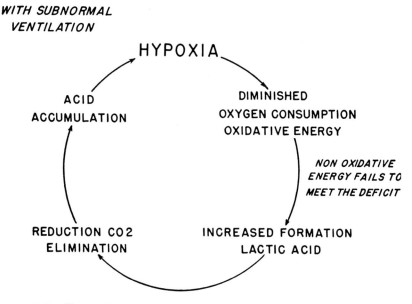

FIGURE 4–8. The tendency toward acidosis due to subnormal ventilation. (From Saklad, M.: *Inhalation Therapy and Resuscitation.* Charles C Thomas, 1953.)

Body Response to Hypoxia

Hypoxia produces a fall in body temperature, probably as a homeostatic reaction which tends to protect the animal. (Traumatic shock is also accompanied by reduction in oxygen consumption.) The time of appearance and degree of response to hypoxia varies greatly in individual patients and is dependent to a large extent upon their condition. Animals with cardiovascular or respiratory disease will often develop hypoxia under conditions which ordinarily would not affect a normal animal. These patients lack ability to compensate by circulatory and respiratory adjustment.

Cellular Effects of Oxygen Deficit

When cell metabolism is reduced by lack of oxygen, there is a short period of stimulation followed by paralysis and finally cell death. During the paralytic stage intracellular electrolytic changes take place which continue to affect the cell even though hypoxia may have ceased. These consist in a loss of intracellular potassium and a rise in intracellular sodium. The latter causes retention of water in the cell or intracellular edema. This edema disrupts normal cell function after the hypoxic insult has been withdrawn, and may be so severe that the cell becomes distended and finally ruptures, producing irreversible cellular changes. Intracellular edema probably does not occur until the hypoxic insult has finished and does not reach its maximum effect for 6 to 8 hours. This may be manifested clinically by return of the patient to consciousness followed by drowsiness and confusion which persist for another 24 hours.

Symptoms of Hypoxia

Symptoms of acute oxygen insufficiency include increased respiratory rate, rise in systolic blood pressure, elevated pulse rate, nausea and vomiting, dilated pupils, muscular incoordination, and twitching followed by convulsions. Cyanosis is not a reliable sign of the extent of hypoxia. Cyanosis is caused by reduced hemoglobin in the capillary blood and a minimum of 5 gm. for each 100 ml. of blood is required to make a visible color change. In anemic animals color changes may not occur until arterial oxygen saturation has fallen to as low as 55%. In very anemic animals cyanosis may never become evident even though the animal dies from hypoxia. Cyanosis is not a prominent characteristic of shock because there is marked capillary constriction.

Since the brain is the organ most sensitive to oxygen deficit, the main characteristic of a hypoxic state is unconsciousness. The severity of the insult will determine the depth of unconsciousness, but as far as the central nervous system is concerned it is impossible to determine what form of hypoxia has caused the insult. Following *severe* hypoxia all reflexes will be absent in the early stages except for the light reflex. Later, the reflexes may become exaggerated. Usually there is a state of vasoconstriction with a fall in blood pressure and increased heart rate, indicating diminished cardiac output. When extensive damage occurs to the vasomotor center the systolic blood pressure will fall to shock levels. Swann (1953) has shown that irreversible cerebral damage occurs in unanesthetized hypoxic dogs approximately 1 minute following circulatory failure or when the blood pressure falls below 55 mm. Hg. With mild hypoxia mental confusion is transitory and recovery may occur after several days of unconsciousness, though neurologic residuals may develop. If a decerebrate state exists for more than 72 hours, complete recovery will not occur and the patient usually dies within 1 to 6 weeks. Hyperpyrexia may develop terminally with temperatures as high as 110° F.

Hyperventilation

From a practical standpoint hyperventilation is no problem. Patients who are hyperventilated cease to breath spontaneously; the color remains good and, as soon as blood carbon dioxide is allowed to accumulate, breathing resumes.

Biddulph *et al.* (1960) hyperventilated dogs with a respirator for 1 hour and reported the arterial blood pH was 7.65. Kanter (1961) in a similar experiment could find no change in glomerular filtration rate, renal plasma flow, hematocrit, rectal temperature, heart rate or total solids in the plasma. In the latter experiment hyperventilation was conducted for 3 hours and the arterial blood pH reached 7.63.

Oxygen Toxicity

When mice were exposed to 100% oxygen at atmospheric pressure for 72 hours most of the animals died, death being attributed to oxygen want (Kaunitz, 1945). At necropsy, rabbits kept in an atmosphere containing 80% oxygen for 8 days had capillary engorgement with hemorrhage, interstitial and alveolar exudate, and hypertrophy and desquamation of alveolar walls with infiltration of mononuclear cells (Binger *et al.*, 1927). These investigators demonstrated that oxygen concentrations greater than 70% led to drowsiness, loss of appetite and weight, dyspnea and cyanosis culminating in death, ironically, from extreme oxygen want.

Administration of over 40% oxygen to premature infants for a long period will cause retrolental fibroplasia with permanent blindness.

Effects of Excess Carbon Dioxide

Carbon dioxide was discovered by Joseph Priestly about 1770, and its anesthetic properties first noted by Hickman in 1824. The latter demonstrated on dogs that the pain of surgery could be abolished by inhalation of this gas; however, strange as it may seem, it was not until 1929 that the anesthetic properties of carbon dioxide were confirmed by Leake and Waters.

Carbon dioxide is the normal physiological respiratory stimulant and is found in a concentration of 0.25% in air. Its administration has been recommended for: (1) replacement therapy, (2) its effect on respiration, (3) its effect on circulation, and (4) for mental conditions in man. As far as replacement therapy is concerned in conditions encountered clinically, carbon dioxide is already retained and further administration is probably detrimental. While carbon dioxide is a powerful respiratory stimulant under normal circumstances, in hypoxia its action becomes reversed and administration may produce respiratory depression. Grodins *et al.* (1946) studied acid-base changes in arterial blood of dogs during fatal hypoxia and successful resuscitation. They concluded that it is unnecessary to add carbon dioxide to the resuscitation mixture in order to maintain a normal carbon dioxide level during artificial respiration.

Many methods for oxygen administration are confined extensions of the respiratory tract resulting in considerable dead space. This tends to cause carbon dioxide accumulation in the patient due to insufficient elimination. Five per cent carbon dioxide can be tolerated by a patient. Higher concentrations produce a rise in pulse rate and systolic blood pressure, increased depth of respiration (often with little increase in rate), and muscular twitching followed by convulsions. The color of the patient may be good. Concentrations of 20 to 30% are sub-anesthetic, 30 to 40% are anesthetic, and over 40% may be fatal (Fig. 4–9).

Biddulph *et al.* (1960) have shown that dogs anesthetized with thiopental and respired with a mixture of 30% carbon dioxide and 70% oxygen had a mean blood pH of 6.78 after 1 hour. Miller *et al.* (1950) found that alveolar carbon dioxide concentrations above 15% depress adrenal function in the dog as evidenced by absence of an eosinopenia following injection of epinephrine. Dogs given a mixture of 30% carbon dioxide and 70% oxygen exhibited a decreased tolerance to thiopental and pentobarbital; in some dogs which subsequently survived the blood pH reached 6.61.

A high incidence of cardiac malformations can be produced in rats by exposure of the mother to carbon dioxide during pregnancy (Haring, 1960). A gas mixture containing 6% carbon dioxide, 20% oxygen and 74% nitrogen was found to produce ventricular septal defects with or without other cardiac abnormalities. For this reason particular care should be exercised to prevent development of high carbon dioxide levels in pregnant animals.

In the past, carbon dioxide has been added to anesthetic gases at the termination of anesthesia, the purpose being to stimulate respiration and thus hasten excretion of anesthetic through the lungs. This practice is detrimental, since most patients already have carbon dioxide retention, and cardiac fibrillation may result.

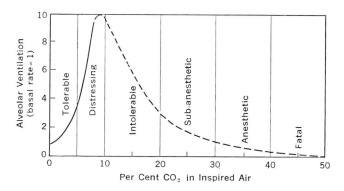

FIGURE 4–9. Effect on alveolar ventilation of breathing carbon dioxide in the inspired air. (Guyton, A. C.: *Textbook of Medical Physiology*, W. B. Saunders Co., 1961 from data of Gray, J. S.: *Pulmonary Ventilation and Its Physiological Regulation*, Charles C Thomas, 1950.)

Pneumothorax

When air enters the pleural cavity the condition known as pneumothorax is produced. Pneumothorax is divided into two types depending upon the cause; in *open* pneumothorax a penetrating wound exists between the pleural cavity and the body surface; in *closed* pneumothorax air enters the pleural cavity through rupture of the lung. The extent and severity of the actions that follow depend upon the size of the opening and the amount of air gaining access to the cavity.

Three events occur in open pneumothorax: (1) There is collapse of the lung on the affected side (Fig. 4–10). The collapsed lung acts as a venous-arterial shunt, since blood passing through the lung is returned unoxygenated to the left side of the heart, and reduces cardiac efficiency. (2) The mediastinum, which forms a fragile barrier between the two halves of the chest cavity, shifts toward the side away from the opening. This causes partial collapse of the other lung. As respiratory movements continue, the mediastinum is drawn toward the closed side of the chest during inspiration and on expiration is forced toward the opening. This action further reduces the effective respiratory volume of the remaining lung. (3) When an open pneumothorax is created the animal will continue to breathe, but the exposed lung instead of moving in the conventional manner becomes smaller on inspiration and larger on expiration. This movement is termed "paradoxical respiration". On inspiration, air pressure in the main bronchus of the exposed lung exceeds that in the trachea,

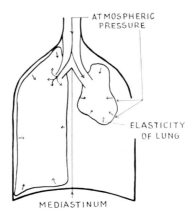

FIGURE 4–10. Forces responsible for collapse of lung when chest wall is opened. (From Wright, J. G. and Hall, L. W.: *Veterinary Anaesthesia and Analgesia.* 5th ed. The Williams & Wilkins Co., 1961.)

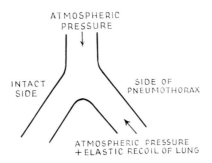

FIGURE 4–11. Forces responsible for "pendulum air" transfer from lung to lung in open pneumothorax. (From Wright, J. G. and Hall, L. W.: *Veterinary Anaesthesia and Analgesia.* 5th ed. The Williams & Wilkins Co., 1961.)

since the pressure is a combination of the elastic recoil of the lung plus the atmospheric pressure (Fig. 4–11). Air drawn into the intact lung comes first from the collapsed lung and then from the exterior, the collapsed lung becoming smaller on inspiration and enlarging on expiration. Consequently, an animal with open pneumothorax has considerable "pendulum air" which transfers from lung to lung and is ineffective in respiratory exchange.

Open pneumothorax is created each time an intrathoracic operation is conducted. For years little chest surgery was done because veterinarians did not have adequate means for respiring animals under these conditions. At the present time, however, many methods are available (Chapter 5, p. 82).

When a thoracotomy is performed, air enters the lungs through the trachea and also the pleural cavity through the wound. The amount of air entering the chest by each route depends on the relationship between the cross-sectional area of the trachea and that of the thoracotomy opening (Wright and Hall, 1961). If a large wound exists, more air enters the thorax by this route and the mediastinum is pushed toward the closed side of the chest. In the dog and cat the mediastinum is very flexible and thin, and changes of intrapleural pressure on one side are immediately communicated to the other. Open thoracotomy in the dog is thus essentially bilateral. The size of the opening determines the length of time the animal can survive without artificial ventilation. With a small aperture, respiration may continue for a long period before asphyxia results.

References

BIDDULPH, C., HOF, H., CLANCY, R., and BROWN, E. B., JR.: Plasma and Tissue Electrolyte Changes Produced in Dogs by Hypercapnia, Hypocapnia, and Hypoxia. Publication 60–83, School of Aviation Medicine, U.S.A.F. Aerospace Medical Center, Brooks Air Force Base, Texas, 1960.

BINGER, C. A. L., FAULKNER, J. M., and MOORE, R. L.: Oxygen Poisoning in Mammals. J. Exper. Med., 45, 849, 1927.

COMBEN, N.: Some Recent Advances in General Anesthesia of the Dog. Brit. Vet. J., 106, 348, 1950.

COMROE, J. H., JR. and SCHMIDT, C. F.: The Part Played by Reflexes from the Carotid Body in the Chemical Regulation of Respiration in the Dog. Am. J. Physiol., 121, 75, 1938.

DAVIS, H. A.: Shock and Allied Forms of Failure of the Circulation. Grune & Stratton, New York, 1949.

DRINKER, C. K.: The Efficiency of the Oxygen-Carbon Dioxide Treatment of Carbon Monoxide Poisoning. J. Indust. Hyg., 7, 539, 1925.

FARHI, L., OTIS, A. B., and PROCTOR, D. F.: Measurement of Intrapleural Pressure at Different Points in the Chest of the Dog. J. Applied Physiol., 10, 15, 1957.

GRODINS, F. S., LEIN, A., and ADLER, H. F.: Changes in Blood Acid-Base Balance During Asphyxia and Resuscitation. Am. J. Physiol., 147, 433, 1946.

HAMILTON, T. B., PHILLIPS, R. A., and HILLER, A.: Duration of Renal Ischemia Required to Produce Uremia. Am. J. Physiol., 152, 517, 1948.

HARING, O. M.: Cardiac Malformations in Rats Induced by Exposure of the Mother to Carbon Dioxide During Pregnancy. Circ. Res., 8, 1218, 1960.

HARRIS, A. S.: Ventricular Fibrillation and Standstill in Coronary Occlusion. Fed. Proc., 5, 41, 1946.

KANTER, G. S.: The Effect of Hyperventilation on Glomerular Filtration and Renal Plasma Flow. Publication 61–48, School of Aviation Medicine, U.S.A.F. Aerospace Medical Center, Brooks Air Force Base, Texas, 1961.

KAUNITZ, J.: Effect of High Oxygen Tension on Respiratory System. J. Mt. Sinai Hosp., 12, 441, 1945.

LEWIS, R. A., THORN, G. W., KOEPF, G. F., and DORRANCE, S. S.: The Role of the Adrenal Cortex in Acute Anoxia. J. Clin. Invest., 21, 33, 1942.

MILLER, F. A., HEMINGWAY, A., NIER, A. O., KNIGHT, R. T., BROWN, E. B., JR., and VARCO, R. L.: The Development of, and Certain Clinical Applications for, a Portable Mass Spectrometer. J. Thoracic Surg., *20*, 714, 1950.

ROMIJN, C.: Respiration in the Dog. II. The Dead Space and Its Variation under Physiological Conditions. Arch. Neerl. Physiol., *27*, 347, 1943.

SAKLAD, M.: *Inhalation Therapy and Resuscitation.* Charles C Thomas, Springfield, Ill., 1953.

STACY, R. W. and WHITEHORN, W. V.: The Comparative Susceptibility of Cats and Dogs to Anoxia. Fed. Proc., *6*, 210, 1947.

SWANN, H. G.: The Principles of Resuscitation. Anesthesiology, *14*, 126, 1953.

TANAKA, R., FUJIMORI, M., and VIRTUE, R. W.: Oxygen Utilization by Dogs after Administration of Potassium Perchlorate During Hypothermia, and at a Pressure of 2 Atmospheres. Anesthesiology, *22*, 20, 1961.

WHITEHEAD, R. W. and DRAPER, W. B.: A Respiratory Reflex Originating from the Thoracic Wall of the Dog. Anesthesiology, *8*, 159, 1947.

WRIGHT, J. G. and HALL, L. W.: *Veterinary Anaesthesia and Analgesia.* 5th ed. The Williams & Wilkins Co., Baltimore, 1961.

OXYGEN ADMINISTRATION AND ARTIFICIAL RESPIRATION

Chapter 5

THE fundamental objectives of respiration are to oxygenate the blood effectively and to eliminate excess carbon dioxide. For this to be accomplished, it is necessary to establish a satisfactory airway and a near-normal tidal exchange. Since this is not always possible, to increase the efficiency of respiration the percentage of oxygen in the inhaled atmosphere is increased.

Oxygen and Carbon Dioxide Production

For many years oxygen was produced by various chemical methods. Today, purified air is liquified by compression and cooling and the oxygen separated by fractional distillation at approximately $-300°$ F. Oxygen produced by this method has a purity exceeding 99.5%.

Following separation it is compressed into cylinders at 1800 to 2400 pounds per square inch (psi). From the standpoint of cost, cylinders containing 244 cubic feet of oxygen should be used since they are most economical. These cylinders hold approximately 6900 liters at 2200 psi (See Fig. 8–3, facing p. 134 for cylinder sizes).

Carbon dioxide can be produced by several methods, among which are: (1) burning of fuels in a special reactor, (2) heating of calcium carbonate, and (3) fermentation of starches or sugars. Car-

5

bon dioxide gas is sold commercially, compressed as a liquid in cylinders or mixed with oxygen in concentrations of 2.5, 5.0, 7.5, and 10%. Higher concentrations depress the central nervous system and ultimately produce asphyxial death.

Determining Oxygen Cylinder Content

A rule of thumb for determining the number of liters of oxygen in commercial cylinders is to multiply the pressure by 3. The length of time a cylinder will last can be estimated by multiplying the pressure times 3 and dividing by the flow in liters per minute.

Example:

> Cylinder pressure 350 pounds and flow 6 liters per minute,
> 350 × 3 ÷ 6 = 175 minutes

Table 5–1 shows the approximate hours of service in standard 244 cubic feet cylinders of oxygen.

Table 5–1.—Approximate Remaining Hours of Service in Standard 244 Cubic Feet Cylinders of U.S.P. Oxygen

	Full Cylinder	Contents at Diminishing Gauge Pressure		
Rate of flow in liters per min.	244 cu. ft. 2,200 lbs. 6,900 liters	183 cu. ft. 1,650 lbs. 5,175 liters	122 cu. ft. 1,100 lbs. 3,450 liters	61 cu. ft. 550 lbs. 1,725 liters
4	28¾ hours	21½ hours	14¼ hours	7¼ hours
6	19 hours	14¼ hours	9½ hours	4¾ hours
8	14¼ hours	10¾ hours	7¼ hours	3½ hours
10	11½ hours	8½ hours	5¾ hours	2¾ hours
12	9½ hours	7¼ hours	4¾ hours	2¼ hours
14	8 hours	6 hours	4 hours	2 hours
16	7 hours	5¼ hours	3½ hours	1¾ hours

Examples—Full cylinder, at 2,200 lbs. pressure, flowing at a rate of 4 liters should last 28¾ hours. A cylinder with 1,100 lbs. pressure flowing at a rate of 6 liters per minute should last 9½ hours.

(Courtesy of Ohio Chemical & Surgical Equipment Company, Madison, Wisconsin.)

Regulators

When using gases from large cylinders, it is necessary that they be reduced to safe pressures. This is accomplished by means of a regulator which may be of one, two, or three stages. Single stage regulators reduce tank pressure to approximately 60 pounds in a single step; two stage regulators reduce tank pressure first to approximately 400 pounds and then to 60 pounds in the second stage;

three stage regulators reduce the pressure to 750 pounds, then 400 pounds, and finally to 60 pounds, following which the gas is metered through a flowmeter.

One and two stage regulators are sometimes hard to distinguish, the former usually being thinner on the lateral view (Fig. 5–1). One stage regulators present certain hazards and disadvantages. If the valve on an oxygen tank provided with a single stage regulator is

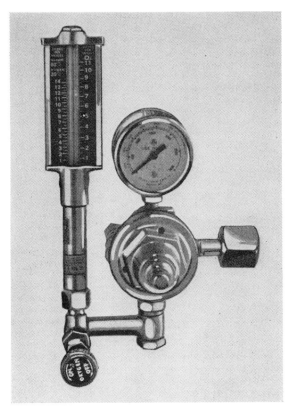

FIGURE 5–1A

opened rapidly and the regulator valve is also open, the regulator may shatter. Single stage regulators do not maintain oxygen pressure as cylinder pressure drops, so frequent adjustments are necessary to produce a uniform delivery of oxygen. With multiple stage regulators, oxygen flow is maintained at a uniform rate until the cylinder is almost exhausted (Fig. 5–2).

After a regulator is attached to the cylinder, the liter-flow mechanism should be turned to the "off" position before the cylinder valve is opened. The cylinder valve should be opened very slowly, oxygen never being permitted to enter a regulator suddenly.

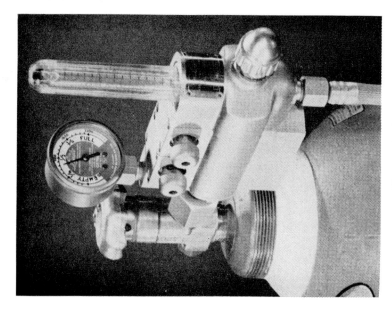

FIGURE 5–1C

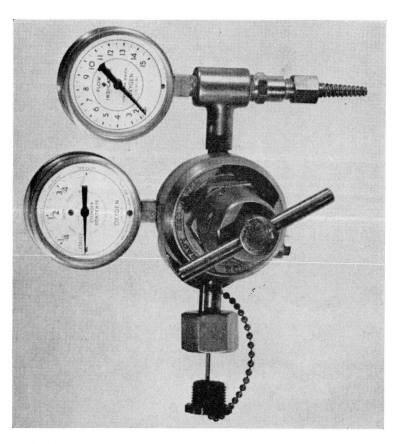

FIGURE 5–1B

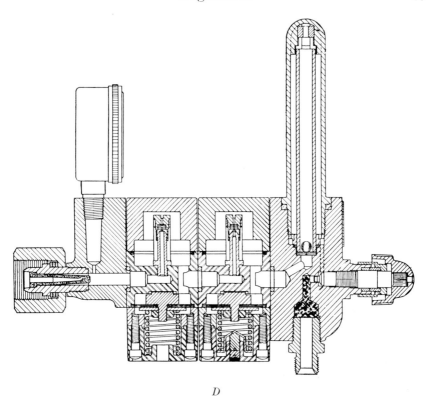

D

FIGURE 5–1. Single stage regulator, kinetic type (*A*), two stage regulator, Bourdon type (*B*), three stage regulator, Thorpe tube type (*C*), and cutaway view of *C*. (From Saklad, M.: *Inhalation Therapy and Resuscitation.* Charles C Thomas, 1953.)

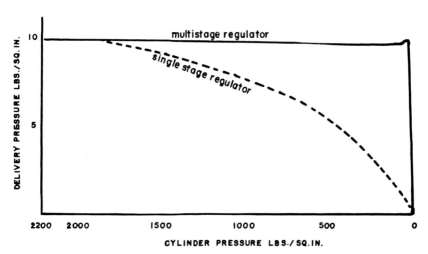

FIGURE 5–2. Comparison of flow characteristics of single versus multi-stage regulators. (From Saklad, M.: *Inhalation Therapy and Resuscitation.* Charles C Thomas, 1953).

The Air Injector Valve

If it is desired to use oxygen at concentrations lower than 100%, an air injector valve can be attached to the regulator (Fig. 5–3). Oxygen entering this apparatus from the regulator passes into a

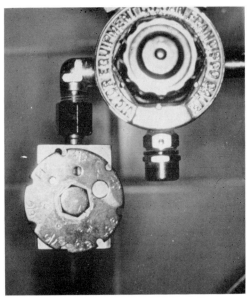

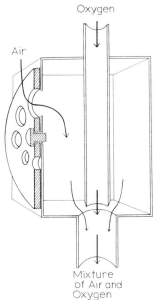

FIGURE 5–3.   An air injector valve (top) for mixing room air and oxygen. The venturi principle is used in its operation (bottom).

chamber through a narrow orifice. This creates a negative pressure
and draws air into the chamber through the port on the front of the
valve. The oxygen-air mixture is then forced out the bottom. The
volume of air aspirated into the chamber depends upon the size of
port in the metal disc.

The disc is marked in per cent of oxygen flowing to the patient.
With the disc set at 40% and an oxygen flow of 3 liters per minute,
approximately 5 liters of air are taken in.

Safety Precautions with Oxygen

At high pressures the oxidizing powers of oxygen are greatly enhanced. Fats, oils, and paints may oxidize with explosive force, producing so-called *flash-flames* or *oxygen-fires*. For this reason grease or
oils should never be used around oxygen cylinders and equipment.
Smoking must be prohibited in areas where oxygen is used. Since
oxygen supports combustion all possible sources should be eliminated.
Candles, open flames, electrical devices such as heating pads or fans,
x-ray equipment, and electrocautery machines are dangerous sources
of combustion.

Oxygen cylinders should be stored so they cannot tip over, otherwise in falling the cylinder valve may be opened or broken. In this
event the cylinder can become jet propelled in the same manner as
a rocket. If stored against a wall, a safety chain should be installed
to hold the cylinder upright.

Permanent Oxygen Supply

In building new hospitals consideration should be given to permanent installation of an oxygen pipeline system (Fig. 5–4). Advantages of such an arrangement include: (1) ability to buy oxygen
in larger tanks with increased economy, (2) removal of unsightly
tanks from operating room and other areas, (3) ability to use oxygen
in several areas of the hospital without duplication of equipment, and
(4) an increased inclination to use oxygen when indicated because of
availability and ease in administration.

Methods of Oxygen Administration

Many types of apparatus are available for administration of oxygen to small animals. Selection of equipment is determined by cost,
convenience, and capabilities desired. In describing equipment for
use in man a definite distinction is made between *inhalators* and
respirators. Inhalators deliver oxygen to a face mask and the patient
through his own respiratory effort draws oxygen into the pul-

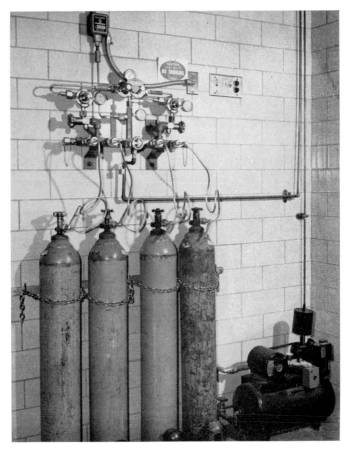

FIGURE 5–4.   Cylinder bank for built-in oxygen pipeline system. A manifold automatically switches flow to full cylinders as ones in use become exhausted. An alarm signals the need for replacing empty cylinders. A vacuum pump (right) provides suction to various parts of the hospital. (Courtesy of Dr. A. R. Evans, Rowley Memorial Hospital, Springfield, Mass.)

monary tree.   Respirators not only deliver oxygen but also, by altering intrapulmonary pressure, forcibly produce an increased tidal and minute volume of respiration. The distinction in equipment for small animals is not so clear. Oxygen can be administered to small animals by the following means:

1. Tent or chamber
2. Nasal catheter
3. Face mask or endotracheal catheter
    a. Diffusion respiration
    b. Non-rebreathing valve
    c. Respirator
    d. Gas machine

The simplest equipment is relatively inexpensive and will prove life-saving in emergencies. Today, the veterinarian who anesthetizes animals without oxygen available is taking an unnecessary risk. If an anesthetic fatality occurred, he could probably be held liable for malpractice.

Tents or Chambers

A simple method for administration of oxygen to man is with an oxygen tent. The canopy of the tent covers the head of the patient's bed and cooled oxygen is pumped into it. The closest approach to this method in veterinary practice has been the use of a transparent plastic bag into which the whole animal or its head is placed. This has not proved very satisfactory for use with small animals because of the restraint problem. For this reason the tendency has been to use oxygen chambers. These are generally of two types: (1) a box with a hinged panel on the top or side which allows access to the interior, or (2) an ordinary hospital cage with solid walls, the door of which has been altered to make it air-tight and to which have been attached the necessary fittings (Fig. 5–5). Equipment for proper use of chambers should include a thermometer, a gauge for determining relative humidity, and an oxygen analyzer.

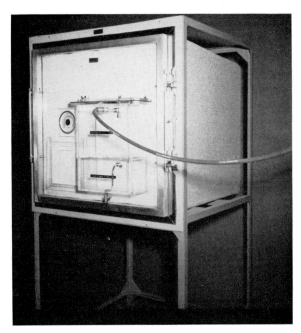

FIGURE 5–5.   Oxygen chamber with oxygen hose entering ice compartment on door. (Courtesy of Kirschner Manufacturing Company, Vashon, Washington.)

Most chambers are built so that oxygen enters at the top, is cooled by passing over ice in a container, and then settles to the patient. Water, produced by the melting ice, is drained to the exterior to prevent a rise in chamber humidity. Warm carbon dioxide rises to the top of the chamber and escapes through vents. The oxygen content should be tested at least 2 or 3 times a day because flow into the chamber is not necessarily an indication of oxygen concentration. Commercial oxygen analyzers for tent or chamber therapy are accurate to within 3 to 5%. Phillips and Burkhardt (1951) have described an analyzer which can be made with a few easily obtainable materials. A recent development in human medicine is the electronic control unit which automatically maintains any desired oxygen level.

Relative humidity within the chamber should be maintained between 40 and 60% in most instances. The carbon dioxide content should not be more than 1.2%. By maintaining a minimum flow of 6 to 8 liters of oxygen per minute with a concentration of 50%, harmful accumulations of carbon dioxide do not take place even in the absence of soda lime. Soda lime should be used when flow rates are less and higher concentrations of oxygen are desired.

A thermometer should be used to determine chamber temperature. Oxygen chambers which are not equipped to cool and dry the air may be detrimental to the patient and even cause death by heat stroke.

In the presence of fever, metabolism is increased and oxygen requirements are thereby increased. When an animal with fever is placed in a chamber, the oxygen flow should be increased to 10 liters per minute, flooding the cage, cooling the ambient temperature, and thereby lowering the animal's temperature.

If desired, a nebulizer can be inserted in the oxygen line and various solutions, such as antibiotics, anti-foaming agents, and bronchodilators, can be vaporized into the oxygen chamber.

Nasal Catheter

For continuous administration of oxygen to animals which are severely depressed, a nasal catheter of small gauge polyethylene (PE 200) or rubber tubing is quite effective. The catheter is held against the animal's head and the distance from the external nares to the pharynx marked on the catheter with adhesive tape. An anesthetic jelly is applied to the catheter and it is inserted along the floor of the nasal passage as far as the mark. Adhesive tape is applied around the catheter and to the nose to hold the catheter in position. Oxygen is then regulated to flow to the patient at the desired rate (Fig. 5–6).

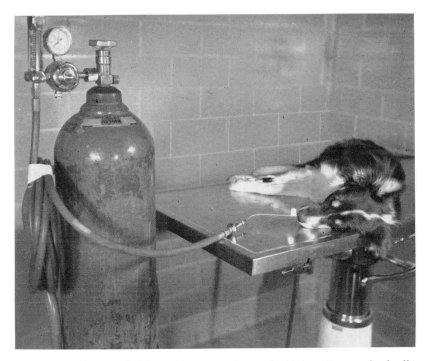

FIGURE 5–6.   Oxygen administered by means of a nasal catheter. Tape marks the distance for proper insertion.

Face Mask

Administration of oxygen by means of a mask is effective during anesthesia and for short periods during emergencies; however, unless the animal is quite moribund or is anesthetized, it probably will fight the mask and reduce its effectiveness.

Endotracheal Intubation

Endotracheal intubation is used for one or more of the following purposes:

1. To maintain an open airway while the patient is under anesthesia.
2. To provide a means for administration of inhalation anesthetics and/or oxygen.
3. To facilitate positive pressure ventilation during open chest surgery.

Endotracheal catheters for use in small animals vary in size from 12 to 44 French,* the former being the smallest diameter and the latter the largest. They are made of rubber, plastic, or metal (Fig. 5–7). A simple tube is sufficient, provided maintenance of an airway is all that is desired, and can be made from ordinary red rubber tub-

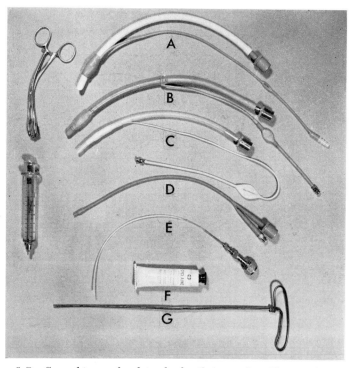

FIGURE 5–7.   Several types of endotracheal catheters and ancillary equipment. From top to bottom they are: (A) Davol plastic catheter with detachable cuff; (B) Magill rubber catheter with built-in cuff and signal balloon; (C) Foregger transparent plastic catheter with Guedel cuff; (D) Bardex catheter, with a tip removed, for use in very small animals; and (E) polyethylene (PE 200) nasal or endotracheal catheter. Water-soluble anesthetic jelly (F) is used to lubricate the catheters. A bent wire (G) is sometimes useful as a stilette to stiffen small catheters on insertion. A syringe and tongue forceps (left) are used to inflate and clamp the cuff.

ing of various diameters. The material is cut into suitable lengths, with the end of the tube which is to be inserted in the patient beveled at a 45° angle. The beveled tip is then put in an open flame until the rubber begins to melt. It is quickly withdrawn and the melted material removed by rubbing with chloroform-soaked cotton. This will produce a smooth, rounded edge on the catheter, preventing trauma to the larynx.

* See Appendix B, p. 409, for comparison of French scale with Davol and Magill catheter numbers.

If the trachea is to be completely occluded except for the catheter lumen, an inflatable cuff is attached to the catheter. The most suitable cuffs have a signal balloon on the opposite end of the inflation tube. When the catheter is inserted in the trachea, the degree of inflation of the hidden cuff can be determined by observation of the balloon.

An inexpensive and effective technique for making new cuffs has been described by Wycoff (1947). The inflation tubing, blunted needle, and signal balloon are salvaged from leaking cuffs. These are then inserted into new cuffs made from Penrose drain tubing. With practice, cuffs can be easily and simply constructed at a fraction of their cost commercially.

To insure longer inflation tube life, a hypodermic needle of suitable size should be blunted on a whetstone and inserted permanently in the tube. A 10 cc. syringe can then be used to inflate the tube. Use of a sharp hypodermic needle for this purpose should be avoided, since the point of the needle frequently will perforate the tube causing it to leak.

If hemostats are used in clamping an inflation tube to keep the cuff distended, they have a tendency to cut the tube. This can be prevented by wrapping the blades with adhesive tape or by use of rubber-shod tongue forceps.

If positive pressure ventilation of the lungs is to be used, a separate metal catheter connector should be purchased for each endotracheal catheter. The connector, which joins the catheter with an adapter on the ventilation apparatus, is inserted into the catheter and never removed. Unless this procedure is followed the correct connector is seldom available when an emergency arises.

Following use, the endotracheal catheter should be washed thoroughly to remove respiratory secretions and anesthetic jelly from the lumen and exterior. It should then be cold sterilized in a suitable solution. Care should be taken to see that antiseptic solutions do not enter the inflation tube since leakage within the patient could burn the respiratory mucosa.

Intubation Procedure

In choosing an endotracheal catheter, the largest diameter which can be introduced without forcing should be selected. Those having a diameter considerably smaller than the natural airway tend to produce a prolonged negative intrathoracic pressure on inspiration. This negative pressure may be high enough to overcome the colloid osmotic pressure of blood in the lung vessels and result in pulmonary edema. It is good practice to have at hand a catheter which is thought to be the correct size and also one larger and one smaller. This insures that the correct size will be available.

When an endotracheal catheter is to be used, *the cuff should be checked by inflating it prior to the time the animal is anesthetized.* After the cuff has been checked to be sure that it is patent, the cuff and tip of the tube are lubricated with water-soluble jelly, preferably one containing an anesthetic. Use of an anesthetic jelly tends to prevent trauma and irritation to the larynx and trachea which otherwise cause postintubation cough.

Endotracheal catheters can be inserted by sight or touch. The sight method depends upon the animal being in a favorable position with sufficient light available to visualize the throat structures. The touch method is by far the most preferable, circumstances sometimes being such that it is impossible to see the epiglottis and larynx.

Once anesthesia has been induced and the jaw muscles have relaxed, the tongue is grasped between the thumb and fingers of the left hand and pulled anteriorly. This brings the larynx into the pharynx for a short distance. The index finger of the left hand is extended to depress the epiglottis, and the tip of the catheter is guided along the finger into the laryngeal opening. The epiglottis and arytenoid cartilages are landmarks for this procedure. When the catheter is properly inserted the arytenoid cartilages can always be felt making an inverted "V" ($\wedge$) over it. It should be emphasized that *the catheter must be placed in this position.* If it is pushed into the animal's pharynx, hoping that it will enter the larynx, it *always* enters the esophagus instead. Holding the open end of the catheter to one's ear is *not* a reliable test of its position and should never be used for this purpose. It will, however, confirm the presence of an open airway once the catheter has been positioned.

The catheter should be inserted so that the cuff is just beyond the larynx. No advantage is achieved by inserting it further. If inserted too far, one bronchus will be intubated and the other occluded, in which event the lung on the occluded side will gradually develop massive atelectasis. In breeds which are not brachycephalic, the endotracheal catheter is fixed to the upper jaw by passing tape around the catheter and the bridge of the nose twice. In brachycephalics the lower jaw is used. An alternate method is to fasten the catheter by means of a heavy rubber band looped about the patient's jaw. If a simple airway is all that is desired, the cuff need not be inflated. If positive pressure ventilation of the lungs is to be employed, the cuff is inflated, the inflation tube clamped, and the intubation procedure is complete (Fig. 5–8).

Following surgery the catheter should be left in position until the animal shows signs of recovery as evidenced by return of the swallowing reflex. If it is removed prematurely, reinsertion will be difficult if the animal is beginning to regain the jaw reflex. Prior to removal the clamp holding air within the cuff should be loosened. Tape fixing the catheter in position is then cut and the catheter carefully removed, taking care to see that the animal does not chew on it.

Advantages of an endotracheal catheter are:

1. It assures a patent airway. This is a *must* with brachycephalic breeds.

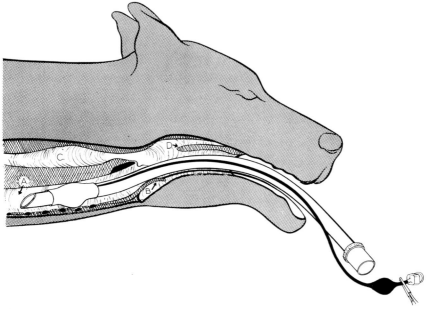

FIGURE 5–8. Schematic drawing of an endotracheal catheter in position: (*A*) trachea, (*B*) epiglottis, (*C*) esophagus, and (*D*) soft palate.

2. It prevents aspiration of vomitus if an inflated cuff is used.
3. It allows administration of oxygen and inhalant anesthetics.
4. Respiration can be easily controlled, enabling open chest surgery.
5. Atelectasis can be prevented.
6. It eliminates dead space, increasing efficiency over a closed system with a mask or cone. (An endotracheal catheter, size 38 French has a volume of 14 cc. A dog's nose, mouth, and pharynx have many times this capacity.)

Unfavorable sequelae which may occur from endotracheal intubation are:

1. Laryngitis and tracheitis due to trauma.
2. Overinflation and rupture of cuff with resultant laryngeal edema.

3. Aspiration or deglutition of the catheter.

4. Massive atelectasis if the catheter is inserted too far.

Diffusion Respiration

The phenomenon of diffusion respiration was first described in the dog by Draper and Whitehead (1944). *Diffusion respiration* may be defined as exchange of oxygen and carbon dioxide between the atmosphere and lung alveoli without respiratory movements. *Mechanical respiration*, occurring as the result of respiratory movements, is much more efficient; however, the anesthetized dog can, for a limited period, obtain sufficient oxygen by diffusion to maintain its metabolic requirements. This phenomenon was first noted during resuscitation of dogs from respiratory arrest produced by thiopental. It was found that artificial respiration could be suspended for a period of up to one-half hour, if there was a high oxygen concentra-

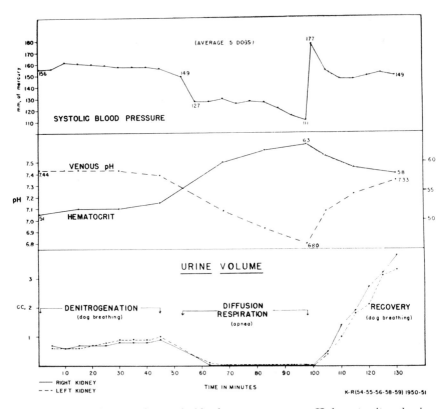

FIGURE 5–9.   Average changes in blood pressure, venous pH, hematocrit and urine volume in 5 dogs during diffusion respiration. Renal innervation intact on both sides. No intravenous fluid given. (From Kopecky, F. A., Rayburn, C. J., Whitehead, R. W., and Draper, W. B.: A Study of Anuria Occurring During Apnea under Diffusion Respiration. Am. J. Physiol., *168*, 131, 1952.)

tion in the respiratory tract and a tube in the mouth delivered 10 liters of oxygen per minute.

Three conditions are necessary for this phenomenon to be successful: (1) replacement of the nitrogen in the respiratory tract and in the atmosphere at the glottis by oxygen, (2) an adequate circulation, and (3) a patent airway.

Diffusion respiration produces a fall in blood pressure and oxygen content of arterial and venous blood with a progressive rise in carbon dixoide content. Concurrently, the pH of arterial and venous blood falls (to 6.72 and 6.84 respectively at 45 minutes). Urine production in dogs during diffusion respiration ceases within a few minutes after arrest of breathing, either with thiopental or muscle relaxants (Kopecky *et al.*, 1952; Irwin *et al.*, 1957) (Fig. 5–9).

Practical application of this phenomenon can be made in hypoxia by insertion of an endotracheal catheter and flow of 5 to 10 liters per minute of oxygen into the respiratory tree. This will temporarily relieve the oxygen want, whether the patient is breathing or not, and is often lifesaving.

Development of the Knowles diffusion respirator was based on this principle (Fig. 5–10). This device consists of an oxygen tank equipped with pressure reducing regulator, a reservoir bag, a water manometer, and tubing connecting these parts with an endotracheal catheter in the patient. In operation the regulator is set to flow so that the lungs are kept under constant positive pressure which can be varied by adjusting the water manometer.

The unit normally operates as an inhalator with the manometer barely immersed in water. Oxygen flow is adjusted to the point where there is a definite rise and fall in the reservoir bag with each respiration. The bag should not be allowed to become fully distended or completely flat.

In open chest surgery the same procedure is followed, except that just prior to opening the thorax the flow rate is increased to 10 to 15 liters and the manometer placed to the 4th calibration (each mark is equivalent to 1 cm. of water pressure). This excess is maintained until the chest is fully opened. The pressure is then reduced by decreasing the flow and if necessary by withdrawing the calibrated plastic manometer partially. Should artificial respiration be required, it can be done manually by rhythmically compressing the reservoir bag or by intermittently closing the expiratory opening. Just prior to closing the chest, the lungs are fully distended to fill the chest cavity. After closure the pressure is withdrawn, the lungs fall to normal atmospheric pressure and a negative pressure develops within the space between lungs and chest wall. In this manner negative pressure is re-established and the animal is able to resume spontaneous respiration.

6

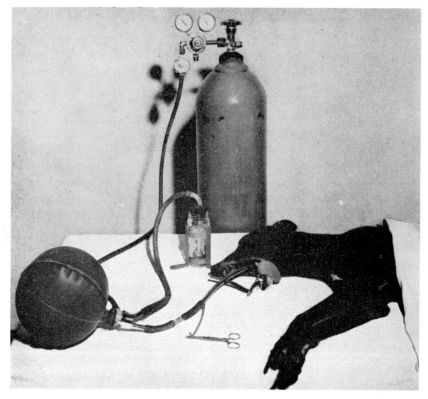

FIGURE 5–10. The Knowles diffusion respirator. Note the metal endotracheal catheter. (Courtesy of Professional Veterinary Services, Inc., Hialeah, Florida.)

Intermittent Positive Pressure Breathing (IPPB)

Though the need for positive pressure ventilation of the lungs has been recognized for a long time, it is only recently that this procedure has become routine in small animal practice. The earliest report of a successful diaphragmatic herniorrhaphy in the dog was by Schneider (1934). Artificial respiration, during the period in which the chest was open, was furnished by an assistant who manipulated an ordinary automobile tire pump attached to a piece of rubber tubing inserted into the trachea. As Schneider stated, "Obviously enough, no measure of the air intake was possible with such an arrangement, but it was variably provided by accelerating and retarding the pumping rate, as the condition of the patient demanded." This procedure while effective, left much to be desired. The mortality rate in diaphragmatic herniorrhaphy using this method of ventilating the lungs was approximately 50%.

As open chest surgery increased, the need for more refined methods of ventilation became apparent; new equipment and techniques resulted, many of them being adapted from human medicine. Most of the equipment will operate either with compressed air (such as an ordinary air compressor-storage tank system) or oxygen from cylinders. Because efficiency is increased by using oxygen there is little tendency for compressed air to be used.

"T" Tube

The simplest apparatus consists of an oxygen cylinder fitted with a reduction valve and flowmeter, a length of rubber tube leading to a T-piece of glass or metal, and a cuffed endotracheal catheter (Fig. 5–11). The endotracheal catheter is connected to one arm of the T,

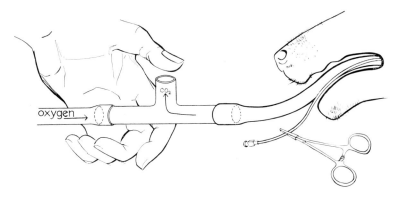

FIGURE 5–11. Oxygen administration with a "T" tube. Positive pressure is produced by intermittently closing the tube with the thumb. Carbon dioxide is exhaled when the thumb is removed.

the oxygen supply to the other, and the third arm is left open. Oxygen flow is started, and the degree of lung inflation and rate of respiration are governed by the anesthetist, who intermittently puts his thumb over the open arm of the T-tube. This method is superior to the tire pump in that 100% oxygen is used rather than room air.

Non-Rebreathing Valves

Several types of non-rebreathing valves originally designed for infant anesthesia, can be employed for positive pressure ventilation of the lungs during open chest surgery. Among these are the Stephen-Slater and Lewis-Leigh valves (Fig. 5–12). An oxygen hose connected to a rebreathing bag is attached to the non-rebreathing valve, which is in turn connected to an endotracheal catheter inserted in the patient. When the chest is closed either valve is automatic, the patient inhaling oxygen from the rebreathing bag and exhaling through the valve into the atmosphere. When the chest is open, it is necessary for an assistant to close the Stephen-Slater valve during inspiration, by placing his finger over the expiratory opening while compressing the rebreathing bag with the other hand. The Lewis-Leigh valve is automatic, squeezing the rebreathing bag automatically closing the exhalation opening; thus the latter has the advantage of being a one-handed operation. With both valves the oxygen regulator is set to flow at a rate which keeps the rebreathing bag approximately two-thirds full.

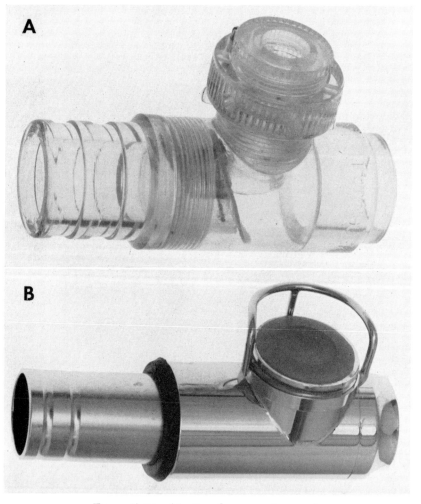

FIGURE 5–12.   (Continued on opposite page.)

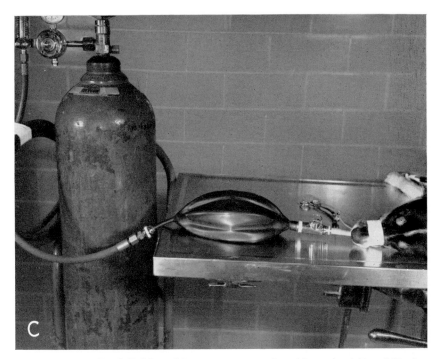

FIGURE 5-12. Lewis-Leigh positive pressure non-rebreathing valve (*A*) and Stephen Slater valve with drapery guard (*B*). (*C*) shows oxygen supply, rebreathing bag, Stephen-Slater valve, and endotracheal catheter in patient. (Courtesy of The Foregger Company, Inc., Roslyn Heights, New York.)

Ambu Resuscitator

The Ambu resuscitator consists of a foam-rubber self-inflating bag, a non-rebreathing valve, and a mask which fits over the patient's face (Fig. 5-13). When the bag is squeezed air is forced into the patient and on release exhaled gases are vented into the room. A connection on the bag enables administration of oxygen if desired, and an endotracheal catheter can be substituted for the mask.

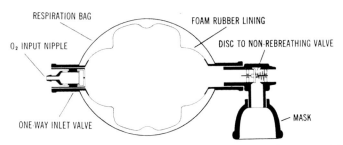

FIGURE 5-13. Schematic drawing of Ambu resuscitator. (Courtesy of Ethical Veterinary Supply Co., Long Island City, N. Y.)

Respirators

A variety of respirators can be made or purchased commercially. In operation these are connected to a mask or endotracheal catheter in the patient, the latter usually being employed. Some of the apparatus are automatic in cycling and produce intermittent positive pressure alone; others have both positive and negative phases. The cycling mechanism is usually activated by the tank pressure. All use 100% oxygen which is detrimental to the patient over long periods of time. In addition, carbon dioxide may be "washed out" of the body producing alkalosis.

Motley *et al.* (1948) studied various types of respirators, determined the pressure curves produced by them, and described the effects on circulation. The latter can be summarized by saying the heart rate tended to increase during the period of negative pressure and no significant electrocardiographic changes were noted. There was little change in blood pressure, the peripheral vascular resistance was increased and, in some, the cardiac output was decreased. The "suck and blow" type of respirator did not produce adverse circulatory effects, though there was no striking increase in right ventricular filling pressure.

With IPPB, intrathoracic pressure is *increased during inspiration*. Intrapulmonary pressure *decreases during expiration*. In the inspiratory phase, when there is increased intrapulmonary pressure, a decreased output from the right side of the heart results, which in turn is made up during the expiratory phase. The effect on the left side of the heart is reversed. During IPPB the pressure should be low during expiration. This period of low pressure should be of sufficient duration that the heart may beat enough times to compensate for reduced output which occurs during the inspiratory period of rising pressure. With several types of respirators there is decreased cardiac output because pressure does not return to that of the atmosphere and the expiratory period is too short.

The ideal pressure curve should increase gradually to a peak not higher than 25 cm. of water.* As expiration begins pressure should drop quickly until atmospheric pressure is reached. Inspiration time should not exceed expiration time (Motley *et al.*, 1948).

Beecher *et al.* (1943) demonstrated that increased intrapulmonary pressure in dogs under anesthesia produces a great rise in venous pressure and a fall in systolic, diastolic, and mean blood pressure. Blood flow through the femoral and carotid arteries was decreased. This was well tolerated by animals in good condition, but those in poor condition were adversely affected and death occurred in some.

During inspiration the normal intrapulmonary pressure is sub-

* 1 mm. Hg = 1.35 cm. H_2O

atmospheric, while during exhalation it is above atmospheric (Fig. 5–14A). Subatmospheric pressure has two functions: (1) to draw air into the lungs, and (2) to draw blood into the thoracic cavity and right heart. If pressure is increased during inspiration alone, a respiratory curve such as Figure 5–14B is produced. This may cause deleterious circulatory effects, since the intrapulmonary pressure is never subatmospheric and may not even reach atmospheric.

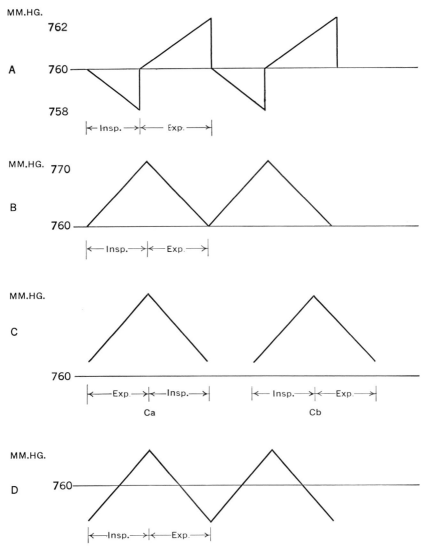

FIGURE 5–14. Graphic representation of intrapulmonary pressures during various types of respiration. Normal (A); inspiratory positive pressure (B); positive pressure on both inspiration and expiration (C, a and b); and "suck and blow" respiration (D). (From Saklad, M.: *Inhalation Therapy and Resuscitation*. Charles C Thomas, 1953.)

Positive pressure during the expiratory phase may be produced during anesthesia if the anesthetist resists the patient's expiratory effort by holding the rebreathing bag during expiration. This is graphically illustrated in Figure 5–14*Ca*.

Some apparatus produces positive pressure throughout the respiratory cycle (Fig. 5–14*Cb*). Positive pressure may occur throughout if a patient under anesthesia is required to breathe against a bag which is too full, or if the anesthetist maintains pressure on the bag during all phases of respiration.

"Suck and blow" apparatus such as the Handy, E & J, Stevenson, and Emerson produce a curve illustrated in Figure 5–14*D*. Using radioactive sodium as a tracer, Thompson (1948) determined that the "suck and blow" respirator produces a circulation of blood in the proper direction without any cardiac activity taking place. This was thought due to filling and emptying of the pulmonary capillaries during artificial respiration. The total volume, however, was quite small. Volpitto *et al.* (1944) concluded that resuscitators producing positive-negative intrapulmonary pressures did not increase the return of blood to the heart effectively, and that any blood flow produced by these resuscitators did not reach the coronary and cerebral arteries but was pushed toward the extremities and cutaneous areas. "Suck and blow" respirators are contraindicated unless they are able to adapt to the patient's spontaneous respiratory efforts; otherwise, the respirator may impede rather than aid respiration. While negative pressure tends to produce congestion, edema, and hemorrhage into the alveoli, Schwerma and Ivy (1945) utilized a "suck and blow" apparatus for 1 to 3 hours and were unable to find lung damage following its use. Orth *et al.* (1945) used eight different methods of artificial respiration on anesthetized dogs. They found that in all, regardless of the anesthetic or duration of artificial respiration, histologic examination showed areas of atelectasis, congestion, and hemorrhagic infiltration. However, in those dogs permitted to recover, these lung lesions were reversible and without sequelae.

Windshield-Wiper Respirator

One of the earliest respirators was made from a truck windshield-wiper control mechanism. This apparatus, which in conventional use is operated by the compressed air system of the truck, is set so that it automatically causes the lungs to inflate at a predetermined rate (Fig. 5–15). There is no synchronization with the patient's respirations which often do not coincide with the respirator. No negative pressure is produced.

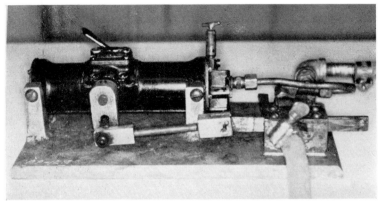

FIGURE 5–15. A respirator made from a truck windshield wiper mechanism. The unit can be operated either by oxygen or compressed air. The tube on the right leads from the gas source and the tube in the foreground leads to the patient.

The PR-3 Resuscitator

The PR-3 resuscitator consists of a high pressure reducing valve containing a cylinder pressure gauge, a low pressure regulator providing a range of 0 to 30 cm. of water, and a differential pressure valve (Burns valve) which converts positive pressure into intermittent positive pressure (Fig. 5–16). At no stage of the cycle is a negative intrapulmonary pressure produced.

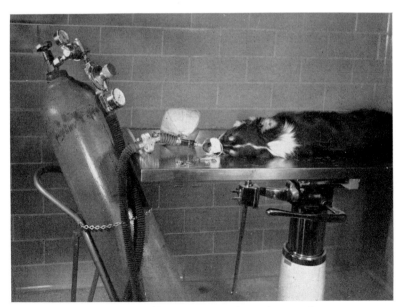

FIGURE 5–16. The PR-3 Resuscitator in operation.

In operation, the low pressure valve is set at 10 to 15 cm. of water; the differential pressure valve then follows the patient's spontaneous respiratory pattern. If breathing stops or the chest is opened, the unit automatically cycles at 12 to 25 times per minute depending upon the pressure used. If the airway becomes blocked, an audible fluttering of the valve warns that corrective measures must be taken.

Dameron and Greene (1950) studied blood oxygen and carbon dioxide levels in dogs after use of the respirator for 1 to $3\frac{1}{2}$ hours and found satisfactory levels of both.

This unit is completely automatic and requires no attendance.

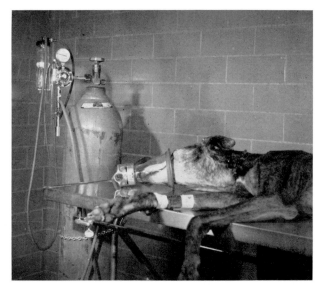

FIGURE 5–17. The Handy resuscitator. This unit consists of a reduction valve connected by a hose to the resuscitator head which is in turn attached to an endotracheal catheter or face mask. An aspirator bottle and sucker tube is on the left of the reduction valve.

The Handy Resuscitator

The Handy resuscitator* is a "suck and blow" unit, exerting alternately 13 mm. Hg positive pressure and 9 mm. Hg negative pressure (Fig. 5–17). It can be used as an inhalator, supplying oxygen for the patient's spontaneous respirations, or as a resuscitator which automatically respires the patient, adjusting depth of respiration to the individual lung capacity of the animal. A valve must be switched to change from one type to the other.

* This is the same as the Stanton Resuscitator used in man.

More expensive models enable adjustment of the high pressure setting to as much as 22 mm. Hg and also to continuous inflation. An aspirator for removing mucus or vomitus from the respiratory tract is available as an accessory.

The Handy resuscitator is a component of the AVR unit used for administration of inhalation anesthetics (Chapter 9, p. 148).

The E and J Resuscitator

The E and J resuscitator has been described by Willis and Weckerly (1952). It is very similar in design and capabilities to the Handy resuscitator.

Gas Machines

Oxygen can also be administered by means of gas machines described in Chapter 9, p. 153.

References

BEECHER, H. K., BENNETT, H. S., and BASSETT, D. L.: Circulatory Effects of Increased Pressure in the Airway. Anesthesiology, 4, 612, 1943.

DAMERON, J. T. and GREENE, D. G.: Use of the Burns Valve as a Simple Respirator for Intrathoracic Surgery in the Dog. J. Thoracic Surg., 20, 706, 1950.

DRAPER, W. B. and WHITEHEAD, R. W.: Diffusion Respiration in the Dog Anesthetized by Pentothal Sodium. Anesthesiology, 5, 262, 1944.

IRWIN, R. L., DRAPER, W. B., and WHITEHEAD, R. W.: Urine Secretion During Diffusion Respiration after Apnea from Neuromuscular Block. Anesthesiology, 18, 594, 1957.

KOPECKY, F. A., RAYBURN, C. J., WHITEHEAD, R. W., and DRAPER, W. B.: A Study of Anuria Occurring During Apnea under Diffusion Respiration. Am. J. Physiol., 168, 131, 1952.

MOTLEY, H. L., COURNAND, A., WERKO, L., DRESDALE, D. T., HIMMELSTEIN, A., and RICHARDS, D. W., JR.: Intermittent Positive Pressure Breathing—A Means of Administering Artificial Respiration in Man. J.A.M.A., 137, 370, 1948.

ORTH, O. S., WILHELM, R. L., and WATERS, R. M.: The Question of Pulmonary Damage with Artificial Respiration. J. Thoracic Surg., 14, 220, 1945.

PHILLIPS, R. L. and BURKHARDT, B. S.: Medical and Surgical Oxygen in Small Animal Practice. Vet. Med., 46, 41, 1951.

SCHNEIDER, R. H.: The Surgical Repair of a Diaphragmatic Hernia in a Dog. Vet. Rec., 14, 1229, 1934.

SCHWERMA, H. and IVY, A. C.: Safety of Modern Alternating Positive and Negative Pressure Resuscitators. J.A.M.A., 129, 1256, 1945.

THOMPSON, S. A.: The Effect of Pulmonary Inflation and Deflation upon the Circulation. J. Thoracic Surg., 17, 323, 1948.

VOLPITTO, P. P., WOODBURY, R. A., and ABREU, B. E.: Influence of Different Forms of Mechanical Artificial Respiration on the Pulmonary and Systemic Blood Pressure. J.A.M.A., 126, 1066, 1944.

WILLIS, T. E. and WECKERLY, L.: An Automatic Means of Controlled Respiration for Open Thoracic Surgery. N. Amer. Vet., 33, 870, 1952.

WYCOFF, C. C.: Manufacture of an Endotracheal Catheter Cuff. Anesthesiology, 8, 643, 1947.

PREANESTHETIC AGENTS

PREANESTHETIC agents are so-called because they are usually given to prepare the patient for administration of an anesthetic agent. In this regard they are used to:

1. Slow the metabolic rate, thereby reducing the amount of general anesthetic needed and increasing the margin of safety.
2. Calm the patient so that anesthesia can be administered without struggling.
3. Reduce secretions of the salivary glands and mucous glands of the respiratory tract, thus maintaining a free airway.
4. Reduce gastric and intestinal motility and prevent vomiting while the patient is under anesthesia.
5. Reduce pain, struggling, and crying during the recovery period.

Many preanesthetic agents are capable of producing analgesia, sedation, or narcosis of the patient to a degree which will enable minor procedures to be carried out without general anesthesia. Their use in combination with local anesthesia helps to restrain the patient and allay apprehension during surgical procedures. By employing such a combination, it is sometimes possible to avoid the dangers of general anesthesia.

Whether preanesthetics are used depends to a degree upon personal preference and the type of practice in which one is engaged. When accustomed to using these agents routinely, the procedure is seldom discontinued. In brachycephalic dogs, it is foolhardy to attempt general anesthesia without administration of a drug to reduce secretions.

A variety of drugs are used as preanesthetic agents. Pharmacologically they fall into the following groups:

A. Anticholinergics   *C*. Morphine and morphine substitutes
B. Tranquilizers   *D*. Miscellaneous agents

Anticholinergics

Atropine Sulfate, U.S.P.

Atropine is obtained by extraction from leaves of the plant *Atropa belladonna*. It is also produced synthetically.

Atropine blocks acetylcholine at the myoneural junction of cholinergic fibers in the autonomic nervous system. This diminishes secretion of mucus in the respiratory tree, dilates the bronchi, and prevents laryngospasm on endotracheal intubation. Motor and secretory activity in the gastrointestinal tract are reduced and vagus inhibition of the heart is prevented. In therapeutic doses atropine does not produce significant blood pressure changes. It blocks the cholinergic fibers of the short ciliary nerves, relaxing the sphincter muscle of the iris and allowing dilation of the pupil. It does not dilate the pupils of birds because their irides are composed of striated muscle (Goodman and Gilman, 1958).

Atropine degradation and elimination varies among animal species. The cat, rat, and rabbit can destroy large quantities of atropine because they have an enzyme, atropine esterase, in the liver (Godeaux and Tonnesen, 1949). In the dog atropine disappears quickly from the blood stream, part being excreted in the urine unchanged or as tropine, and part being unaccounted for.

The dose of atropine sulfate is rather arbitrary. Jones (1957) recommends 0.02 mg./lb. or $\frac{1}{200}$ to $\frac{1}{100}$ gr. for dogs. A convenient weight-dose relationship is as follows:

$\frac{1}{300}$ gr. up to 10 lb.

$\frac{1}{150}$ gr.—10 to 40 lb.

$\frac{1}{75}$ gr. above 40 lb.

Atropine may be given subcutaneously, intramuscularly, or intravenously, the latter method being used when a quick effect is desired. Since its action is rapid it can be given at any time prior to induction of anesthesia or even mixed with intravenous anesthetic agents (thiamylal is an example). Atropine sulfate is inexpensive and results obtained from its use more than justify the time and expense of administration.

Methylatropine Nitrate (Eumydrine; Metropine)

Methylatropine nitrate is a quaternary amine possessing the peripheral actions of atropine, but is devoid of central effects. Its peripheral parasympatholytic actions are similar to atropine but are more potent. This is particularly true in regard to suppression of salivary secretions and blockage of cholinergic stimulation of the intestine and vascular system. The autonomic ganglia are also blocked.

Methylatropine nitrate has been shown to have a potency 1.9 times greater than atropine in depressing the salivary secretion of cats (Bülbring and Dawes, 1945). Its toxicity when injected intraperitoneally in white mice is 3 times that of atropine (Graham and Lazarus, 1940).

The preanesthetic dose for cats is 0.02 mg./lb. of body weight.

Scopolamine Hydrobromide, U.S.P. (Hyoscine Hydrobromide)

Scopolamine is another alkaloid of belladonna. Chemically it is closely related to atropine. It occurs as colorless or white crystals, or as a granular powder which is quite water soluble.

Its actions are similar to atropine in that it blocks the action of acetylcholine on the viscera. It is not as potent as atropine in its action on the cardiac vagus but is a more potent mydriatic. In man it has been used in combination with morphine, since it is thought scopolamine potentiates the action of morphine on the brain. In England, Wright (1957) described its use in dogs combined with morphine and atropine as a preanesthetic agent. When used in this manner a dose of $\frac{1}{200}$ gr./20 lb. of body weight was administered.

In the United States, Hall (1953) reported a combination of methadone, scopolamine, and nembutal anesthesia in dogs. All three drugs were given intravenously, methadone first and, after a variable period, scopolamine and nembutal together in rapid succession. Hall indicated that $\frac{1}{200}$ gr. of scopolamine is sufficient for all but the heaviest dogs, larger doses producing quick shallow respirations. Knowles (1957a) advocates the use of scopolamine intravenously prior to cataract surgery, since it has better mydriatic action than atropine.

Dogs react erratically to the effects of scopolamine; small doses produce drowsiness and hallucinations; larger doses produce marked restlessness, hallucinations, ataxia, and frequently emesis. The same effect has been shown to occur with rats and rabbits.

A combination of morphine and scopolamine has been used in human obstetrics to produce amnesia or so-called "twilight sleep." This combination in proportions of 25 to 1 has been used for pre-anesthesia in dogs by Knowles (1957a). Because of the erratic effects produced by scopolamine alone, its use in small animals is not as universal as atropine.

Tranquilizers

One of the important pharmacological advances of recent years has been the development of tranquilizers or *ataraxic* agents. These have proved useful in a wide variety of conditions in small animals, namely:

1. As preanesthetic sedatives.
2. To relieve anxiety in hospitalized animals.
3. To restrain refractory animals during examination.
4. To prevent animals from licking wounds, chewing bandages and splints.
5. As an antiemetic for carsickness and prior to administration of anthelmintics.

Tranquilizers have been classified according to their chemical structure and pharmacological properties. According to chemical structure they can be divided into four groups: (1) the phenothiazine derivatives, (2) reserpine and related alkaloids, (3) the diphenylmethane derivatives*, and (4) the propanediol derivatives. Berger (1957) has pointed out that no pharmacological test has been developed to which all tranquilizers show a positive response. For this reason in the pre-tranquilizer era these drugs would have been classified according to their more pronounced pharmacological actions. Chlorpromazine would have been called a hypnotic; reserpine would have been considered a true sedative; meprobamate would have been a muscle relaxant and anticonvulsant.

Based on several testing procedures tranquilizers can be divided according to their pharmacological properties into two broad classes: (1) the *autonomic suppressants* which includes the phenothiazines, reserpine, and the diphenylmethanes, and (2) the *central relaxants* containing meprobamate, mephenesin, and similar compounds. The

* None of these are used to any extent in small animals.

autonomic suppressants antagonize such substances as acetylcholine, histamine, and serotonin which serve to regulate certain functions of the autonomic nervous system. In this respect, these suppressants have many common pharmacological properties with atropine, scopolamine, and the antihistamines. They are like atropine and scopolamine in that they produce a sleep pattern in the electroencephalogram, without producing sleep, and block avoidance and conditioned reflexes perhaps by interfering with memory, learning, and performance. They prolong barbiturate anesthesia, as do the antihistamines, probably by interfering with the enzyme acting on the barbiturate. Strychnine hyperexcitability is increased, and the electroconvulsive threshold lowered.

Conversely, the central relaxants do not affect the autonomic nervous system. Barbiturate anesthesia is prolonged only in large doses, and strychnine hyperexcitability is counteracted. A marked relaxant effect is exerted on spastic muscles. Both groups reduce aggressiveness and hostility in monkeys. The autonomic suppressants, however, produce withdrawal, listlessness, anorexia, and catatonia. These animals exhibit an "isolation from environment." Monkeys given central relaxants, on the other hand, retain their appetite and interest in their environment.

When used as preanesthetic agents the tranquilizers are usually administered intravenously, although the intramuscular and oral routes may be used. The latter two are not as fast or reliable. Intravenous injection should be made at least 5 minutes prior to administration of a general anesthetic agent. This allows time for the animal to receive the full effect prior to induction of anesthesia. An exception is reserpine which is slow and requires 1 to 2 hours.

Injection should be made slowly. As it occurs, the animal will show signs of relaxation, slumping to the table if previously erect. The eyes usually assume a glazed appearance with the membrana nictitans protruding. Occasionally acute toxic symptoms will be seen. Among these are extreme depression, hypotension, tremors, dyspnea, and ataxia. Epinephrine is contraindicated in treatment of the hypotension, norepinephrine or phenylephrine being the drugs of choice. While there are few reports of small animals dying from intravenous administration of tranquilizers, deaths have occurred. An occasional animal may become aggressive or show other evidence of central nervous stimulation. Generally these agents are not as effective in cats as in other animals.

Advantages of preanesthetic tranquilizers are:

1. The animal is easier to handle during induction of anesthesia.
2. The required amount of general anesthesic is reduced.
3. The antiemetic action inhibits vomiting.

4. Recovery from anesthesia is smooth and free from thrashing and crying.
5. Little delay is necessary between administration of preanesthetic and anesthetic agent.
6. No narcotic license is needed.

Disadvantages of tranquilizer administration are:

1. The cost is many times greater than combined morphine and atropine.
2. Tranquilizers do not produce true analgesia.
3. Persons handling tranquilizers may become sensitized resulting in urticaria and pruritus.

Phenothiazine Derivatives

Chlorpromazine Hydrochloride (Thorazine)

Chlorpromazine can be considered the prototype of the phenothiazine derivatives. It is a whitish-grey water-soluble powder marketed for oral use in 10, 25, and 50 mg. tablets, and for intramuscular and intravenous injection in sterile solution containing 25 mg./ml. A syrup containing 10 mg./ml. is also available.

Chlorpromazine possesses three main pharmacologic properties: (1) antiemetic action, (2) central depressant action, and (3) enhancing effect on the activity of analgesics, anesthetics, and sedatives. The central depressant activity probably is on the ascending reticular formation of the midbrain which controls the centers for vomiting and temperature. It also influences the activity of the central nervous system, including the autonomic nervous system, muscle tone, and pituitary gland. Its antiemetic action is believed due to depression of the emetic chemoreceptor trigger zone and the vomiting reflex centrally. In addition, the volume of gastric secretion is lowered and the small intestine, bladder, and uterus are relaxed.

Intravenous injection of 2 to 5 mg./kg. of chlorpromaxine in anesthetized dogs causes a decrease in the respiratory rate, increased tidal volume, and an over-all decreased oxygen consumption (Bourgeois-Gavardin et al., 1955). No consistent changes in renal function occur in dogs when given 50 mg. of chlorpromazine intravenously except for a moderate increase in urine volume and sodium excretion.

Chlorpromazine produces effects similar to a stressing agent, in that blood eosinophils and lymphocytes decrease and a simultaneous decrease in adrenal ascorbic acid content occurs.

The hypotensive effect of chlorpromazine may produce shock. It antagonizes and sometimes reverses the pressor and vasoconstrictor

7

action of epinephrine and other sympathomimetic amines (ephedrine, methamphetamine, methoxamine, mephentermine, amphetamine, and others). Epinephrine should not be used under these circumstances because it may result in further lowering of the blood pressure. Norepinephrine or phenylephrine are the most suitable vasopressor agents for use in this situation.

Paradoxically, it has been reported that dogs were completely protected against the lethal effect of hemorrhagic shock by intravenous administration of chlorpromazine at a rate of 2 mg./kg., before or immediately after hemorrhage. Treated dogs exhibited none of the usual signs of shock. In addition, shock resulting from injection of irritants into the cerebral peduncles of dogs was modified and mortality reduced by intravenous chlorpromazine, either before or after the procedure.

The fate of chlorpromazine in the body is not completely clear but the main metabolite appears to be chlorpromazine sulfoxide which can be found in the urine of dogs. The sulfoxide undergoes further metabolism to an unidentified product. The biological half-life is estimated to be 6 hours (Salzman and Brodie, 1956).

Chlorpromazine when used in surgery is expected to (1) make the patient easier to restrain during administration of the anesthetic, (2) reduce the volume of general anesthetic required, (3) prevent vomiting, (4) produce muscle relaxation, and (5) eliminate struggling and crying on recovery. Some veterinarians using chlorpromazine as a preanesthetic believe it to be superior to morphine or meperidine for this purpose. A dosage schedule for various species is listed in Table 6–1.

No deaths occurred in dogs given 50 mg./kg. (22.6 mg./lb.) of body weight subcutaneously or 100 mg./kg. (45.4 mg./lb.) orally

Table 6–1.—Chlorpromazine: Route of Administration and Dose Range (mg./lb.)

				Average Dose		
	I.V. Range	I.M. Range	Oral Range	I.V.	I.M.	Oral
Dog	0.25 to 2.0	0.5 to 3.0	0.25 to 4.0	0.5	1.0	1.5
Cat	0.25 to 2.0	1.0 to 3.0	1.0 to 4.0	0.5	1.0	1.5
Chinchilla			1–3 drops syrup			1–3 drops
Birds						
Parakeets			1 drop syrup			1 drop
Large birds			0.25			0.25

Dosing varies from 1 to 4 times daily depending on the type of case and the desired results.

(Data obtained from Pitman-Moore Company, Indianapolis, Indiana.)

(Courvoisier *et al.*, 1953). It has no ill effect on fetuses in utero (Macko *et al.*, 1958). In another study, when 200 mg. was given orally to pregnant bitches for 7 days prior to whelping, normal full-term pups were delivered.

Estrada (1956) reported a reaction in a 25 lb. terrier given 6 mg./lb. at a rapid rate; opisthotonus, urination, and collapse occurred. The animal regained its ability to stand about 30 minutes after injection but remained depressed for several hours. According to Burch (1957) perivascular infiltration of chlorpromazine solution in dogs will cause swelling and pain.

Promazine Hydrochloride (Sparine)

Promazine has the same basic structure as chlorpromazine but lacks a chlorine atom on the phenothiazine nucleus. It is a white crystalline salt, readily soluble in water and alcohol. Solutions are stable indefinitely. It is supplied in solution for intravenous and intramuscular injection and in tablets of 25, 50, and 100 mg. for oral therapy.

In general, the effects of promazine are similar to those of chlor-promazine, though less hypnosis and fewer side effects have been reported.

Clifford (1957) has reported favorably on the use of combined promazine-meperidine-pentobarbital anesthesia in the cat. A solution of 5 mg./ml. of promazine was given subcutaneously at a rate of 2 mg./lb. of body weight. One ml. of 2% procaine was added to the syringe containing the appropriate dose to reduce pain from the injection. Five mg. of meperidine per pound of body weight was also given subcutaneously. Approximately 1 hour later pento-barbital was given intravenously "to effect." The result was a marked reduction in sleeping time when compared with cats anesthetized with pentobarbital alone. Cats receiving preanesthetic were also easier to restrain for venipuncture.

The intravenous dose of preanesthetic promazine in the dog is 1 to 2 mg./lb. of body weight. The amount of barbiturate necessary for anesthesia is thereby reduced $\frac{1}{3}$ to $\frac{1}{2}$.

Promazine has proved to be a safe and efficient preanesthetic agent for dogs (Weberlein *et al.*, 1959; Knowles, 1957b; Krawitz, 1957). It is probably the most widely used tranquilizer in small animal practice.

Triflupromazine Hydrochloride (Vetame)

Triflupromazine is a phenothiazine-type tranquilizer containing fluorine. The pH of a 2% solution is 4.1; it precipitates from aqueous solutions at a pH of 6.4. The parenteral form is marketed in brown bottles to protect it from decomposition by light. It is also available in 10 and 25 mg. tablets for oral administration.

Triflupromazine has about 10 times the antimetic effect of chlorpromazine and 3 to 5 times the tranquilizing potency. Its side effects are essentially equivalent to chlorpromazine. On rare occasions it may stimulate dogs to chew on any object close at hand. This effect though alarming is transitory.

The recommended intravenous dose for the dog is 0.5 to 1 mg./lb. When triflupromazine is used as a preanesthetic, the dosage of barbiturate is generally $\frac{1}{2}$ to $\frac{2}{3}$ that usually required. The intravenous LD_{50} for the dog is 16.7 ± 4.2 mg./kg.

In clinical practice triflupromazine has proved to be comparable to promazine in its effects.

Propiopromazine Hydrochloride (Tranvet)

Propiopromazine, a phenothiazine derivative, is a yellow odorless powder which is readily soluble in water and alcohol. Its effects are similar to other phenothiazine derivatives in that it has an antiemetic effect, causes epinephrine reversal, and lowers blood pressure in animals under pentobarbital anesthesia. It is somewhat more sedative, produces greater potentiation of barbiturates, and a greater degree of motor deficit than chlorpromazine.

An intravenous dose of 1 mg./lb. in dogs will produce ataxia, pupillary constriction, decreased activity, and slight prolapse of the nicitating membrane. The same effects are produced in cats and monkeys. If administered prior to thiopental or pentobarbital anesthesia the amount of anesthetic required will be reduced and the sleeping time prolonged.

Propiopromazine has proved clinically to be a safe and efficient tranquilizer with effects lasting in some instances as long as 2 to 3 days.

Mepazine (Paxital, Pacatal)

Mepazine contains the basic phenothiazine structure but differs from chlorpromazine in that the side chain contains a heterocyclic (piperidine) ring. It is an odorless white crystalline substance, similar pharmacologically to the other phenothiazines.

Mepazine has a relatively low acute animal toxicity (Table 6–2). Lethal doses cause central nervous depression, reduced muscle tonicity, paralysis, and terminal convulsions.

The fate of mepazine in the body is not clear; 4% is eliminated unchanged or as sulfoxide in the urine and 11% is degraded in the liver.

Ripps (1957) and Knowles *et al.* (1957) reported its use clinically in over 400 dogs. The latter authors stated that 2 mg./lb. appeared to be the optimum preanesthetic dose. When it was given intravenously, 10 minutes prior to pentobarbital, the dose of anesthetic was reduced 20 to 30%. These authors also reported the use of mepazine to prolong anesthesia. When used in this fashion, it was given slowly, intravenously, to effect. If used as a preanesthetic it was not used postanesthetically. Neither Ripps nor Knowles *et al.* experienced any undesirable side effects.

Table 6–2.—Mepazine Toxicity

Species	Route of Administration	LD_{50}
Mouse	I.V.	50 mg./kg.
	Oral	700 mg./kg.
Rat	Oral	1200 mg./kg.
Rabbit	I.V.	20 mg./kg.

Perphenazine (Trilafon)

Perphenazine is an amino derivative of chlorphenothiazine. It is available in solution for parenteral injection and in 4 and 8 mg. tablets for oral use.

It possesses 5 to 10 times the potency of chlorpromazine in its suppression of behavioral activity and 24 times the antiemetic effect (Roth *et al.*, 1959). Perphenazine potentiates barbiturate anesthesia effecting a reduction of $\frac{1}{4}$ to $\frac{1}{3}$ in the anesthetic required. The intravenous dose for preanesthesia in the dog is 0.25 to 1 mg./lb. of body weight. It should be injected intramuscularly or intravenously, *never subcutaneously*. Its toxicity is comparable to chlorpromazine and deaths have occurred following its use. In lethal doses tonic or tonic-clonic convulsions lead to death by respiratory arrest. The intravenous LD_{50} for the dog is 51 mg./kg. (Irwin *et al.*, 1959).

Ethyl Isobutrazine (Diquel)

Ethyl isobutrazine is a phenothiazine derivative with properties similar to other members of this group. It potentiates anesthesia and analgesia, reducing the dose of pentobarbital approximately 30% in recommended dosage.

Ethyl isobutrazine is available in solution containing 25 mg./ml. and in tablets of 10 and 50 mg. For small animals the oral and intramuscular doses are 2 to 5 mg./lb.; the intravenous dose is 1 to 2 mg./lb.

Reserpine and Related Alkaloids

Reserpine (Serpasil; Reserpoid)

Reserpine is a pure active alkaloid isolated in 1952 from the root of *Rauwolfia serpentina Benth,* a shrub found in India. Indians for many years have ground the root and used it as treatment for a variety of conditions. Reserpine possesses the antihypertensive and tranquilizing properties characteristic of the whole root. The tranquilizing effect appears to be due to depression of the sympathetic centers in the hypothalamus with little or no cortical depression. Other effects include myosis, relaxation of the nictitating membrane, and hypothermia.

Reserpine has been suggested for restraint in surgical procedures by Earl (1956). However, the onset of action is slow regardless of the route of administration. When given intravenously the maximum effect is obtained in about 2 hours. This feature limits the usefulness of the drug.

Reserpine probably should not be used in the dog because of species sensitivity. Connor and Haas (1955) reported anorexia, nausea, vomiting, diarrhea, muscular weakness, tremors, incoordination, and depression as toxic symptoms. In this species other drugs are more suitable preanesthetic agents.

The dose for dogs must be adjusted for each individual; 0.025 mg./kg. orally is well tolerated. Intravenously 0.05 to 0.1 mg./kg. is effective, while 0.5 mg./kg. can result in death due to superpurgation. According to Earl (1956) the intramuscular dose for wild turkeys is 0.2 mg./kg. The effective dose range was noted to be very narrow. In chinchillas daily doses of 1.0 to 2.0 mg. produce tranquilization. Rats are said to tolerate a daily dose of 2.0 mg./kg. orally without weight loss. Monkeys have been maintained on daily oral doses of up to 3.0 mg./kg. for long periods.

Propanediol Derivatives

Meprobamate (Equanil; Miltown)

Meprobamate is a long-acting propanediol derivative with muscle relaxant and anticonvulsant actions. The muscle relaxant action is similar to mephenesin (Chapter 12, p. 231) but of greater potency and longer duration. Its usefulness is limited since it is only slightly soluble and for this reason is available only in tablet form. For preanesthetic use, it must be administered at least 1 hour before induction of general anesthesia. According to Huebner (1956) it is effective in small animals for (1) anxiety and tension states, and (2) conditions associated with muscle spasm.

Dose for the dog is 100 to 400 mg. 2 to 4 times daily.

Morphine and Morphine Substitutes

Morphine Sulfate, U.S.P.

The chief pharmacologic effect of morphine is analgesia, which is due to depression of the sensory area of the cerebral cortex. Morphine also affects the medullary centers, the respiratory, cough, and vasomotor centers being depressed, while the vomiting center is stimulated. With therapeutic doses there is a reduction in the basal metabolic rate resulting in a temperature drop of 1 to 3° F.

Depression of the respiratory centers results in decreased respiratory minute volume and increased alveolar carbon dioxide tension. Depression of the vasomotor center produces lowered blood pressure. According to Krantz and Carr (1951), when morphine is given intravenously to the dog and cat, leg volume increases indicating capillary bed dilatation and accounting for blood pressure fall. In the dog there is also a marked bradycardia.

A useful action of morphine is its direct stimulatory effect on the vomiting center. The sphincters of the gastrointestinal tract are stimulated causing an over-all action that is constipating; increased intestinal peristalsis tends to combat this effect. Dogs given parenteral morphine usually defecate soon after administration.

The reflex centers of the spinal cord are stimulated. This should be remembered when the use of pentylenetetrazol or other cord stimulants is contemplated since spinal convulsions will result. Morphine is contraindicated in strychnine poisoning for the same reason (Jones, 1957). Morphine produces an irregular effect on the brain depending upon the species in which it is administered. Individual variations will also occur among members of the same species. In the cat morphine produces mania with tonic convulsions which may last for hours and terminate fatally. Stimulation is also seen in the mouse. Because of its irregular effects, the use of morphine as a preanesthetic agent is confined almost entirely to the dog.

According to Krantz and Carr (1951) the liver is capable of destroying morphine. Morphine is excreted in the urine (65% in 24 hours and another 20% during the next few days). Morphine stimulates the secretion of antidiuretic hormone from the posterior lobe of the pituitary and is contraindicated in uremia, since it has been shown that urine production may be reduced as much as 90%.

Morphine Toxicity

There is a wide variation in the toxicity of morphine for the dog, depending upon age and condition of the animal. According to Jones (1957) the fatal subcutaneous or intravenous dose of morphine sulfate varies from 50 to 100 mg./lb. of body weight. Booth (1961) states that doses of 400 to 500 mg./kg. of body weight have been given to the dog without fatality, provided pentobarbital sodium has been given intravenously to counteract the spinal convulsions which resulted. Fatal doses of morphine sulfate in the dog cause death from respiratory depression. Morphine is contraindicated in dogs suffering from traumatic shock and will often prove fatal if this rule is ignored. Death is due to severe depression of blood pressure, cardiac output, and lowered oxygen consumption (Powers *et al.*, 1947). The action of morphine can be reversed by the narcotic antagonists, nalorphine or levallorphan (Chapter 16, p. 352).

Advantages of morphine as a preanesthetic agent in the dog are:

1. The animal is quieted and more tractable.
2. It causes vomition and defecation.
3. The amount of general anesthetic needed is reduced.
4. It prevents excitement on recovery (crying, thrashing).
5. It reduces postoperative pain and helps prevent shock.

Disadvantages are:

1. Respiration and blood pressure are depressed.
2. It cannot be used on cats.
3. A narcotic license is required and records of administration must be kept.
4. It is contraindicated in shock (lowers blood pressure, oxygen intake, cardiac output).
5. Vomiting and defecation are occasionally undesirable as in intestinal obstruction, diaphragmatic hernia.

Administration of Morphine

Hypodermic tablets containing $\frac{1}{4}$ gr. of morphine sulfate are the form commonly used. These are dissolved in sterile distilled water and injected subcutaneously or intramuscularly. The dose for dogs varies widely, the following schedule being convenient when using $\frac{1}{4}$ gr. tablets.

1– 5 lb. — $\frac{1}{16}$ gr.
5–10 lb. — $\frac{1}{8}$ gr.
10–20 lb. — $\frac{1}{4}$ gr.
20–30 lb. — $\frac{1}{2}$ gr.
30–40 lb. — $\frac{3}{4}$ gr.
over 40 lb. — 1 gr. or more depending upon body weight

Booth (1961) has recommended the use of 2.5 mg./lb. of body weight as a preanesthetic. Four and one-half mg./lb. of body weight reduces the dose of pentobarbital sodium to $\frac{1}{3}$ that usually given.

Since morphine administered subcutaneously or intramuscularly does not produce its effect immediately, it should be given at least 30 minutes prior to induction of anesthesia. Following administration dogs should be put on a run so they can eliminate.

Morphine is widely used as a preanesthetic agent for dogs, usually in combination with atropine. The dose remains the same whether given with atropine, scopolamine, or alone. From the standpoint of cost, morphine is much cheaper to use as a preanesthetic agent than are the tranquilizers. The dose of morphine for some other species and its effects are listed in Table 6–3.

Table 6–3.—Effect of Morphine in Various Species

Species	Dose and Route of Administration	Effect
Mouse	0.1 mg./gm. S.Q.	Excitement
Rat	5 mg./kg. S.Q.	Soporific
Rabbit	5 mg./kg. S.Q.	Soporific
	20 mg./kg. S.Q.	Narcotic
Cat	0.5 mg./kg. I.V., I.M., S.Q., Oral	Excitatory
Monkey (*Macacus rhesus*)	2 mg./kg.	Soporific
	10 mg./kg.	Narcotic
	20 mg./kg.	May be lethal
Chimpanzee	4 mg./kg.	Soporific
Dog	10 mg./kg. S.Q.	Narcotic
	50 mg./kg. S.Q.	Deep narcosis (24 hours)

(From data of Krueger, H., Eddy, N. B., and Sumwalt, M.: *The Pharmacology of the Opium Alkaloids*. Part I. U. S. Public Health Service, 1941.)

Morphine Narcosis for Cesarean Section

To avoid the dangers of general anesthesia, morphine has been used as the sole analgesic and narcotic agent in cesarean section in the bitch. When used for this purpose, morphine sulfate is given at a rate of $\frac{1}{15}$ gr./lb. of body weight. In old or debilitated animals, which are poor risks, this dose should be reduced. Morphine narcosis produces hypersensitivity to noise and spinal reflexes are easily stimulated causing rigidity of the limbs. For this reason loud noises should be avoided. The bitch can be placed in sternal recumbency immediately following the operation and will hold her head up and look around. This is desirable if she is to be sent home.

Fetal respiration is slightly depressed but the puppies are quickly able to nurse. The bitch, however, is ataxic for as long as 18 hours postoperatively and will not care for the puppies. Care must be exercised to see that she does not lie on them and crush them. When this procedure is used, therefore, nalorphine or levallorphan (Chapter 16, p. 352) should be given to speed recovery of the mother and puppies. It is also best to send them home with the owner so that they can be well attended.

Morphine-Apomorphine Narcosis

A combination of morphine sulfate and apomorphine hydrochloride can be given for deep narcosis in the dog, thus allowing painful surgical procedures to be undertaken without general anesthesia. One of the chief uses for this mixture has been in cesarean section, though it is quite effective in many other situations.

A conventional dose of morphine is administered and followed in 30 minutes with $\frac{1}{40}$ to $\frac{1}{10}$ gr. of apomorphine, depending upon the size of the dog. The two drugs may be given simultaneously if desired though more strenuous vomiting is produced. The pharmacological action of the mixture has not been well explained; however, it appears to be a synergism. Little has been written regarding this technique and its safety though no fatalities have been reported (——, 1952).

Apomorphine in the above dose can also be given to potentiate and prolong anesthesia in dogs beginning to recover from morphine-pentobarbital.

Meperidine Hydrochloride, U.S.P. (Demerol; Isonipecaine; Pethidine)

Meperidine hydrochloride was synthesized by Eisleb and Schaumann in 1939. It is a white crystalline powder, the free base exhibiting a strong alkaline reaction, the hydrochloride being neutral. It is commonly marketed as a solution containing 50 mg./ml. or as 50 mg. tablets.

The analgesic effect of meperidine is not as great as that of morphine. It has a spasmolytic effect similar to atropine and reduces salivary and respiratory secretions. Meperidine is used as a preanesthetic narcotic agent to quiet the animal and make it more tractable on induction. It decreases the amount of general anesthetic needed and reduces postoperative pain and tendency toward shock. It does not cause nausea, vomiting, or defecation in most animals. However, Scott et al., (1947) report it stimulates the small bowel. It is destroyed for the most part in the liver, a small amount being excreted in the urine.

When given intravenously to dogs, there is a fall in blood pressure due to peripheral vasodilation (Gruber et al., 1941). This effect is occasionally utilized to reduce hemorrhage during such operations as ear cropping. Rapid intravenous administration must be avoided since the drug stimulates the central nervous system and will cause convulsions.

The subcutaneous dose of meperidine as a preanesthetic agent for dogs is 10 mg./kg. to 10 mg./lb. One hundred mg. is equal to the analgesic effect of $\frac{1}{6}$ gr. of morphine sulfate. Meperidine administered as a preanesthetic agent should be given 30 minutes prior to anesthesia in order for its full effect to develop prior to induction.

Another use for meperidine is in animals that prematurely begin to arouse from pentobarbital anesthesia. When administered intramuscularly to these animals (5 mg./kg.), anesthesia will be prolonged and recovery will be free of struggling and crying. Meperidine can also be used as the sole agent for cesarean section in dogs. The dose for this purpose is 15 mg./lb.

The action of meperidine is reversed by nalorphine or levallorphan.

Booth and Rankin (1954) in a study of the effects of meperidine in the cat, indicate that the dose is 5 to 10 mg./kg. of body weight administered subcutaneously. Animals so treated were tractable and easier to handle though the depression produced was not marked. With doses of 30 to 50 mg./kg., a marked rise in rectal temperature occurred. At this dose level there was a decided increase in pulse rate along with a moderate increase in respiratory rate. Doses of 10 mg./kg. at times produced restlessness, and at dose levels of 30 to 50 mg./kg. generalized muscular spasms occurred in some animals. Convulsive seizures were observed at the higher dose levels. Using the technique of Ercoli and Lewis to measure the pain threshold, it could not be proved that analgesia was produced in the cat.

Advantages of preanesthetic meperidine are:

1. It is an efficient analgesic and narcotic with a wide margin of safety.
2. It can be used alone or combined with local or regional anesthesia to alleviate pain and minimize restraint.
3. When used as a preanesthetic agent, recovery from anesthesia is smooth and free from excitement.
4. It can be used in cats.

Disadvantages are:

1. It is more expensive than morphine.
2. It is a respiratory depressant.
3. It requires a narcotic license and records of administration must be kept.

Methadone Hydrochloride, U.S.P. (Methadone; Amidone; Dolophine)

Methadone hydrochloride is a synthetic analgesic and narcotic agent unrelated to morphine. It is a white odorless crystalline compound, which is water-soluble. A 1% aqueous solution has a pH of 5.8 and under ordinary conditions its solutions are stable. It is active orally and parenterally. Toxicity by the oral, subcutaneous, and intravenous routes is approximately in the ratio of 3:2:1 respectively (Table 6–4). Nalorphine or levallorphan will reverse the toxic action.

Table 6–4.—Summary of Acute Toxicity Studies of Methadon in Dogs

Administration	Animals (No.)	S.A.D.[1] (mg./kg.)	M.T.D.[2] (mg./kg.)	L.D.$_{50}$[3] (mg./kg.)
Oral	21	35.0	50.0	75.0
Subcutaneous	22	15.0	25.0	50.0
Intravenous	27	10.0	17.5	27.0

[1]Surgical anesthetic dose. [2]Maximum tolerated dose, survival of 100% of the animals. [3]Lethal dose, 50, death of 50% of the animals.
(From Reutner, T. F., and Gruhzit, O. M.: Methadon, A New Analgesic. J.A.V.M.A., *113*, 448, 1948.)

Vomiting, salivation, incoordination, and muscular weakness are observed in dogs receiving high doses for extended periods. There is no disturbance in hematopoesis, non-protein nitrogen, or bromsuphalein liver function values and the urine is free of albumin and sugar (Reutner and Gruhzit, 1948). Metabolism of the drug is obscure, about one-fourth being excreted in the urine.

Both clinical and experimental studies indicate that methadone stimulates the respiratory rate. Burroughs (1953) states that on intravenous administration in dogs there follows relaxation with partial to complete loss of postural control, generalized depression, copious salivation, and frequently defecation within a few minutes. Generalized depression accompanied by an increase in the pain threshold is seen for 2 to 6 hours. During this period high pitched noises stimulate the animal to attempt to regain postural control.

The dose of methadone is 1 mg./kg. administered intravenously or subcutaneously. When the latter route is used at least $\frac{1}{2}$ hour should elapse before induction of anesthesia. The barbiturate dose is reduced approximately one-half. When given at the above rate, methadone alone can be used for analgesia and narcosis for many minor surgical procedures and for restraint.

Burroughs (1953) recommends its use for cesarean section, supplementing methadone analgesia with epidural procaine and local infiltration at the incision site. Depression of the fetuses is minimal and the bitch remains conscious throughout the procedure. This method can also be used for hysterectomies on adult dogs affected with pyometra.

Advantages of methadone are:

1. It is an efficient analgesic and narcotic with a wide margin of safety.
2. It can be used alone or combined with local or regional anesthesia to alleviate pain and minimize restraint.
3. When used as a preanesthetic agent, recovery from anesthesia is smooth and free from excitement.

Disadvantages are:

1. It produces salivation, defecation, and increased sensitivity to sharp noises.
2. It produces the typical morphine response in cats and therefore cannot be used in this species.
3. It is more expensive than morphine.
4. A narcotic license and records of its administration must be kept.

Anileridine (Leritine)

Anileridine is a synthetic narcotic with a potency between that of meperidine and morphine. When injected subcutaneously in rats, it is 12 times as active as meperidine and equal to morphine; in dogs it is 3 to 6 times more potent than meperidine, but somewhat less active than morphine. The duration of action in dogs is 5 to 6 hours. Peak concentrations in the plasma of dogs are observed $1\frac{1}{2}$ to 3 hours after oral administration and within 1 hour following subcutaneous injection. Small amounts are present in the plasma 24 hours after administration.

Anileridine has a mild and indirect hypnotic action, is antitussive, and is spasmolytic in action on the small intestine. In dogs it does not produce nausea or vomiting and will antagonize apomorphine and morphine-induced vomiting. It does not have the constipating effect of morphine. The degree of respiratory depression produced is comparable to that of meperidine. Its use intravenously is contraindicated since it produces severe respiratory depression by this route. In anesthetized cats anileridine produces less depression of blood pressure than equal doses of morphine or meperidine.

There is a wide margin of safety with both oral and subcutaneous administration. Several investigators have reported tonic and clonic convulsions in animals with a dose of 20 mg./kg. either intramuscularly or subcutaneously. This is greatly in excess of therapeutic dosage. Other signs of acute toxicity in animals include salivation, lacrimation, loss of righting reflex, dyspnea, hypnosis, and catalepsy. Nalorphine readily reverses the effects of anileridine in rats, cats, and dogs.

Anileridine is a white crystalline powder. It is very soluble in water, producing a solution with a pH of approximately 3. It is available in 25 mg. tablets for oral administration and as a sterile solution containing 25 mg./ml. for parenteral use. In dogs, 1 to 3 mg./lb. subcutaneously or intramuscularly has been used with good results. Heard (1962) has advocated its use as the sole agent in cesarean section, particularly in toy breeds. One ml./5 lb. of body weight is administered subcutaneously. As with morphine, the bitch is sensitized to noise; however, there is less hypnosis and fetal depression. Following surgery she can be placed on her feet and will walk.

References

BERGER, F. M.: The Chemistry and Mode of Action of Tranquilizing Drugs. Ann. N. Y. Acad. Sci., 67, 685, 1957.

BOOTH, N. H.: Personal Communication. Colorado State University, Fort Collins, Colorado, 1961.

BOOTH, N. H. and RANKIN, A. D.: Evaluation of Meperidine Hydrochloride in the Cat. Vet. Med., 49, 249, 1954.

BOURGEOIS-GAVARDIN, M., NOWILL, W. K., MARGOLIS, G., and STEPHEN, C. R.: Chlorpromazine: A Laboratory and Clinical Investigation. Anesthesiology, 16, 829, 1955.

BÜLBRING, E. and DAWES, G. S.: A Method for the Assay of Atropine Substitutes on the Salivary Secretion. J. Pharm. & Exper. Therap., 84, 177, 1945.

BURCH, G. R.: Quoted in Laboratory and Clinical Reports on Thorazine. Pitman-Moore Company, Indianapolis, Indiana, 1957.

BURROUGHS, H. E.: Methadon Narcosis in Dogs. J. Small Animal Med., 1, 301, 1953.

CLIFFORD, D. H.: Effect of Preanesthetic Medication with Chlorpromazine, Meperidine, and Promazine on Pentobarbital Anesthesia in the Cat. J.A.V.M.A., 131, 415, 1957.

CONNOR, N. D. and HAAS, K. B.: Effects of Reserpine in the Dog. J.A.V.M.A., 126, 137, 1955.

COURVOISIER, S., FOURNEL, J., DUCROT, R., KOLSKY, M., and KOETSCHET, P.: Pharmacodynamic Properties of 10-(2-Dimethylaminopropyl)-2-Chlorophenothiazine Hydrochloride. Arch. int. pharmacodyn., 92, 305, 1953.

EARL, A. E.: Reserpine (Serpasil) in Veterinary Practice. J.A.V.M.A., 129, 227, 1956.

ESTRADA, E.: Clinical Uses of Chlorpromazine in Veterinary Medicine. J.A.V.M.A., 128, 292, 1956.

GODEAUX, J. and TONNESEN, M.: Investigations into Atropine Metabolism in the Animal Organism. Acta Pharmacol. et Toxicol., 5, 95, 1949.

GOODMAN, L. S. and GILMAN, A.: The Pharmacological Basis of Therapeutics. 2nd ed., The Macmillan Co., New York, 1958.

GRAHAM, J. B. P. and LAZARUS, S.: The Actions of Methyl-Atropine Nitrate (Eumydrin). J. Pharm. & Exper. Therap., 70, 165, 1940.

GRUBER, C. M., HART, E. R., and GRUBER, C. M., JR.: The Pharmacology and Toxicology of the Ethyl Ester of 1-Methyl-4-Phenyl-Piperidine-4-Carboxylic Acid (Demerol). J. Pharm. & Exper. Therap., 73, 319, 1941.

HALL, H. C.: Methadone, Scopolamine, and Nembutal Anesthesia in Fifteen Dogs. J.A.V.M.A., 122, 289, 1953.

HEARD, W. T.: Personal Communication. Denver, Colorado, 1962.
HUEBNER, R. A.: Meprobamate in Canine Medicine: Summary of Seventy-seven Cases. Vet. Med., *51*, 488, 1956.
IRWIN, S., SLABOK, M., DEBIASE, P. L., and GOVIER, W. M.: Perphenazine (Trilafon), A New Potent Tranquilizer and Antiemetic: I. Behavior Profile, Acute Toxicity and Behavioral Mode of Action. Arch. int. pharmacodyn., *118*, 358, 1959.
JONES, L. M.: *Veterinary Pharmacology and Therapeutics.* 2nd ed. The Iowa State College Press, Ames, Iowa, 1957.
KNOWLES, J. O.: Small Animal Anesthesia. Univ. Penn. Bull., *148*, 4, 1957.
KNOWLES, J. O.: Clinical Experience with Tranquilizing Agents. J.A.V.M.A., *130*, 10, 1957.
KNOWLES, A. T., KNOWLES, J. O., KNOWLES, R. P., and YOPP, G. F.: Clinical Experience with Mepazine. J.A.V.M.A., *131*, 379, 1957.
KRANTZ, J. C., JR. and CARR, C. J.: *The Pharmacologic Principles of Medical Practice.* 2nd ed. The Williams & Wilkins Co., 1951.
KRAWITZ, L.: A Safer Technique for the Induction of General Anesthesia in Small Animals. Vet. Med., *52*, 442, 1957.
MACKO, E., SCHEIDY, S. F., and TUCKER, R. G.: Chlorpromazine in the Dog. Vet. Med., *53*, 378, 1958.
POWERS, S., REED, C., and GREGERSEN, M. I.: The Effects of Morphine on Dogs in Hemorrhagic and Traumatic Shock. Am. J. Physiol., *148*, 269, 1947.
REUTNER, T. F. and GRUHZIT, O. M.: Methadon, A New Analgesic. J.A.V.M.A., *113*, 448, 1948.
RIPPS, J. H.: Some Clinical Uses of Mepazine in the Dog. N. Amer. Vet., *38*, 189, 1957.
ROTH, F. E., IRWIN, S., ECKHARDT, E., TABACHNICK, I. I. A., and GOVIER, W. M.: Perphenazine (Trilafon), A New Potent Tranquilizer and Antiemetic: II. General Pharmacology. Arch. int. pharmacodyn., *118*, 375, 1959.
SALZMAN, N. P. and BRODIE, B. B.: Physiological Disposition and Fate of Chlorpromazine and a Method for Its Estimation in Biological Material. J. Pharm. & Exper. Therap., *118*, 46, 1956.
SCOTT, C. C., CHEN, K. K., KOHLSTEADT, K. G., ROBBINS, E. B., and ISRAEL, F. W.: Further Observations on the Pharmacology of Dolophine (Methadon, Lilly). J. Pharm. & Exper. Therap., *91*, 147, 1947.
WEBERLEIN, M. K., MCCLUMPHA, C. A., BRENGLE, L. A., LICKFELDT, W. E., and DAWSON, H. A.: Promazine in Canine Medicine. J.A.V.M.A., *134*, 518, 1959.
WRIGHT, J. G.: *Veterinary Anaesthesia.* 4th ed. The Williams & Wilkins Co., Baltimore, 1957.
————.: Morphine-Apomorphine Analgesia. A Clinical Review. J. Small Animal. Med., *1*, 220, 1952.

GENERAL ANESTHESIA

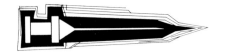

Chapter 7

GENERAL anesthesia may be defined as complete unconsciousness. Commonly used drugs capable of producing this state fall in three broad categories:

1. The inhalation anesthetics
2. The barbiturates
3. Miscellaneous agents

The Stages of General Anesthesia

For descriptive purposes general anesthesia has been divided into four stages depending upon neuromuscular signs exhibited by the patient (Table 7–1). It should be emphasized that no clear division exists between stages, one blending into the next. In addition, variation in response among patients is to be expected. Preanesthetic medication, adequacy of oxygenation, carbon dioxide retention, and physical status of the patient will all modify the signs. Patient response is also governed by the anesthetic which is being administered, considerable variation existing between agents.

Stage I. This is termed the stage of analgesia or voluntary movement. If an irritant gas is being administered, the animal from fear and excitement will struggle violently, cry, and temporarily refuse to breathe, then will breathe deeply and rapidly. Epinephrine is released causing a strong rapid heartbeat and dilation of the pupils. The corneal reflex is still present. Frequently the patient salivates profusely and voids urine and feces. The animal is still conscious and, while analgesia is present to some degree, is not a fit subject for painful procedures.

Stage II. This is called the stage of delirium or involuntary movement. As the cortical centers become depressed the patient loses consciousness. This feature marks the change from Stage I. The patient reacts to external stimuli by violent reflex struggling, breath holding, tachypnea, and hyperventilation. Continued epinephrine release causes a fast strong heartbeat, and the pupils may be widely dilated. Whining and crying are common. Excessive saliva-

Table 7–1.—Characteristics of the Stages of Anesthesia Without Premedication

Stages of Anesthesia	Depression of Central Nervous System	Nerves Depressed	Mucous Membrane Color (1)	Pupil Size (2)	Eyeball Activity (3)	Muscle Tone	Respiration	Pulse and Blood Pressure (B.P.)	Reflexes						Miscellaneous
									Lid	Corneal	Skin	Swallowing	Cough	Pedal	
I Analgesia (stage of voluntary movement)	Sensory cortex		Normal / Flushed		Voluntary		Rapid and irregular	Rapid pulse and elevated B.P.	+	+	+	+	+	+	Pain abolished
II Delirium (stage of involuntary movement)	Motor cortex / Decerebrate rigidity (4)		Flushed		++++		Very irregular (erratic)	Rapid pulse and elevated B.P.	+	+	+	+	+	+	Unconscious, Swallowing, emesis, may occur
III Surgical — Plane 1	Midbrain	III	Flushed / Normal		+		Slow and regular	Normal pulse and normal B.P.	+ / −	+	+	−	+	−	
Plane 2	Spinal cord (increased depression)	V / X	Normal		Fixed		Slow and regular	Normal pulse and normal B.P.	−	+ to −/−	−	−	+	−	
Plane 3	Spinal cord (increased depression)	VI	Normal / Pale		3rd eyelid relaxed		Delayed thoracic / Chiefly abdominal	Rapid pulse and fall in B.P. (5)	−	−	−	−	−	−	Smooth muscle depressed, Pedal reflex absent (6)
Plane 4	Spinal cord (severe depression)		Pale				Abdominal (shallow)	Rapid, weak pulse and fall in B.P.	−	−	−	−	−	−	Anal reflex present
IV Paralysis (death follows)	Medullary paralysis		Pale and cyanotic			None	None (diaphragm paralyzed)	Shock level	−	−	−	−	−	−	Anal and bladder sphincters relaxing

1. Cyanosis occurs in any stage of oxygen want.
2. Pupil size in the etherized dog is so inconsistent that it is not a reliable sign.
3. Nystagmus is not prominent in the dog as it is in some other species.
4. Decerebrate rigidity (extension of the limbs) is frequently observed in the dog just before entering Stage III. Relaxation occurs on entering Plane 1.
5. It has been estimated that 15 minutes in Plane 3 is as shock producing as 2 hours in Plane 2.
6. Pedal reflex activity as ether in Plane 1 but may persist as long as Plane 3 when barbiturate anesthesia is employed.

(From Booth, N. H. and Rankin, A. D.: *Laboratory Outline for Pharmacology.* 2nd ed. Colorado A & M College, Fort Collins, Colorado, 1954; Jones, L. M.: *Veterinary Pharmacology and Therapeutics.* 2nd ed. The Iowa State College Press, Ames, Iowa, 1957, with additions.)

tion and swallowing movements take place. In the dog and cat reflex vomiting may occur, particularly if the animal has been recently fed.

Stage III. This is the stage of surgical anesthesia and is characterized by unconsciousness with progressive depression of the reflexes. Muscular relaxation develops and respirations become slow and regular. Vomiting and swallowing reflexes are lost.

In human anesthesiology this stage has been further divided into Planes 1 to 4 to give finer differentiation. A simpler and probably as effective method is to divide this stage into *light surgical anesthesia* (Planes 1 and 2) and *deep surgical anesthesia* (Planes 3 and 4). Most surgical operations are carried out in the former.

In light surgical anesthesia the eyelids remain open, the palpebral and corneal reflexes being slowed but still responsive to stimulation. The pedal reflex disappears in this part of Stage III. The skin and muscle becomes unresponsive to severe stimuli such as cutting with a knife. The respirations are smooth, regular, and deep and are produced by both diaphragmatic and intercostal muscle contractions. The iris constricts slightly early in Stage III and then gradually dilates as deep surgical anesthesia is approached.

In deep surgical anesthesia the corneal, palpebral, and pedal reflexes are completely suppressed. The skeletal muscles begin to lose tone and intercostal respiration begins to decline progressively. This makes the respiratory movements shorter and gasping in character and is a sign of dangerously deep anesthesia. On cessation of intercostal breathing the diaphragm continues to carry on respiratory function. Complete suppression of diaphragmatic movement indicates the end of Stage III and the entrance of the patient into Stage IV. In deep surgical anesthesia the heat-regulating mechanism in the hypothalamus is inactivated and the patient's temperature drops. The pulse gradually weakens.

Stage IV. In this stage the nervous system is extremely depressed and respirations cease. The heart will continue to beat only for a short time. Blood pressure is at the shock level with mucous membranes blanched and the pupils widely dilated. The anal and bladder sphincters relax. Death quickly intervenes unless immediate resuscitative steps are taken.

If the anesthetic is withdrawn and artificial respiration initiated before heart action stops, these effects may be overcome and the patient go through the various stages in reverse.

The stages described above are best seen when ether is administered, probably because considerable time is required for an anesthetic concentration to accrue in the central nervous system. This allows the various signs to become apparent. With intravenous anesthetics the time between stages is so short that many signs are often inapparent.

Maynert (1960) has conducted an extensive study of the reflexes exhibited by dogs as they arouse from pentobarbital, thiopental, trichlorethanol, paraldehyde, and ethanol anesthesia. The first reflex to reappear was ranked number one and as others appeared they were ranked consecutively (Table 7–2). No individual reflex

Table 7–2.—*Return of Reflexes in Dogs Following Large Intravenous Doses of Various Anesthetics**

	Sodium Pentobarbital 35 mg/kg	*Sodium Thiopental* 30 mg/kg	*Trichlor-ethanol* 160 mg/kg	*Paraldehyde* 850 mg/kg	*Ethanol* 2.6–3.5 gm/kg
Wink reflex	2.0 (1–3)	2.3 (1–3)	5.0 (2–9)	3.3 (1–5)	2.7 (1–4)
Corneal reflex	4.1 (2–7)	4.6 (2–8)	4.6 (2–7)	5.5 (3–8)	4.8 (1–8)
Swallowing reflex	7.7 (6–9)	7.2 (6–8)	7.8 (5–9)	5.6 (4–8)	6.7 (6–8)
Endotracheal reflex	4.6 (3–6)	3.7 (2–4)	2.8 (2–5)	3.4 (1–5)	2.2 (1–3)
Patellar reflex	1.3 (1–3)	1.3 (1–3)	1.0	2.3 (1–7)	3.2 (1–8)
Respiratory reflex	3.2 (2–4)	3.6 (2–5)	3.6 (2–5)	3.3 (2–6)	4.0 (2–5)
Movement reflex	6.5 (5–8)	6.2 (5–7)	5.6 (4–7)	6.0 (4–8)	6.0 (4–8)
Spontaneous movement	6.7 (5–8)	7.6 (6–9)	6.8 (4–8)	6.8 (6–9)	7.2 (5–9)
Head-righting reflex	8.9 (8–9)	8.5 (8–9)	7.8 (6–9)	8.8 (8–9)	8.2 (7–9)
Walking	10.0	10.0	10.0	10.0	10.0
Freedom from ataxia	11.0	11.0	11.0	11.0	11.0

* Mean rank is indicated in the first column and range in the second.

Wink reflex—contraction of orbicularis oculi induced by a tap on the inner canthus of the eye.

Corneal reflex—contraction of the orbicularis oculi when the cornea is touched with cotton.

Swallowing reflex—swallowing movement produced by separating the jaws and pulling the tongue.

Endotracheal reflex—Coughing produced by vigorous movement of an endotracheal tube within the trachea.

Patellar reflex—extension of the leg when the quadriceps tendon is tapped.

Respiratory reflex—a change in the respiratory pattern produced by forceful and rapid dilation of the anal sphincter.

Movement reflex—movement of an extremity produced by forceful and rapid dilation of the anal sphincter.

Spontaneous movement—movement of an extremity without a provoking stimulus.

Head-righting reflex—ability of the animal to maintain its head in an upright position without support.

(From Maynert, E. W.: The Usefulness of Clinical Signs for the Comparison of Intravenous Anesthetics in Dogs. J. Pharm. & Exper. Therap., *128*, 182, 1960.)

was always found to reappear in the same order when all were tested. From this investigation Maynert concluded that the intensity of neurological derangement could best be estimated using a scale containing six levels of depression:

Level 0—Freedom from ataxia.
Level 1—Ability to walk though ataxic.
Level 2—Presence of the head-righting reflex.
Level 3—Presence of spontaneous movement, the movement reflex, or the swallowing reflex.
Level 4—Presence of one or more of the following reflexes: wink, corneal, endotracheal, or respiratory.
Level 5—Only the patellar reflex present.

The question of how best to judge the various stages of anesthesia arises, particularly when so many modifying factors must be taken into account. *The experienced anesthetist finds himself relying less on classical signs of anesthesia and more on the patient's response to stimuli.* These stimuli may be produced by the surgeon or the anesthetist himself and may produce responses in respiration, circulation, or muscle tone. Needless to say, effective anesthesia is that which just obliterates the patient's response to painful stimuli without depressing vital functions.

References

MAYNERT, E. W.:   The Usefulness of Clinical Signs for the Comparison of Intravenous Anesthetics in Dogs. J. Pharm. & Exper. Therap., *128*, 182, 1960.

THE
INHALATION
ANESTHETICS

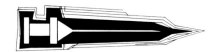

Chapter 8

Advantages and Disadvantages of
Inhalation Anesthesia

INHALATION anesthesia has two distinct advantages: (1) The agents used are not metabolized within the body but are exhaled through the lungs; therefore, recovery from anesthesia is not dependent upon body detoxification mechanisms. In poor-risk patients this is particularly helpful. (2) Because these agents are rapidly exhaled, the anesthetist has good control of the level of anesthesia and can quickly alter the depth at any time.

Certain disadvantages also are inherent with these agents: (1) They require constant surveillance by an anesthetist during administration, (2) most of them are explosive and inflammable, and (3) many are irritant to body tissues.

Methods of Administration

Inhalation anesthetics are divided into volatile liquids and gases according to their physical state. The common liquids are ethyl ether, vinyl ether, chloroform, halothane, methoxyflurane, ethyl chloride, and trichloroethylene (Table 8–1). The common gases are nitrous oxide, ethylene, and cyclopropane. All of the gaseous agents are administered by means of a closed system (see below). Volatile

Table 8-1.—Historical and Clinical Data on the Inhalation Anesthetic Agents

Agent (Chemical Name)	Ethylene	Acetylene	Nitrous Oxide	Cyclo-Propane	Ethyl Chloride	Divinyl Ether	Diethyl Ether	Ethyl Vinyl Ether	Trifluoro-Ethyl Vinyl Ether	Trifluoro-Chlorobromo Ethane	Chloroform	Trichloro-Ethylene
Chemical Formula	$CH_2=CH_2$	$CH\equiv CH$	N_2O	CH_2 CH_2-CH_2	C_2H_5Cl	$(CH_2=CH)_2O$	$(C_2H_5)_2O$	$C_2H_5OCH=CH_2$	$CF_3CH_2OCH=CH_2$	$CF_3CHBrCl$	$CHCl_3$	$CCl_2=CHCl$
Discovery	1779 by Ingenhousz	1836 by Davy	1772 by Priestley	1882 by Freund	1648 by Glauber	1887 by Semmler	1540 by Cordus	1930 by Fraenkel	1951 by Shukys	1956 by Suckling	1831 by Guthrie, Liebig, and Soubeiran independently	1864 by Fisher
First Observation of Narcotic Properties	1864 by Herman	1922 by Wieland	1799 by Davy	1929 by Lucas and Henderson	1847 by Flourens	1930 by Leake and Chen	1796 by Beddoes	1930 by Leake	1953 by Krantz	1956 by Raventos	1847 by Flourens	1915 by Plessner
First Used Clinically in Man	1923 by Luckhardt and Carter and, independently, by Herb	1923 by Wieland and Gauss	1844 by Wells	1933 by Waters	1894 by Carlson	1933 by Gelfan and Bell	1842 by Long 1846 by Morton	1947 by Krantz	1953 by Sadove	1956 by Johnson	1847 by Simpson	1934 by Jackson
Type of Compound	Unsaturated hydrocarbon	Unsaturated hydrocarbon	Oxide of nitrogen	Cyclic hydrocarbon	Halogenated hydrocarbon	Unsaturated ether	Saturated ether	Unsaturated ether	Unsaturated halogenated ether	Halogenated hydrocarbon	Chlorinated hydrocarbon	Unsaturated chlorinated hydrocarbon
Molecular Weight	28.05	26.04	44.02	42.08	64.52	70.09	74.12	72.10	126.04	197.39	119.39	131.4
Boiling Point °C.	-103.9	-88.5	-89.5	-32.8	12.57	28.4	34.6	35.8	43.2	50.2	61.3	86.7
Vapor Density (Air = 1) at 25°C.	0.97	0.90	1.53	1.48	2.22	2.42	2.56	2.49	4.4	6.9	4.12	4.53
Vapor Pressure, mm.Hg., at 20°C.	38,110 737 p.s.i.	Completely gaseous state at 20° C.	Completely gaseous state at 20° C.	4,256 82.3 p.s.i.	1,003 19.4 p.s.i.	558	444	401	286	235	166	57
Commercial Preparation	Dehydration of ethanol—cracking of fuel gases	Hydrolysis of calcium carbide	Decomposition of ammonium nitrate by heat	Treatment of 1 chloro,-3-bromo-propane with zinc for ring closure	Addition of hydrogen chloride to ethylene. Treatment of ethanol with hydrogen chloride	Dehydrochlorination of di(chloroethyl) ether with potassium hydroxide	Dehydration of ethanol with sulfuric acid	Reaction of acetylene and ethyl alcohol	Reaction of acetylene and trifluoroethyl alcohol	Stepwise halogenation of trichloroethylene	Chlorination of acetone or alcohol	Dehydrochlorination of tetrachloroethane with lime

(Courtesy of Dr. Wm. H. L. Dornette and Ohio Chemical and Surgical Equipment Company)

Impurities which may be Present in Crude Product	Ethano Ether Polymerized hydrocarbons Carbon monoxide	Arsine Phosphine Hydrogen sulphide	Higher oxides of nitrogen Nitrogen Ammonia	Propylene Hydrogen Halogenated hydrocarbons	Halogenated hydrocarbons Ethanol Ethylene	Polymers Formaldehyde Formic acid Acetic acid Peroxides	Peroxides Aldehydes	Acetaldehyde Non-volatile matter	Trifluoroethanol bis-trifluoro-ethyl acetal trifluoro-acetaldyde	HCl, HBr, other halogenated hydrocarbons	Phosgene Hydrogen chloride Acetone	Dichloroacetylene Phosgene Hydrogen chloride
Stabilizing Agent Added	None	Stored in acetone solution	None	None	None	0.01% phenyl alpha naphthalamine and 3.5% ethanol	None. Trace C_2H_5OH present from manufacture	0.01% phenyl alpha naphthalamine and 3.5% ethanol. Less than 2% diethyl ether present from manufacture	0.01% phenyl alpha naphthalamine	0.01% thymol	0.01% phenyl alpha naphthalamine	0.01% thymol
Reaction with Soda Lime	Stable		Stable	Stable	Alcoholic sol. of KOH may be hydrolyzed into HCl and C_2H_5OH	Stable	Traces of aldehydes may be formed	Stable	Stable	Stable	Converted to salt of formic acid when warmed	Dehydrochlorination to Dichloroacetylene
Cell/Plasma Ratio	8:1		1:1	2.5:1							6.5:1	
Oil/Water Distribution Ratio at 37° C.	14.4	2.2	3.2	34.43		41.3	3.2	45 ± 5	94 at 25°C.	330	100	
Potency (ethyl ether = 1)	0.25:1	0.5:1	0.15:1	1:5	1:1	1:1	1:1	1.5:1	1.5:1	4:1	3:1	5:1
% Conc. of Inhaled Mixture for: Analgesia	20-35	60-80	35-40	3-5	—	0.2	—	—	1.0-2.0	—	—	0.28
Anesthesia	80-90	—	85-90	20-25	3.0-4.5	4	3.5-4.5	3.0	2.4-8.2	0.8-1.2	1.35-1.65	0.55-0.7
Respiratory Arrest	—	—	—	35-39	—	10-12	6.7-8	—	12.9	3.6-4.0	2	—
mgm % Conc. in Blood For: Anesthesia	140	—	—	16-20	20-30	28	90-130	25	9.3	—	20-30	—
Respiratory Arrest	—	—	—	—	40	68	140-180	—	38.7	—	40-60	—
Inflammable Range in % — Air	3.05-28.6	2.5-81	Will support combustion only	2.40-10.3	4.0-14.8	1.70-27.0	1.85-36.5	—	Dry 4.2	Nonflammable	Oxidized by flame $2CHCl_3 + O_2 \triangle 2COCl_2 + 2HCl$	Below 32°C. nonflammable, above 32°C. 15%
O2	2.90-79.9	2.8-91		2.48-60.0	4.05-67.2	1.85-85.5	2.10-82.0	2.1 (lower limit)	Sat. with H_2O 4.0-80 7.5-78			10.3-64.5
Ignition Temperature in °C. — Air	490°	305°	Will support combustion only	498°	517°	360°	304°	—	—	Nonflammable	Oxidized by flame $2CHCl_3 + O_2 \triangle 2COCl_2 + 2HCl$	419°
O2	485°	296°		454°	468°	327°	182°	—	—			

liquid agents are administered by a variety of methods which include the following:

1. *The Open Drop Method.* A mask constructed of wire mesh covered with gauze is used. It is placed over the patient's nose without completely occluding the edges so that a free exchange of air can occur around them. Anesthetic is dripped on the gauze.

2. *The Semi-Open Drop Method.* This is the one most commonly employed by veterinarians. A mask is again used but the edges are occluded, by a towel or similar substance, so that inhaled air must pass through the gauze, vaporizing the anesthetic agent which is dripped on it. This method results in higher anesthetic concentrations than the open drop method and also tends to produce hypoxia and increased carbon dioxide retention. Greater caution must therefore be exercised.

3. *Anesthetic Chambers.* These are used for small dogs, cats, and other species. Following induction in the chamber the animal is removed and anesthesia is maintained by some other method.

4. *Endotracheal Insufflation.* With this method gas is introduced into the trachea, which is not completely occluded so that exhalation can occur around the tube.

5. *The Semi-Closed System.* Oxygen and anesthetic are administered to the patient by means of an apparatus connected to a mask or endotracheal catheter with inflated cuff. An expiratory valve allows escape of carbon dioxide and excess gases into the surrounding atmosphere.

6. *The Closed System.* This system, employing a gas machine, delivers oxygen and anesthetic to the patient through a mask or endotracheal catheter with inflated cuff. Anesthetic and enough oxygen to meet the patient's metabolic requirements are introduced into the system, and carbon dioxide is removed by absorption with soda lime. The patient rebreathes the exhaled anesthetic since none is allowed to escape from the system.

A more detailed discussion of methods and equipment for administration of inhalant anesthetics is given in Chapter 9.

Volatile Liquid Anesthetics

Ether, U.S.P. (Ethyl Ether; Diethyl Ether; $(C_2H_5)_2O$)

Ethyl ether was synthesized by Valerius Cordus in Germany in 1540. Ether, as it is commonly called, is a colorless highly volatile liquid with a pungent odor and irritating vapor. For practical purposes it is *always* explosive. Ether oxidizes in the presence of air or oxygen to form peroxides and aldehydes which are toxic. In addition peroxides may, on rare occasions, cause explosions. Because light causes oxidation, ether is stored in sealed metal containers coated inside with copper or other metal which combines with oxygen. This preferential absorption by the metal prevents oxidation.

Ether may be administered by open drop, semi-open drop, semi-closed, closed, or chamber methods. With the exception of methoxyflurane, it has the longest induction time of the inhalation anesthetics, varying from 3 to 10 minutes depending upon the concentration administered, premedication, physical status of the patient, and other variable factors. The concentration necessary for anesthesia is 3.5 to 4.5% by volume in the inhaled mixture; 6.7 to 8.0% will cause respiratory failure. For rapid induction higher concentrations are necessary to saturate the blood. Ether is absorbed and excreted unchanged from the body, 80 to 92% being exhaled, the remainder being eliminated in urine and other body fluids. Complete desaturation of the body is slow, requiring about 8 hours.

Ether is irritant to all tissues, and this accounts for many of the effects seen during and after anesthesia. Because it irritates the mucous membranes of the respiratory tract, breath-holding by the patient is common during induction. When ether is administered by the semi-open drop method, this leads to inhalation of high concentrations of vapor with paralysis of the respiratory centers. Removal of the mask and artificial respiration will resuscitate most of these patients; however, most deaths from ether anesthesia occur during induction. There is marked increase in the flow of saliva and mucus which may interfere with respiration. This also lowers resistance of the lung tissue to infection and increases susceptibility to postoperative pneumonia.

Ether irritates kidney tissues and reduces urine output during anesthesia. McNider (1920, 1921, 1922) has shown that the effect varies with age, dogs 4 to 11 years old having marked reduction in urine output or even complete anuria after 1 hour of anesthesia. Ten per cent dextrose solution injected intravenously before ether administration has a protecting effect. Albuminuria and tubular casts are common in the postanesthetic period.

The effect on the liver is minimal. Histologically, centrilobular glycogen depletion and slight fatty changes have been noted in dogs anesthetized for 3-hour periods on 5 consecutive days (Stephen *et al.*, 1958). Bromsulphalein tests in these animals were unaltered.

Cardiac output is increased during induction because of epinephrine release. During light surgical anesthesia output is increased about 20% above normal and blood pressure is normal or slightly elevated (Blalock, 1928). Deep surgical anesthesia is accompanied by a progressive fall in blood pressure due to beginning paralysis of the vasomotor centers and decreased cardiac output. In the stage of medullary paralysis the centers are affected in the following order: respiratory, vasomotor, and cardiac.

There is no demonstrable effect on cardiac muscle histologically. However, disturbances of rhythm and extrasystoles frequently occur, particularly on induction. The blood pressure is usually unchanged or slightly elevated unless anoxia, hypercapnea, or other factors are present. Anemia and icterus are occasionally seen after anesthesia. It is not certain whether this is due to the effect upon the blood or liver. The most obvious change in the blood is a hyperglycemia which may be sufficiently high to produce glycosuria. There is hemo-concentration with an increase in the red cell count and hemoglobin, accompanied by a decrease in plasma volume. Leukocytosis also occurs, the polymorphonuclear leukocytes increasing relatively and absolutely. Progressive acidosis develops through loss of bicarbonate (due to excretion of sodium with acetone bodies) and loss of carbon dioxide through increased respiration.

Contraindications for ether anesthesia are acute or chronic respiratory infections, acidosis, kidney or liver disease, shock, and surgery requiring use of electrocautery.

The advantages of ether are that it gives good muscular relaxation, has a wide margin of safety, is a respiratory stimulant, and does not depress the circulation at the usual level of anesthesia. It is stable, easily preserved, relatively inexpensive, and can be administered with a minimum of equipment.

The disadvantages include a long induction period accompanied by excitement, slow recovery, irritation to all tissues, and flame and explosion hazards.

For the patient, ether is the *safest volatile agent* in the hands of the inexperienced anesthetist. It is the most commonly used inhalation anesthetic.

Vinyl Ether, U.S.P. (Divinyl Ether; Divinyl Oxide; Vinethene; $(CH_2:CH)_2O$)

Vinyl ether was first prepared by Semmler in Germany in 1887. Its anesthetic properties were first described by Leake and Chen in 1930 in the United States.

Vinyl ether is a highly volatile clear fluid with an ethereal non-pungent odor. It is an unstable compound decomposed by heat, light, and air, forming peroxides and aldehydes. For this reason it is stored in dark bottles containing an amine as anti-catalyst.* Opened bottles should be discarded after 10 days and solutions in

---

* Merck's Vinethene contains vinyl ether, 4% absolute alcohol to prevent freezing of exhaled water vapor on a mask, and 0.01% phenyl-alpha napthalamine as a stabilizer. The fluorescent tinge of vinethene is due to the stabilizer.

unopened containers should be discarded after the expiration date on the label. Vinyl ether is highly inflammable and explosive when mixed with air and oxygen.

Vinyl ether may be administered by open, semi-open, or closed techniques. A concentration of 4% in inspired air produces anesthesia. Respiratory arrest occurs with concentrations of 10 to 12%. Vinyl ether is eliminated unaltered from the body, the major portion through the lungs with small amounts in urine and other body secretions.

Induction and recovery are more rapid than with ethyl ether, averaging 2 to 4 minutes. Vinyl ether is also less irritant to the mucous membranes, therefore the excitement stage is less pronounced. It has a greater margin of safety than ethyl ether but this is offset by its greater potency, hence administration is more difficult. Anesthesia is characterized by fair muscular relaxation; in some animals characteristic running movements are made with the hind or all four extremities. There is good oxygenation and no cyanosis. The best indication of the stage of anesthesia is the rate, depth, and smoothness of respiration.

Liver necrosis due to vinyl ether has been reported in dogs and mice (Jones et al., 1958). Liver damage is much greater if there is low liver glycogen and hypoxia during the anesthetic period. With prolonged use there is impairment of urea clearance in the kidney. Vinyl ether has also been shown to cause cardiac fibrillation in dogs. There is little effect on blood pressure. The salivary glands are stimulated during the induction period.

Chief advantages of vinyl ether are rapid induction and recovery with a minimum of equipment necessary for administration. Disadvantages include the relative high cost of the agent, the danger of fire and explosion, unsatisfactory muscle relaxation, and the hazard of cardiac fibrillation. Divinyl ether has been demonstrated to be more dangerous for the patient than either diethyl or ethylvinyl ethers (Mörch et al., 1956).

Possible uses for vinyl ether include induction prior to other agents, anesthesia of short duration, and operations not requiring good muscular relaxation. It is contraindicated for anesthesia of more than 15 to 20 minutes, in operations requiring good muscle relaxation, in hepatic or renal disease, or in hypoxia. Because of its inherent disadvantages vinyl ether is not used to anesthetize small animals outside of the laboratory.

Chloroform, U.S.P. ($CHCl_3$)

The anesthetic properties of chloroform were discovered in animals by Flourens in 1847.

Chloroform is a clear sweet noninflammable liquid with a pleasant odor and nonirritating vapor. When heated with air, it forms phosgene gas. For this reason 1% ethyl alcohol is added which combines to form ethyl carbonate and ethyl chloride.

Chloroform may be administered by either open or closed techniques. It is a very potent anesthetic; for light anesthesia the inhaled concentration is 1.35%, for deep anesthesia 1.65%, and respiratory arrest 2%. As much as 4% may be needed for induction. Chloroform is not altered within the body, the major part being eliminated through the lungs with small amounts in urine and other body secretions.

During induction respirations are deep and accelerated due to struggling. As anesthesia develops, however, chloroform gradually depresses respiration and breathing becomes slow and shallow. The respiratory center becomes progressively less sensitive to carbon dioxide.

An undesirable feature of chloroform is its effect on the heart, liver, and kidneys. Chloroform is directly toxic to the heart in concentrations commonly employed for induction. This causes dilatation of the left atrium particularly, since it is exposed first to the agent in high concentration. The entire heart may be affected, however, with reduced force of contraction and generalized dilatation resulting. Such a heart is more susceptible to arrest from vagus stimulation. Fatal poisoning of the heart results in progressive atrial and ventricular dilatation until contractions stop.

Blood pressure rises during induction because of struggling, but as anesthesia deepens, it is markedly lowered due to toxic action on the heart, depression of the vasomotor center, and dilatation of the splanchnic vessels. Chloroform is thought to have a direct relaxing effect on blood vessel musculature. In the cat, chloroform increases the susceptibility to vasodilation of the blood vessels by histamine. If the latter is released due to tissue injury from chloroform, the capillary bed may dilate and blood pressure fall.

Chloroform anesthesia of any duration produces central necrosis of the liver which starts to develop 6 to 10 hours following administration. Liver function in the dog is greatly decreased as indicated by bromsulphalein tests. Fifteen minutes of anesthesia may cause dye retention 8 days later and 2 hours of anesthesia may even cause retention 6 weeks later. Dogs which are fasted 24 hours will develop more severe lesions than those which have been fed. A high protein diet and high oxygen intake with a closed system will help protect against liver damage.

There is a tendency for anuria to develop during anesthesia due to decreased kidney function; this is followed by polyuria and albuminuria after recovery.

Deaths from chloroform may occur during induction, after a prolonged period of anesthesia, or 24 to 48 hours after recovery. Death during induction usually occurs in animals which are highly excited and is due to ventricular fibrillation. These animals inhale large amounts of chloroform and suddenly collapse without warning. Premedication with a narcotic or tranquilizer will lessen the struggling and atropine will block the cardioinhibitory effect of vagus stimulation.

After prolonged chloroform anesthesia death may occur due to progressive respiratory failure, the respiratory center becoming increasingly less sensitive to carbon dioxide. This type of fatality may be prevented by decreasing the concentration as the anesthetic period progresses. Premedication will also aid in preventing this type of fatality. Draper and Whitehead (1942) gave various anesthetics to dogs to the point of respiratory arrest and then used artificial respiration as the *sole* means of resuscitation. In more than 600 anesthetic periods their failure to resuscitate the animal was:

Anesthetic	Failure to Resuscitate
Ether	0.8%
Vinyl ether	2.9%
Chloroform	10.3%

Deaths which occur postanesthetically are due to central necrosis of the liver and fatty degeneration of the heart, kidneys, and liver. If sufficient damage is done to these organs that their normal functions cannot be maintained, death occurs. These fatalities usually happen 24 to 48 hours following anesthesia but occasional deaths are reported up to 10 days.

Chloroform anesthesia is contraindicated in patients with cardiac, renal, or hepatic disease. Anoxia aggravates the harmful effects of chloroform; hence, patients with severe anemia should not be subjected to this type of anesthesia. Because of its toxicity and narrow margin of safety, chloroform is not used for small animal anesthesia in the United States. Its use continues, however, in other countries.

To reduce the potency and toxicity of chloroform early workers formulated ACE mixture which consisted of 1 part alcohol, 2 parts chloroform and 3 parts ether. This mixture has been abandoned and is only of historical interest.

Halothane (Fluothane; Halsan; $CF_3CHClBr$)

Halothane is a clear colorless volatile liquid with a nonirritating odor. Some decomposition occurs when it is exposed to light, so the liquid is stabilized by the addition of 0.01% (w/w) thymol and stored in amber glass bottles. It is unaffected by warm soda lime and can be used in closed systems. Halothane is *nonexplosive* and *noninflammable* when mixed in high concentrations with oxygen. It is the most expensive of the volatile liquid anesthetics.

Halothane vapor in concentrations of 2 to 4% produces Stage III, Plane 2–3 anesthesia in dogs and monkeys in 2 to 5 minutes. Surgical anesthesia is maintained by inhalation of 0.8 to 1.2% mixtures, depending on whether preanesthetic agents are administered. On this basis, it is estimated that halothane is about twice as potent as chloroform and 4 times as potent as diethyl ether. Recovery occurs rapidly and, with prolonged anesthesia, is frequently complete in 10 to 20 minutes (Fig. 8–1).

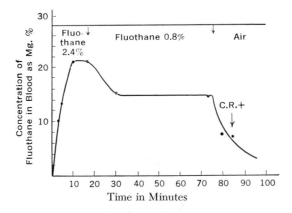

FIGURE 8–1. Concentration of halothane (Fluóthane) in the blood of a dog during anesthesia. C. R. = Corneal reflex. (From Raventos, J.: The Action of Fluothane— A New Anesthetic. Brit. J. Pharmacol., *11*, 394, 1956.)

The action of halothane on the cardiovascular system is somewhat controversial. All investigators agree that a definite hypotension is produced (20 to 40 mm. Hg decline in the dog) but the mechanism is in question. It has been explained as (1) a ganglionic blocking action, (2) a central vasomotor depression, and (3) a direct depression of the myocardium. Following reduction in concentration of the drug the blood pressure rapidly returns to normal levels, indicating lack of permanent damage to the cardiovascular system. Dogs under anesthesia have hyperemic mucous membranes but bleeding in the operative field is not excessive. Various authors have commented on the complete absence of shock in both man and animals anesthetized with this agent.

Bradycardia follows the administration of halothane. This can be counteracted by atropine and its administration is advised. The heart is sensitized to intravenous epinephrine, and arrhythmias may follow its use (Hall and Norris, 1958). Methoxamine or phenylephrine are vasopressors of choice with halothane since they have been shown to produce a blood pressure rise without alteration in cardiac rhythm.

In dogs, both the amplitude and frequency of respiratory movements are decreased with halothane. This results in progressive respiratory acidosis. Inhalation of high concentrations produces apnea which is easily reversible, but deaths in dogs and monkeys have been reported. Respiratory failure precedes cardiac failure by a considerable margin. Because of its potency the depth of anesthesia can be altered with several respirations.

Salivary, mucous, and bronchial secretions are absent during halothane anesthesia. Laryngospasm is not produced and vomiting is rarely a complication.

Minimal pathological changes have been found in the livers of dogs and monkeys anesthetized for long periods but nothing comparable to those seen following chloroform. Results of liver and kidney function tests following 3 hours of halothane anesthesia for 5 consecutive days were within normal limits (Stephen et al., 1958). Fatalities due to liver necrosis have been reported in man.

Halothane can be administered by open mask, but it is difficult to control the level of anesthesia since small changes in concentration markedly change the depth. Both open and semi-open systems are wasteful of the agent and therefore almost prohibitive in cost. Halothane is best used in a closed system with special metering equipment to give exacting control of the anesthetic concentration. Induction is accomplished by direct administration of vapor with a mask, or by intravenous injection of a thiobarbiturate, followed by maintenance with halothane through an endotracheal catheter. The latter method of induction is usually preferred.

Halothane has been used in dogs in combination with a wide variety of preanesthetic and anesthetic agents (Lumb, 1959). Both succinylcholine and d-tubocurarine have been administered, the former with good and the latter with variable results (Stephen et al., 1958). Nitrous oxide may be given concurrently to potentiate analgesia.

Halothane has been widely accepted in human anesthesiology as evidenced by the fact it is the anesthetic of choice for intracardiac operations at the Mayo Clinic (Dawson et al., 1960).

Methoxyflurane (Penthrane; $CHCl_2CF_2OCH_3$)

Methoxyflurane is a clear colorless liquid which will not explode in any concentration at room temperature. It will explode at higher temperatures and at concentrations above those used clinically. It can be used safely with the electric cautery.

Methoxyflurane has a boiling point above that of water, but vaporizes much more readily because of its low latent heat of vaporization. The concentration attainable during administration is limited by the vapor pressure and efficiency of the vaporizer to a maximum of approximately 4% at 23° C. The concentration necessary for maintenance is less than 2%. Respiratory arrest is difficult or impossible to produce under clinical conditions unless mechanical ventilation is used.

Good muscular relaxation is produced. The action of curariform drugs is potentiated to about the same degree as with diethyl ether.

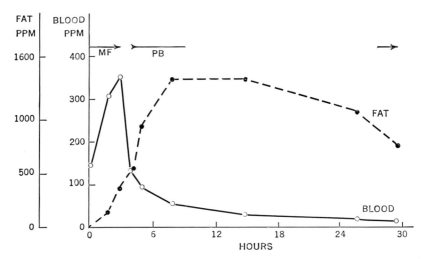

FIGURE 8–2. Methoxyflurane concentrations in blood and fat of a dog during and following 3 hours of anesthesia. MF = methoxyflurane (Penthrane), PB = Pentobarbital sodium. (From Chenoweth, M. B., Robertson, D. N., Erley, D. F., and Golhke, R.: Blood and Tissue Levels of Ether, Chloroform, Halothane and Methoxyflurane in Dogs. Anesthesiology, *23*, 101, 1962.)

The classical eye signs are of no value in determining the stages of anesthesia; the pupils change very little and the eyeballs become fixed early. Respiratory rate, pulse, and degree of reflex activity are the best criteria.

Induction with methoxyflurane alone is slow, requiring approximately 10 minutes. Salivation is not stimulated. Respirations are at first slightly increased followed by a progressive decrease in rate and minute volume with deepening anesthesia. This leads to acidosis if anesthesia is maintained over long periods.

The heart is sensitized to epinephrine but to a much smaller degree than with cyclopropane. Blood pressure falls progressively and is directly related to the depth of anesthesia. During long periods of anesthesia shock levels will be reached.

The tone and motility of the gastrointestinal tract are decreased; vomiting has not been observed in dogs fed prior to anesthesia.

No change in blood cells or coagulation time has been reported. The blood sugar is slightly reduced when breathing is augmented.

Methoxyflurane concentrations in the blood rise and fall fairly rapidly in direct relationship to the amount administered. The fat concentration rises for about 2 hours after administration even though the blood level falls. Thirty hours later there is still a measurable amount of methoxyflurane in the blood and the fat concentration is still high (Fig. 8–2). The odor of the drug can be detected in the breath for many hours since all but a trace is eliminated through the lungs.

Advantages claimed for methoxyflurane are lack of explosive capability and good muscle relaxation with freedom from side effects and toxicity. Disadvantages are long induction and slow recovery, with depression of blood pressure and respiratory acidosis during long periods of anesthesia.

Ethyl Chloride, U.S.P. (C_2H_5Cl)

Ethyl chloride was first produced by Basil Valentine in the 17th century, and its anesthetic properties discovered by Pierre Flourens, a French physiologist, in 1847. Its local anesthetic properties when used as a spray were discovered by P. Redard of Switzerland in 1888.

Ethyl chloride is a gas at room temperature, but at low temperature or under pressure is a colorless liquid with an ethereal odor. Its vapors mixed with air are potentially explosive, and it should not be used with the electric cautery. However, the minimum ignition temperature of this mixture is $936°$ F. It burns with a green flame producing hydrogen chloride.

Ethyl chloride is a potent general anesthetic, mixtures of 3.0 to 4.5% producing anesthesia, and a 6% mixture producing respiratory failure. Since ethyl chloride vapor is nonirritating, induction is easy and rapid, requiring 1 or 2 minutes. It is difficult to maintain prolonged anesthesia safely because of its adverse effect on circulation.

Ethyl chloride depresses the respiratory center and death, if it occurs, is usually from respiratory arrest. It also directly depresses the myocardium and death from ventricular fibrillation may occur. The heart is sensitized to epinephrine to the same degree as with cyclopropane (Morris *et al.*, 1953). Peripheral vasodilation, cardiac slowing, and a direct depressant action on the vasoconstrictor center, all tend to produce a fall in blood pressure. Hepatitis and renal damage have occurred following its use. In the dog ethyl chloride does not produce good muscle relaxation. Maintenance of anesthesia is difficult because of persistent running movements, muscle twitching, and tremors even with deep anesthesia. It possesses a narrow margin of safety.

Because of the disadvantages associated with the use of ethyl chloride as a general anesthetic, its use for this purpose has been restricted to anesthesia of birds and very short anesthetic periods in cats.

For information concerning ethyl chloride as a local anesthetic see Chapter 13, p. 252.

Trichloroethylene, U.S.P. (Trichlorethylene; Trilene; Trimar; Chlorylene; Westrosol; $CCl_2 = CHCl$)

Trichloroethylene was first discovered in 1864 and was studied as an anesthetic by Jackson and co-workers in the United States in 1934. It is a clear colorless fluid with a characteristic odor resembling that of chloroform. It is decomposed by light in the presence of moisture. For this reason it is stored in amber bottles and 0.01% thymol is added to retard decomposition. Methylene blue may be added to distinguish it from chloroform. It can be administered using the open, semi-open, insufflation, or semi-closed techniques. *It cannot be used with soda lime in the closed technique.* It is not stable in the presence of alkaline absorbents and forms dichloroacetylene, which is explosive, and phosgene, both of which are toxic if inhaled. The concentration necessary for anesthesia in inspired air is between 0.5 and 0.75%.

It is not inflammable with air or oxygen in concentrations below 10%. Vapor mixed with pure oxygen may ignite above 68° F., but not if mixed with air.

Most of the drug is eliminated unchanged through the lungs and in body fluids. A small percentage may be decomposed in the body. Butler (1949) has shown that in the dog trichloroethylene is probably converted into chloral hydrate, which is then transformed into trichloroethanol and trichloroacetic acid. These are excreted in the urine.

Trichloroethylene frequently causes auricular fibrillation and ectopic ventricular systoles in cats (Johnson *et al.*, 1958). In addition it sensitizes the hearts of both dogs and cats to epinephrine. Excretion of bromsulphalein by the liver is impaired and cloudy swelling and necrosis can be found in the liver after prolonged or repeated use.

In both dogs and cats induction is accomplished slowly ($1\frac{1}{2}$ to 5 minutes) with a brief period of excitement. Trichloroethylene anesthesia is unique in that as anesthesia deepens the respiratory rate and depth increase. Rapid deep respirations are a sign of deep anesthesia and indicate the concentration should be reduced. Trichloroethylene provides poor muscle relaxation in the dog, and overdosage easily occurs if the depth of anesthesia is increased to provide relaxation. To overcome this deficiency Hansson (1956) suggests the use of combined succinylcholine and trichloroethylene. In cats, muscular contractions of the legs sometimes are seen. Hyperactivity may occur in the cat during recovery, if the animal is disturbed. The recovery period is of approximately 30 minutes duration.

Trichloroethylene anesthesia has not met with approval in the dog because of the reasons mentioned above. In the cat its use has been more widespread, the advantages being easy induction which can be accomplished by one person, analgesia, lack of objectionable odor, and absence of fire and explosion hazards.

Disadvantages of tricholoroethylene anesthesia include cardiotoxicity and sensitization to epinephrine, hepatotoxicity, poor muscle relaxation, unsuitability for use in a closed system, and poor vaporization.

Anesthetic Gases

Nitrous Oxide, U.S.P. (N_2O)

Nitrous oxide is a colorless sweet-tasting nonirritating gas which is 1.53 times heavier than air. It is noninflammable though it will support combustion. The gas is produced by heating ammonium nitrate to about $250°$ C.

$$NH_4NO_3 \xrightarrow[\triangle]{} N_2O + 2H_2O$$

It is compressed into liquid at a pressure of about 30 atmospheres and marketed in cylinders at 650 to 800 psi. Nitrous oxide is administered with a semi-closed technique or a closed system with oxygen.

Nitrous oxide is exhaled unaltered from the lungs. It is an innocuous agent when used with adequate oxygen and has no ill effect on any organ of the body, dogs having been anesthetized as long as 72 hours without harm. It is considered the safest of the inhalant anesthetics. The only demonstrable change is a mild leukocytosis which persists less than 24 hours after administration has ceased. Nitrous oxide must be given in at least 80% concentration to produce anesthesia. Symptoms and lesions which have developed following anesthesia have been attributed to hypoxia and asphyxia.

Nitrous oxide because of its properties (nonexplosive, nonirritating, quickly absorbed and eliminated without effect on any organ of the body) is one of the best available gaseous agents if used with sufficient oxygen. In this respect it should be pointed out that the body must have at least 15% oxygen or progressive hypoxia develops. Its chief disadvantage is lack of potency.

Following Horace Wells' introduction of nitrous oxide as an anesthetic agent in exodontia, its use became widespread in America and Europe for both dental and surgical procedures. During its early use, oxygen was not administered concurrently, and it was generally believed that the patient in some way split off and utilized the oxygen of the nitrous oxide molecule. Hewitt, in 1886, found that nitrous oxide anesthesia could be maintained if oxygen was given in a concentration equal to that of air. He recommended a 7% oxygen mixture for rapid induction and dental anesthesia of less than 1 minute, little realizing that his recommendation would be adopted for operations lasting more than 1 hour.

As gas machines were developed, the standard recommendation for nitrous oxide was that it be administered in a mixture with 5 to 10% oxygen. Cyanosis and hypoxia were considered essential to nitrous oxide anesthesia. McKesson, in 1911, introduced the saturation technique in which 100% nitrous oxide gas was used for induction. It was continued almost to the point of complete anoxia and respiratory arrest, at which time oxygen was given under sufficient pressure to inflate the lungs. The anesthetist then administered a mixture of nitrous oxide-oxygen which was adequate for maintenance. In the event this did not provide muscular relaxation the administration of 100% nitrous oxide was repeated as before. In the light of present day knowledge this technique has been shown to be unnecessary and dangerous.

In man nitrous oxide is used in conjunction with intravenous anesthetic agents such as thiopental or thiamylal in so-called "balanced anesthesia". The concentration is generally from 50 to 70% nitrous oxide and 50 to 30% oxygen. This is of particular advantage when explosive agents must be avoided as with the use of electrocautery. Other combinations commonly used are thiopental-curare-nitrous oxide, halothane-nitrous oxide, and nitrous oxide-oxygen-ether (G-O-E). The latter receives its name from the sequence of administration, gas-oxygen-ether, and provides a pleasant induction with nitrous oxide followed by deep anesthesia and good muscle relaxation with ether.

Because few veterinarians possess the necessary equipment, and because nitrous oxide alone does not provide adequate anesthesia except for the most minor surgery, it is seldom used in veterinary medicine. Moreover, because of these limitations it is highly doubtful that its use will ever increase.

Cyclopropane, U.S.P. (Trimethylene; C_3H_6)

Cyclopropane was first prepared by the German chemist August von Freund in 1882. Its anesthetic property for animals was discovered by Lucas and Henderson of Toronto in 1929.

Cyclopropane is a colorless nonirritating gas with a sweet odor and taste. It is heavier than air and its mixtures with air or oxygen are inflammable and explosive. Cyclopropane is the most expensive of the common anesthetic gases and is marketed as a liquid under pressure in steel cylinders. It is the most potent of all anesthetic gases in clinical use and is administered only in a closed system.

Induction is quickly accomplished using 20 to 25% cyclopropane mixed with oxygen. The induction period is usually only 2 to 3 minutes in duration. Light anesthesia may be maintained by a 10 to 15% mixture; concentrations above 25% may produce respiratory arrest. Following induction the cyclopropane is shut off and the patient rebreathes the existing mixture.

The depth of anesthesia is best determined by the respiratory movements which are progressively depressed. In respiratory arrest the heart will continue to beat for a short time, allowing artificial respiration to be instituted. If anesthesia lightens, more cyclopropane is added to the mixture as needed. Very small amounts are used during the average anesthesia, 1 gallon per hour being the maximum in most instances. Open or semi-closed systems are too costly of anesthetic gas and are hazardous from the explosion standpoint.

Cyclopropane is not irritating to the mucous membranes, therefore induction is easy. The respiratory center is directly depressed and respiration is not reflexly stimulated as with ether. For this reason preanesthetic morphine is contraindicated. Under cyclopropane anesthesia the heart rate is depressed. Cardiac arrythmias are common; vagal escape, A-V block, and ventricular tachycardia may all occur, particularly when anesthesia is deep. The heart of the dog is reflexly sensitized to epinephrine and ventricular fibrillation frequently follows its administration. Cyclopropane causes hypertension during anesthesia, followed in some instances by hypotension when anesthesia has been prolonged. Methoxamine has been shown to be a safe vasopressor agent for use during cyclopropane anesthesia (Stutzman et al., 1949).

Cyclopropane does not significantly affect either the liver or the kidneys. Changes in body functions include depression of metabolism and elevation of the blood sugar level. These are slight, however, and promptly return to normal following anesthesia.

There are no histological changes in any organ, including the heart, which are characteristic of cyclopropane.

Advantages of cyclopropane are rapid induction with lack of irritation, rapid recovery, and wide margin of safety. The chief disadvantages are lack of profound abdominal relaxation, sensitization of the heart to adrenalin and most other sympathomimetic amines, the expense of the gas and special equipment, and the explosion hazard.

Cyclopropane has been used for small animal anesthesia in both the United States and Great Britain. The necessity for closed system equipment and the hazard of explosion have limited its application.

Ethylene, U.S.P. ($CH_2 = CH_2$)

Ethylene was introduced in 1923 as an anesthetic for animals and man by Luckhardt and Carter of Chicago. It is a colorless nonirritating gas with an ethereal odor and taste. It is marketed in liquified form under pressure in steel cylinders.

Ethylene alone is noninflammable, but when mixed with air or oxygen it is highly inflammable and explosive. This is its chief drawback. Because ethylene is slightly lighter than air it will hang in the operating room in an inflammable layer several feet above the floor. Ethylene mixed with nitrous oxide forms a violently explosive mixture, and the two should never be used simultaneously. Administration is accomplished by means of apparatus equipped with a flowmeter and either semi-closed or closed inhalers. Because of the fire and explosion hazard, closed methods are advised.

Induction is usually accomplished with a 90% ethylene-10% oxygen mixture; maintenance is with an 85–15 mixture which in long operations can be gradually reduced to 80–20.

Ethylene approaches the ideal anesthetic gas in that it has little effect upon respiration, circulation, or other systems or organs of the body. It is one of the safest of all general anesthetics for the patient, since it is practically impossible to kill with an overdose. The chief disadvantages are that it produces incomplete muscular relaxation, must be used in concentrations which produce hypoxia, and is highly inflammable and explosive. Ethylene is used in the more moribund human patients because of its great safety.

Ethylene, like nitrous oxide, will probably never be used to any extent in animals because of equipment limitations and explosion hazards.

Physical Properties of Medical Gases

Pressure in cylinders containing liquified compressed gas and vapor in equilibrium is determined by the vapor pressure of the liquid at the existing temperature, and has no relation to the amount of liquid remaining in the cylinder. At a constant temperature, pressure in a cylinder filled with liquified compressed gas will remain approximately constant until all the liquid has been exhausted, at which time the pressure drops as the remaining gas is withdrawn. Pressure in a cylinder containing liquified compressed gas, therefore,

Fig. 8–3. Net Contents of Cylinders for all Gases*

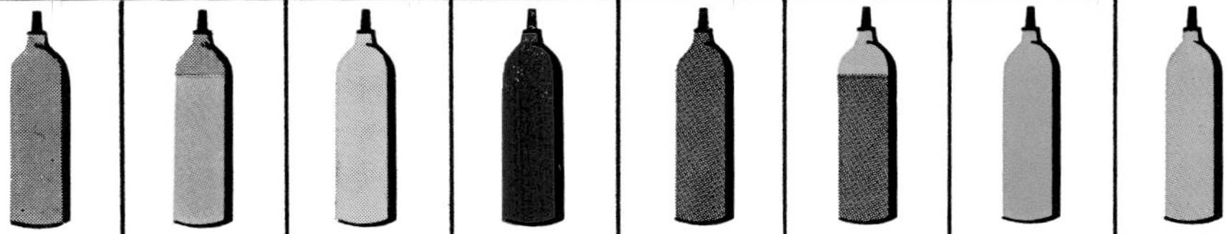

Size	CO_2	CO_2-O_2	$(CH_2)_3$	C_2H_4	He	He-O_2	N_2O	O_2	Cylinder Dimensions	Weight of Empty Cylinder (lbs.)
G	3200 gals.	1400 gals.		2800 gals.	1100 gals.	1126 gals.	3655 gals.	1400 gals.	$8\frac{1}{2} \times 55''$	100
M		800 gals.		1600 gals.			2000 gals.	800 gals.	$7 \times 47''$	66
E		165 gals.		330 gals.			420 gals.	165 gals.	$4\frac{1}{4} \times 29\frac{3}{4}''$	15
D	250 gals.	95 gals.	230 gals.	200 gals.	80 gals.	82 gals.	250 gals.	95 gals.	$4\frac{1}{4} \times 20\frac{1}{4}''$	$10\frac{1}{4}$
B		40 gals.		100 gals.			100 gals.	40 gals.	$3\frac{1}{4} \times 16\frac{1}{2}''$	$5\frac{3}{4}$
A	50 gals.	20 gals.		40 gals.	15 gals.	15 gals.	50 gals.	20 gals.	$3 \times 10\frac{3}{4}''$	$2\frac{1}{2}$
†DD			230 gals.						$3\frac{3}{4} \times 23\frac{1}{4}''$	$8\frac{3}{4}$
†BB			100 gals.						$2\frac{3}{4} \times 19\frac{3}{4}''$	4
†AA			40 gals.						$2\frac{3}{4} \times 11''$	3

Cylinder Color Code

* Courtesy of Ohio Chemical & Surgical Equipment Co.
† Cyclopropane cylinders may be chrome plated and bear orange labels.

is not an indication of the amount of remaining gas. This can be determined only by weighing the cylinder.

The pressure in cylinders charged with non-liquified compressed gas is related to the temperature and the amount of gas remaining in the cylinder. With the temperature constant, if the pressure is reduced by one-half the cylinder will be approximately one-half full.

Gases which are liquified when compressed in cylinders are nitrous oxide, cyclopropane, and carbon dioxide. Gases which are non-liquified include oxygen, helium, carbon dioxide-oxygen mixtures, helium-oxygen mixtures, and ethylene.

Cylinder sizes and approximate contents for the various gases are shown in Figure 8–3.

Regulations Concerning Medical Gases

Interstate shipment of compressed gases is regulated by the United States Government under the provisions of an Act of Congress dated March 4, 1921. This Act states that cylinders containing medical gases which are shipped in commerce are subject to the jurisdiction of the Interstate Commerce Commission and must comply with ICC specifications.* In addition medical gases are also regulated by the Federal Food, Drug and Cosmetic Act. This Act states that medical gases must conform to the standards of the *Pharmacopeia of the United States* and must be appropriately labeled.

A cylinder color code entitled *Simplified Practice Recommendation R176-41 of the Bureau of Standards* has been published by the U. S. Department of Commerce. The code stipulates a cylinder color for each gas to enable quick recognition of cylinder content.

Kind of Gas	*Cylinder Color*
Oxygen	Green
Carbon Dioxide	Gray
Nitrous Oxide	Light Blue
Cyclopropane	Orange
Helium	Brown
Ethylene	Red
Carbon Dioxide and Oxygen	Gray and Green
Helium and Oxygen	Brown and Green

It should be remembered, however, that the above color code is to be used only as a guide. The primary identification of the cylinder content is always the label.

* The ICC cylinder specifications and regulations have been reprinted by the Bureau of Explosives of the Association of American Railroads as "Interstate Commerce Commission Regulations for Transportation of Explosives and Other Dangerous Articles by Land and Water in Rail Freight Service and by Motor Vehicle (Highway) and Water Including Specifications for Shipping Containers". This pamphlet is available from the Bureau of Explosives, 30 Vesey Street, New York 7, New York.

References

BLALOCK, A.: The Effects of Ether, Chloroform, and Ethyl Chloride Anaesthetics on the Minute Cardiac Output and Blood Pressure. Surg., Gynec. & Obst., *46*, 72, 1928.

BUTLER, T. C.: Metabolic Transformations of Trichloroethylene. J. Pharm. & Exper. Therap., *97*, 84, 1949.

DAWSON, B., THEYE, R. A., and KIRKLIN, J. W.: Halothane in Open Cardiac Operations. Anesthesia & Analgesia, *39*, 59, 1960.

DRAPER, W. B. and WHITEHEAD, R. W.: Chances of Resuscitation after an Overdose of Ether, Divinyl Ether and Chloroform. Lancet, *1*, 442, 1942.

HALL, K. D. and NORRIS, F. H., JR.: Fluothane Sensitization of Dog Heart to Action of Epinephrine. Anesthesiology, *19*, 631, 1958.

HANSSON, C. H.: Succinylcholine Iodide as a Muscular Relaxant in Veterinary Surgery, J.A.V.M.A., *128*, 287, 1956.

JOHNSON, V. L., KLAVANO, P. A., WRIGHT, R., and SAX, D.: Some Effects of Trichlorethylene on the Electrocardiogram of the Cat. Vet. Med., *53*, 375, 1958.

JONES, W. M., MARGOLIS, G., and STEPHEN, C. R.: Hepatotoxicity of Inhalation Anesthetic Drugs. Anesthesiology, *19*, 715, 1958.

LUMB, W. V.: Closed-Circuit Halothane Anesthesia in the Dog. J.A.V.M.A., *134*, 218, 1959.

MACNIDER, W. DEB.: A Study of the Anurias Occurring in Normal Animals During the Use of the General Anesthetics. J. Pharm. & Exper. Therap., *15*, 249, 1920.

MACNIDER, W. DEB.: A Preliminary Paper on the Relation Between the Amount of Stainable Lipoid Material in the Renal Epithelium and the Susceptibility of the Kidney to the Toxic Effect of the General Anesthetics. J. Pharm. & Exper. Therap., *17*, 289, 1921.

MACNIDER, W. DEB: Naturally Nephropathic Animals: The Ability of an Alkaline Solution to Influence the Amount of Stainable Lipoid Material that Appears in the Kidney Following the Use of a General Anesthetic. J. Pharm. & Exper. Therap., *20*, 365, 1922.

MÖRCH, E. T., AYCRIGG, J. B., and BERGER, M. S.: The Anesthetic Effects of Ethyl Vinyl Ether, Divinyl Ether, and Diethyl Ether on Mice. J. Pharm. & Exper. Therap., *117*, 184, 1956.

MORRIS, L. E., NOLTENSMEYER, M. H., and WHITE, J. M., JR.: Epinephrine Induced Cardiac Irregularities in the Dog During Anesthesia with Trichloroethylene, Cyclopropane, Ethyl Chloride and Chloroform. Anesthesiology, *14*, 153, 1953.

STEPHEN, C. R., MARGOLIS, G., FABIAN, L. W., and BOURGEOIS-GAVARDIN, M.: Laboratory Observations with Fluothane. Anesthesiology, *19*, 770, 1958.

STUTZMAN, J. W., PETTINGA, F. L., and FRUGGIERO, E. J.: Cardiac Effects of Methoxamine (Beta-(2, 5-Dimethoxyphenyl)-Beta-Hydroxyisopropyl Amine HCl) and Desoxyephedrine During Cyclopropane Anesthesia. J. Pharm. & Exper. Therap., *97*, 385, 1949.

EQUIPMENT AND METHODS FOR ADMINISTRATION OF INHALATION ANESTHETICS

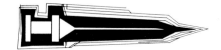

Chapter 9

In recent years many types of equipment have become available for administration of inhalation anesthetics. All have advantages and disadvantages; some have glaring faults. Equipment described in this chapter is representative of that in common use today.

Masks

One of the earliest methods of anesthetic administration was by means of a mask (also termed cone in veterinary medicine). A volatile liquid anesthetic is dripped onto gauze or other porous substance incorporated into the wall of the mask, and respiratory gases passing through the gauze hasten volatilization. A high concentration of anesthetic is thus confined under the mask for the patient to inhale. The usefulness of this equipment is attested by the fact that it is still widely employed today.

The simplest mask consists of an ordinary hand towel folded to fit the patient's face (Fig. 9–1).

Another inexpensive method for making a mask is to remove both ends from a tin can. This is then wrapped with gauze, by repeatedly running the gauze through the center hole and around the outside, until the can is covered (Fig. 9–2). A piece of cotton is placed in one end and the anesthetic is dripped on it.

A variety of masks are available commercially. Most are made of metal, plastic, or leather, clear plastic having the advantage that the patient's face is visible to the anesthetist. If anesthetics are to be administered by the open or semi-open drop methods, one end is covered with gauze or cotton onto which the anesthetic is dripped,

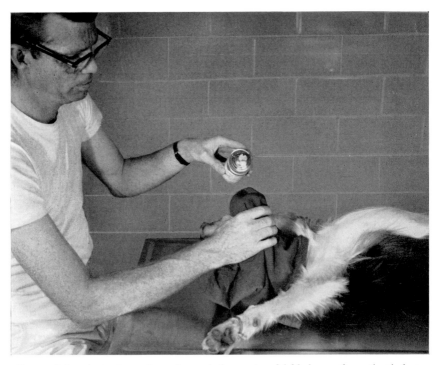

FIGURE 9–1.   A simple mask can be made from a towel folded over the patient's face.

while the opposite end is applied over the patient's muzzle. With the semi-open drop method the connection between mask and patient is made air-tight by means of a rubber gasket or towel.

A dripper is helpful in maintaining a steady even flow of anesthetic onto the mask. The simplest is probably made by notching a cork (usually provided with ether cans) on opposite sides before inserting it and a piece of gauze in the anesthetic container (Fig. 9–3).

Administration of Ether or Other Volatile Agent with a Mask

In anesthetizing animals with a mask, preanesthetic narcotic administration or tranquilization is of great benefit to prevent struggling and enable a smooth induction. Atropine should always be administered to prevent excessive salivation and vagus arrest of the heart. Ophthalmic ointment (any kind is effective) should be instilled in the conjunctival sacs to protect the eyes from high concentrations of anesthetic vapor. The animal should be restrained by means of ropes or held tightly by an assistant. Induc-

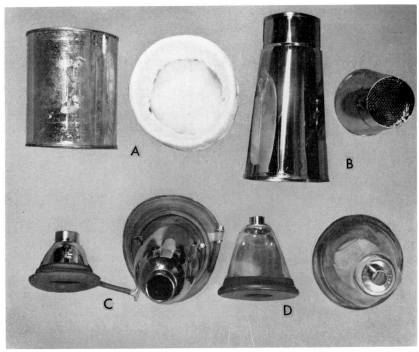

FIGURE 9–2. Four types of masks are shown left to right. (*A*) A mask made by wrapping gauze around a tin can. Cotton fills the lumen at one end. (*B*) Stainless steel masks with a screen across the lumen on which gauze or cotton is placed. (*C*) Foregger masks with inflatable face cushion for use with a gas machine. (*D*) Transparent plastic masks with rubber face gasket for use with the AVR unit.

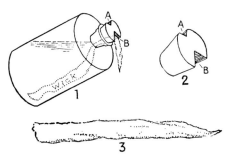

FIGURE 9–3. Equipment for open drop administration. (1) Container of anesthetic liquid; (2) cork with small notch (*A*) and large notch (*B*); (3) wick, strip of gauze, cotton, or piece of pipe cleaner long enough to reach to bottom of container. (From American Medical Association: *Fundamentals of Anesthesia*. 3rd ed. W. B. Saunders Co., 1954.)

tion is started by holding the patient's head and the mask firmly in one hand, and dripping anesthetic on the mask with the other.

The tendency is to push the anesthetic to the patient rapidly in order to pass quickly through the stage of reflex activity. This often results in dangerously high concentrations of anesthetic. In addition, hypoxia and high carbon dioxide levels are produced in the patient. Anesthesia induced by the semi-open drop method is usually a combination of anesthesia and asphyxia. To overcome hypoxia, various methods of introducing air or oxygen under the mask have been devised and will be described later in this chapter.

Once the patient passes through Stage II, the drip is slowed. Anesthesia is maintained by administration at a slow rate, the mask remaining on the patient during the maintenance period. If anesthesia becomes too deep, the mask should be completely removed.

Administration of Ethyl Chloride to Cats

Ethyl chloride administered by the open drop method has been used as the sole anesthetic agent for short operations in cats. Administration can be accomplished by removing the bottom from a paper cup and inserting a plug of cotton in its place. Ethyl chloride is sprayed on the cotton and the cup is held in front of the cat's nose. Because ethyl chloride vapors are non-irritating, little restraint is required, the cat frequently being unaware that it is breathing vapor.

Relaxation usually occurs within 2 minutes following initial administration. At this point the cup can be applied closely over the muzzle to produce the desired depth of anesthesia. Once the surgical procedure is completed and the cup removed, recovery is very rapid, the animal usually being ambulatory in 5 minutes.

Boxes or Chambers for Anesthetization of Small Animals

A wide variety of boxes and chambers for administration of volatile liquid anesthetic agents have been used. They vary from the simple bell jar, under which a cotton pledget soaked with anesthetic is inserted along with the patient, to elaborate chambers which provide constant circulation of gases and carbon dioxide absorption. The advantages of a chamber are:

1. It requires no restraint, therefore, anesthesia can be induced without an assistant.
2. It presents a professional appearance to the owner.
3. Anesthetic emergencies are almost completely eliminated.
4. The danger of explosion is remote.

Hardenbergh and Mann (1927) used an "etherizing cabinet" and asserted that dogs and cats pass into a state of anesthesia with a minimal amount of struggling and without relaxation of the bladder or anal sphincters. Initial administration of ether, which is ordinarily the most dangerous part of the procedure, is safely accomplished since animals rarely become over-anesthetized in a cabinet. The usual struggle during induction, with its attendant noise and unpleasantness, is eliminated.

Most boxes or chambers are made of glass or transparent plastic. This allows visualization of the patient during induction and maintenance of anesthesia. Stiles (1959) has described an ether box made from an aquarium (Fig. 9–4). An elaborate chamber for anesthetizing animals from the size of mice to that of cats has been described by Zauder and Orkin (1959) (Fig. 9–5). This chamber, which was designed principally for experimental testing of anesthetic agents, provides for constant circulation of gases and carbon dioxide absorption. In addition it is air-tight, has ports for sample removal, and is vented to the outside by means of rubber tubing.

Boxes and chambers have their greatest application in anesthesia of cats, laboratory animals, and various species of wild animals, such as skunks. Their chief disadvantage lies in the fact that maintenance of anesthesia must be achieved by some other means, since it is impossible to perform manipulative procedures within the box while anesthetic is being administered. In addition more ether may be required than with a mask and induction may take slightly longer.

Insufflation

An insufflation system delivers anesthetic gas into the pharynx or trachea for the patient to inhale, while exhalation occurs *around* the delivery device. The classical example is that described by Hardenbergh and Mann (1927) in which ether vapor is delivered to the patient via endotracheal catheter (Fig. 9–6).

This device, which can be simply made, consists of a 1-pound ether can into the top of which two small metal tubes are soldered. One tube is connected to a perforated sleeve which, when open, allows entrance of room air. This is, in turn, connected to an endotracheal catheter. The other tube in the top of the can is unobstructed allowing room air to enter. As the patient inhales, air is drawn into the can, picks up ether vapor and passes through the endotracheal catheter to the patient. The concentration of ether can be altered by adjusting the opening in the perforated sleeve. A small piece of paper pasted over the open tube in the top of the can flutters to indicate respiration.

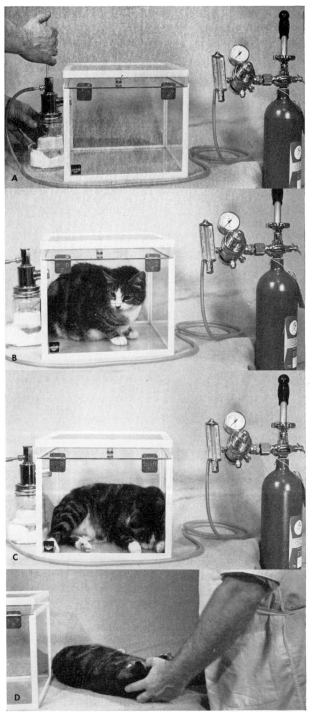

Figure 9–4. *(Legend on opposite page)*

In operation, the animal is anesthetized either in a chamber or by intravenous injection of a thiobarbiturate. The ether can is filled to not over two-thirds of its capacity, the endotracheal catheter is inserted, connected to the can, and the valve adjusted. Once regulated, anesthesia can be maintained for hours with little attention.

The Trimar Inhaler

The Trimar inhaler is designed to administer trichloroethylene (Trimar) or ether anesthesia to cats (Fig. 9–7). To operate the inhaler the following procedure is used:

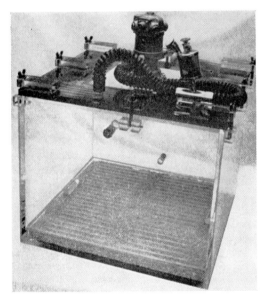

FIGURE 9–5. An elaborate anesthetic chamber which provides for constant circulation of gases and carbon dioxide absorption. (From Zauder, H. L., and Orkin, L. R.: Chamber for Anesthetization of Small Animals. Anesthesiology, *20*, 708, 1959.)

FIGURE 9–4. Induction of anesthesia with an ether box. (*A*) The equipment consists of a plastic box, nebulizer, and oxygen cylinder with reduction valve and flowmeter. Inside the pint jar below the nebulizer is a 3-oz. bottle containing 20 cc. of ether, with a plastic suction tube extending from the bottom of the nebulizer into the bottle containing the ether.

B. Cat is placed in the box and the lid closed. They seldom offer resistance, usually remaining quiet in a crouching position. Oxygen is allowed to flow for approximately 2 minutes at a rate of 3 to 4 liters per minute, or until the ether is gone from the bottle. Salivation may occur but is seldom excessive.

C. Induction of anesthesia is complete approximately 9 minutes after the start of oxygen flow.

D. The cat is removed from the box and anesthesia is continued with an ether cone.

(From Stiles, S. W.: Induction of Ether Anesthesia in Cats. J.A.V.M.A., *134*, 275, 1959.)

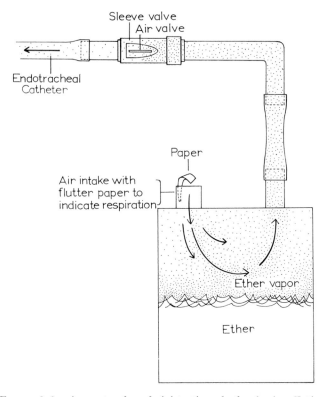

FIGURE 9–6.   Apparatus for administration of ether by insufflation.

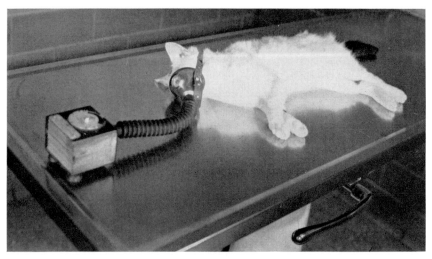

FIGURE 9–7.   The Trimar inhaler. Anesthetic is poured through the perforated screen.

1. The inhaler is assembled, being sure that the mask valves are functioning.
2. Approximately 1 ounce of trichloroethylene is poured through the perforated screen on the end of the vaporizer. The air mixer valve is set to "full" concentration.
3. The animal is restrained. If working alone, this can be accomplished by taping the forelimbs and hindlimbs to each other with adhesive tape.

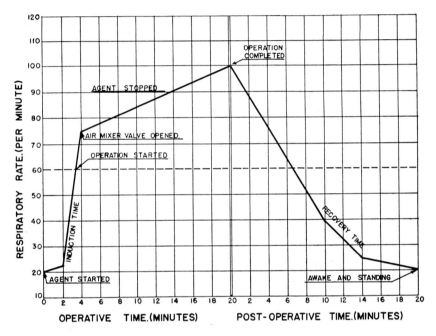

FIGURE 9–8. Respiratory rate, induction and recovery time of a cat with trichlorothylene anesthesia. The cat was spayed and declawed. (From Candlin, P. T.: Trimar Anesthesia for Cats. J.A.V.M.A., *132*, 105, 1958.)

4. The mask is placed in position over the patient's face.
5. Induction usually requires 1 to 3 minutes. After the cat is anesthetized, the retainer strap is fixed behind the ears to hold the mask in position.
6. The stage of anesthesia is determined by the rate and depth of respirations; other signs are not reliable. Increased rate and depth indicate deepening anesthesia (this is true *only* with trichloroethylene).
7. Following induction, the air mixer valve is opened (usually to 1, 2, or 3). Further adjustment may be necessary to maintain the desired level of anesthesia.

10

8. Recovery from trichloroethylene usually occurs within 30 minutes (Fig. 9–8). Cats may salivate and make chewing movements during and after recovery.
9. Following use, the mask, tubing, and vaporizer are disassembled, the mask rinsed in water, and the component parts left disassembled until used again.

Several precautions should be observed with trichloroethylene anesthesia. (1) High concentrations should be avoided, since these predispose to vagal arrest of the heart. (2) Epinephrine and norepinephrine are contraindicated. (3) Trichloroethylene should be stored in a cool place and protected from light, since toxic decomposition products may result. (4) Trichloroethylene should not be used with soda lime, since toxic products will develop.

Ethaire Unit

The Ethaire unit is a combination of the Ambu resuscitator with a bubble-type ether vaporizer (Fig. 9–9). The unit is so constructed that anesthetic mixed with air can be delivered by auto-inhalation to the patient by means of a face mask or endotracheal catheter. Brooks et al. (1962) have reported the use of ether, halothane, and chloroform in the unit, although they indicate a preference for the former.

Under normal circumstances the patient activates the unit by his own respiratory efforts. As the patient inhales, air enters the system through a port in the self-inflating bag, bubbles through the vaporizer, and passes into the patient via the non-rebreathing valve. On exhalation the gases are vented through the non-rebreathing valve into the room. An adjustable control allows all or part of the gas to bypass the vaporizer.

A simple respiratory monitor emits an audible whistle as the patient exhales. In the event breathing ceases the surgeon or anesthetist is thus alerted to the emergency. If this occurs, the rebreathing bag can be rhythmically compressed to ventilate the patient until spontaneous breathing resumes. If oxygen is needed, a hose from the reducing valve on an oxygen tank can be attached directly to the adapter of the self-inflating bag.

Induction is usually accomplished with a thiobarbiturate, such as thiamylal, following which the animal is intubated and attached to the unit.

The unit has the advantage of being lightweight and very portable. Because air is used rather than oxygen, the cost of anesthesia is reduced over apparatus utilizing oxygen. Use of air with ether reduces the explosion hazard. On the other hand, hypoxia with its resultant dangers may occur more easily.

The plastic non-rebreathing valve is rather delicate and will dissolve with some anesthetic agents (methoxyflurane is an example); therefore, care must be taken to prevent any liquid from flowing into the valve from the vaporizer.

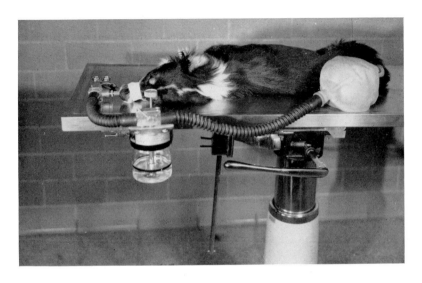

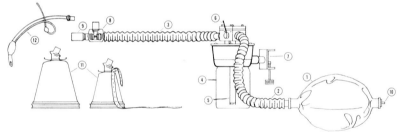

FIGURE 9–9.   The Ethaire unit in use (top) and component parts (bottom).
(1) Self-inflating bag. (2,3) Conductive (anti-static) corrugated tubing. (4) Anesthetic jar. (5) Anesthetic vaporizer assembly. (6) Selector switch for variable anesthetic mixture control. (7) Connecting clamp on swivel. (8) Non-rebreathing valve. (9) Small animal respiratory monitor (audible). (10) Oxygen input adaptor. (11) Animal face masks. (12) Endotracheal catheter with connector.

Halsan Apparatus

A semi-closed apparatus for administration of halothane has been described by Singleton (1961). This unit consists of an oxygen regulator with flowmeter, F.N.S. vaporizer, breathing bag, and a Lewis-Leigh non-rebreathing valve connected to an endotracheal catheter (Fig. 9–10). In operation the vaporizer is set at 2.8 to 3.2% for approximately 3 minutes and then reduced to a maintenance

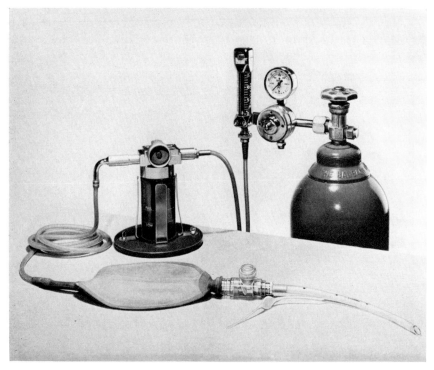

FIGURE 9–10.   A semi-closed system for administration of halothane. Exhaled gas is vented through the non-rebreathing valve (Courtesy of Fort Dodge Laboratories, Fort Dodge, Iowa).

level of 0.8 to 1.2%. Oxygen flow is adjusted to maintain a stable tension in the breathing bag. Because halothane is vented from the system and not reused, this is not economical in operation.

The AVR Unit

A combined anesthetizer-vaporizer-resuscitator (AVR) unit has been developed which, as the name implies, not only is a mechanical resuscitator but also, by incorporation of a vaporizer, is capable of administering volatile liquid anesthetic agents (Fig. 9–11).   Ether

FIGURE 9–11.   AVR units with ether vaporizer (A) and halothane vaporizer (B). A hose connects the oxygen tank with the resuscitator mechanism. Oxygen flows from the resuscitator unit through the vaporizer to the inhaler body which is connected to an endotracheal catheter in the patient. A schematic drawing (C) illustrates oxygen flow through a unit when oxygen-ether positive-negative ventilation is used. (1) Oxygen control valve. (2) Adjustable positive pressure valve. (3) Vaporizer control valve. (4) Exhalation valve. (5) Continuous inflation valve.

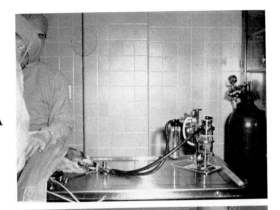

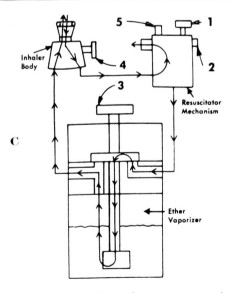

FIGURE 9–11.   *(Legend on opposite page)*

has been the agent recommended for use with this equipment. A special vaporizer is required for halothane.

Basically, the unit consists of a Handy resuscitator connected to a vaporizer from which tubing leads to a piston-toggle-diaphragm. The latter is connected to an endotracheal catheter or mask. The AVR unit is adjusted to function on 50 psi of oxygen and this pressure energizes the system.

Three methods of ventilating the patient may be employed depending upon the desires of the anesthetist. They are:

1. Automatic ventilation
2. Insufflation (spontaneous inhalation by the patient)
3. Continuous inflation

1. *Automatic Ventilation.* With automatic ventilation the re-suscitation cycle has two phases. During the *inhalation phase* oxygen flows to the patient until intrapulmonary pressure reaches 13 mm. Hg. When this pressure is reached the piston-toggle-diaphragm moves to the exhalation position and a negative or *expiratory phase* commences. Oxygen flow is diverted to a venturi which withdraws used gases from the lungs and discharges them into the room. The expiratory phase continues until a negative pressure of 9 mm. Hg is reached, at which point the piston-toggle-diaphragm shifts to the inhalation phase and the flow of oxygen into the animal's lungs is resumed. This alternating sequence of positive and negative pressure produces the inhalation and ex-halation phases of breathing for a non-breathing patient.

When operating effectively the unit produces a rhythmic clicking sound with each respiratory cycle. A rapid clicking is indicative of ineffective ventilation due to:

a. Obstruction of airway by mucus or improper position of animal.
b. Obstruction in mask.
c. Pulmonary collapse (atelectasis).

Absence of clicking indicates mechanical difficulty due to lack of oxygen pressure somewhere within the unit.

Irregular clicking occurs when the animal breathes spontaneously at a rate different than that of the respirator. This is an indication to change the setting of the unit to the insufflation position.

Two safety release valves are incorporated, the positive pressure safety releases at 19.5 mm. Hg and the negative pressure safety releases at 13 mm. Hg negative pressure. Excessive positive or negative intrapulmonary pressures are thus avoided.

2. *Insufflation.* If desired, the unit can be used to supply oxygen to the patient through his own respiratory efforts. This setting conserves oxygen and can be used except when the chest is open or the animal is not breathing spontaneously.

3. *Continuous Inflation.* On completion of open chest surgery it is sometimes desirable to inflate the lungs continuously for a short period of time during final chest closure. This inflates collapsed lobes and prevents pneumothorax. To accomplish this, the unit is set at continuous inflation while the last sutures are tied.

The foregoing paragraphs apply to use of the AVR unit as a resuscitator; it also has the capability to induce and maintain ether anesthesia. If the unit is used for induction, a mask is attached to the inhaler body. Preanesthetic morphine-atropine is administered to reduce struggling and inhibit secretion, and the animal is restrained by fastening his limbs to the table. The valve on the oxygen cylinder is opened and the unit is set to run on oxygen-ether automatic ventilation. The mask is then applied to the patient and held in position. The unit control valve is adjusted to the "medium" or "fast" range and the control valve on the vaporizer to the "on" position, causing oxygen to bubble through the ether. Once induction is complete, maintenance can be continued by using the mask or an endotracheal catheter can be inserted and connected to the unit. If induction is accomplished with a thiobarbiturate, an endotracheal catheter is inserted and attached to the inhaler body.

For maintenance of anesthesia, the vaporizer is turned to a lower setting. This may need to be adjusted from time to time. The unit is designed to administer ether continuously during the maintenance period and should not be used intermittently if a constant plane of anesthesia is desired.

When anesthesia is to be terminated, the vaporizer control valve is turned off and oxygen flow is continued to eliminate ether vapor from the patient. If the unit is turned to "resuscitation", ether vapor will be eliminated more quickly. As soon as the animal shows evidence of consciousness, oxygen administration can be stopped.

In the event anesthesia becomes too deep, the vaporizer control valve is turned off and the unit is turned to "resuscitation". The respirations produced quickly eliminate excessive ether from the patient, and the depth of anesthesia is lightened.

By adjusting the positive pressure valve various degrees of lung inflation can be produced and, when desirable, inflation can be reduced to improve access to and vision of the surgical site.

Standard oxygen cylinders used to operate the AVR unit will be effective for the following periods of time

Cylinder	Operating Period
D	24 to 36 minutes
E	60 to 95 minutes
H	8 to 10 hours

Advantages of the AVR unit are:

1. It is versatile. It can be used for oxygen insufflation, for positive pressure ventilation of the lungs, and for administration of ether anesthesia (or halothane with a special vaporizer).
2. It is almost completely automatic and can be operated by the surgeon, if necessary.
3. When used as a respirator, the negative intrapulmonary pressure facilitates carbon dioxide removal and prevents hypercarbia in the patient when undergoing prolonged anesthetic periods.

Some disadvantages of the AVR unit are:

1. It uses relatively large quantities of oxygen and ether or halothane.
2. The ether-oxygen mixture is expelled into the room and thus presents an explosion hazard.
3. When used as a respirator it may, under certain conditions, be difficult to tell when the patient is dead, since the unit automatically continues respiring the animal regardless of its status.

The Closed System of Administration

The apparatus described so far have all been of the open or semi-closed type, so-called because all gases exhaled by the patient have been vented into the surrounding room air. Another type is called the *closed system* because gases, instead of being vented, are recirculated to the patient. This method, which allows no escape of anesthetic mixtures, is known as the *rebreathing technique*. Oxygen is administered at a rate just sufficient to meet the metabolic requirements of the patient, and carbon dioxide produced by the patient is absorbed by soda lime. Anesthetic gases are added to the oxygen in measured amounts to produce and maintain anesthesia. Some advantages of the closed system are:

1. There is better control of the anesthetic agent.
2. It provides a warm moist vapor for the patient to breathe.
3. Anesthetic agents are reused; therefore, it is more economical than open systems.
4. There is less danger of explosion because inflammable gases are not vented in great quantities into the surrounding room.

Gas Machines

Devices for administration of anesthetic gases by the rebreathing technique are termed *gas machines*. Most will also administer vapors of volatile liquid anesthetic agents, thus greatly increasing their capabilities. Gas machines are usually operated as a closed system; however, they may be used as a semi-closed system, an

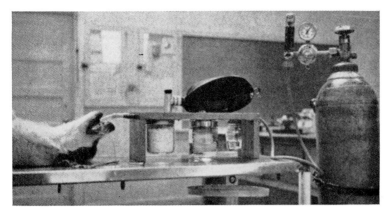

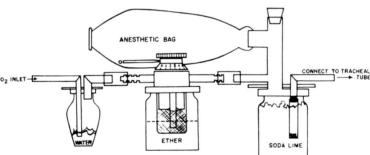

FIGURE 9–12. A simple gas machine. (Booth, N. H., Rankin, A. D., and Will, D. H.: Simplified Apparatus and Method for Administering Oxygen and Ether to the Dog. J.A.V.M.A., *137*, 114, 1960.)

expiratory valve allowing escape of a portion of the anesthetic mixture.

Gas machines vary considerably in cost and capabilities. In general, expensive models are more accurate in metering anesthetics and give better control of anesthesia. They also enable a wider choice of anesthetic agents.

Booth *et al.* (1960) have described a very simple gas machine which can be constructed inexpensively (Fig. 9–12). More refined devices produced specifically for small animal anesthesia are shown in Figures 9–13 and 9–14.   The most elaborate machines, made for use on man and equipped with connections for several anesthetic gases, are generally too expensive for veterinary use (Fig. 9–15). However, when these are employed they give excellent service.

While many gas machines are rather formidable in appearance, they all possess most of the following basic components:

1. An oxygen tank.
2. Tanks of anesthetic gases, for example, nitrous oxide.
3. Reduction valves for the tanks.
4. Flowmeters to indicate flow rate of gases.

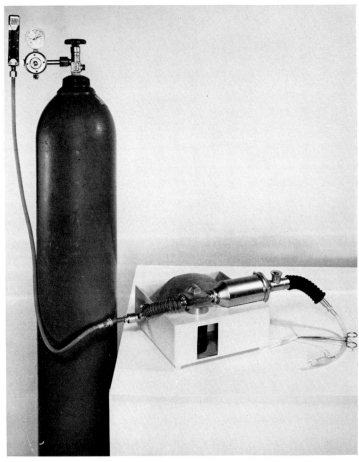

FIGURE 9–13. The PVS fluothane anesthesia apparatus consists of a source of oxygen and a FN Shalothane vaporizer, which is in turn connected to a to-and-fro system composed of a rebreathing bag, soda lime canister, and endotracheal catheter. It can be used either as a semi-closed system or as a closed system with carbon dioxide absorption. (Courtesy of Professional Veterinary Services, Inc., Hialeah, Florida.)

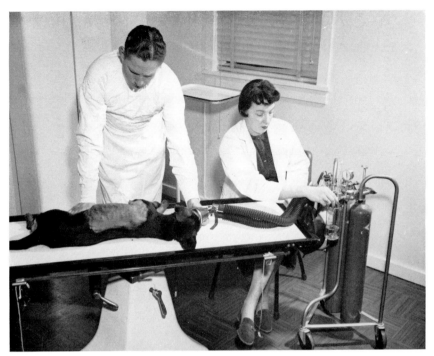

FIGURE 9–14. The Ohio ether-oxygen machine, model 950, designed specifically for small animal anesthesia. (Courtesy of Ohio Chemical and Surgical Equipment Company.)

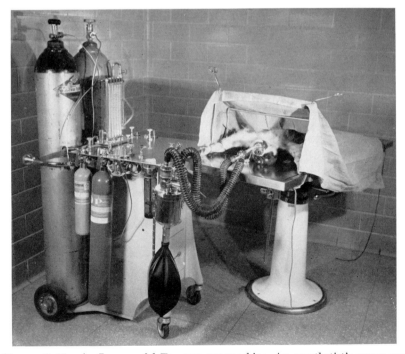

FIGURE 9–15. An Iowa model Foregger gas machine. An anesthetist's screen supports the drape over the dog's head.

5. A vaporizer to volatilize liquid anesthetics such as ether.
6. A canister containing soda lime.
7. A rebreathing bag.
8. An endotracheal catheter (or mask) connecting the system with the patient.
9. An expiratory or "pop-off" valve.

Some of these components are described in the following paragraphs.

Flowmeters

Flowmeters indicate the rate at which anesthetic gases and oxygen flow to the patient. Those commonly used are either (1) the fixed orifice flowmeter, or (2) the variable orifice flowmeter.

With the first type, gas under pressure is forced through a standard orifice. This causes a pressure differential on either side of the orifice. If a manometer is placed so that one limb is upstream to the orifice and the other limb downstream, the pressure drop across the orifice can be measured on the manometer. The so-called "wet flowmeter" which has been standard equipment on Foregger apparatus is an example of this type (Fig. 9–16F). Depression of water in the upstream limb of the manometer is calibrated as flow rate on the manometer tube. This type of flowmeter is highly efficient provided the orifice is kept clean and the water level remains constant.

Variable orifice flowmeters are of several types, but the basic principle in their operation is the same. The differential between upstream and downstream pressures remains constant, while the diameter of the orifice varies. The rate of flow is directly proportional to the size of the orifice, the larger the size, the greater the flow and *vice versa*.

The variable orifice flowmeter, sometimes called the Thorpe tube, consists of a tapered glass tube containing a ball, bobbin, rotor, or other type of float. The inside diameter of the tube enlarges from the bottom upward, so that when gas enters at the bottom the rotor is elevated to the point where gas escapes around the rotor. The rotor then floats free in the tube suspended by the flow of gas. If gas flow is increased, the float rises within the tube. The tube is calibrated and the float height indicates flow rate.

As gas flows through the tube and passes the float, a pressure drop occurs. The difference in the upstream and downstream pressure is equal to the weight of the float and an equilibrium is reached. If the flow rate is increased, the float again rises until the pressure differential equals the weight of the float, at which point a new equilibrium is established.

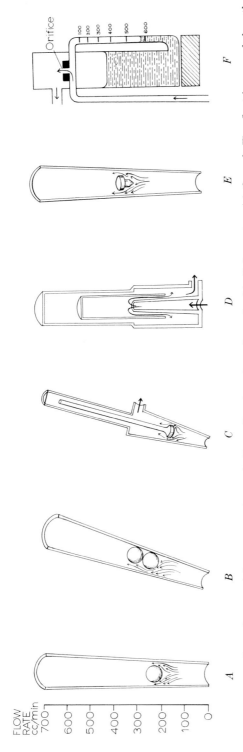

FIGURE 9–16. Several types of flowmeters. Arrows indicate direction of gas flow. In "dry" flowmeters (*A* through *E*) a float is suspended on the stream of gas. As flow increases the float rises. Calibration of the tube enables measurement of flow rate. *F* is a "wet" flowmeter containing distilled water. As gas flows through the orifice a pressure differential is created on the two columns of water. This differential is measured as gas flow on the small calibrated tube.

(157)

Some flowmeters are calibrated to function with the tube placed at an angle, compensation being made for the effect of friction between float and tube wall. Others are accurate only when the tube is vertical and the float rotates freely in the tube. Gas machines equipped with the latter usually have a built-in leveling device which must be adjusted each time the equipment is moved.

Vaporizers

If volatile liquid anesthetic agents are used in a gas machine, it is necessary to have some form of vaporizer to volatilize them.

Oxygen flowing through the vaporizer becomes partially saturated with anesthetic vapor, which is then carried to the patient. Oxygen thus acts as a transport mechanism for these agents, in addition to satisfying the patient's oxygen requirements.

Four types of vaporizers are commonly employed for anesthetic liquids. Listed in order of increasing potency they are surface, wick, bubble, and drip (Fig. 9–17).

In surface vaporizers oxygen passes over the liquid anesthetic and in the process displaces vapor rising from the liquid. This reduces the partial pressure of the vapor and liquid begins to evaporate to restore the vapor pressure. Heat required for vaporization (latent heat of vaporization) is extracted from unevaporated liquid and the vaporizer jar itself, thus lowering their temperature and reducing the vapor pressure of the remaining liquid. For this reason, simple vaporizers are reduced in efficiency as time elapses and the liquid anesthetic cools.

Wick vaporizers contain cotton fibers partially immersed in the anesthetic, which increases the area of contact between gas and liquid. The cotton fibers have greater affinity for water than for anesthetic and absorb exhaled water vapor, if present, to the exclusion of anesthetic liquid.

Bubble vaporizers direct the gas flow through the anesthetic and thus increase the amount of vapor entrained. These also tend to develop a falling output due to cooling of the anesthetic liquid.

The drip method employs a reservoir containing the anesthetic agent. A valve controls the release of liquid and the rate of flow can be seen in a drip chamber. The agent is allowed to drop at a metered rate onto a copper screen from which it evaporates. The screen is usually incorporated in a soda lime canister and absorption of carbon dioxide produces heat which in turn vaporizes the anesthetic.

To overcome the loss of efficiency which occurs in vaporizers during prolonged periods of anesthesia, some refinements have been developed. These include immersion of the vaporizer in a second

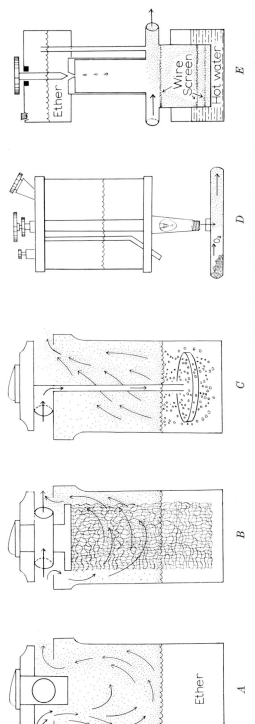

FIGURE 9-17. Vaporizers in order of increasing efficiency: (A) surface, (B) wick, (C) bubble, and (D, E) drip. Arrows indicate direction of gas flow.

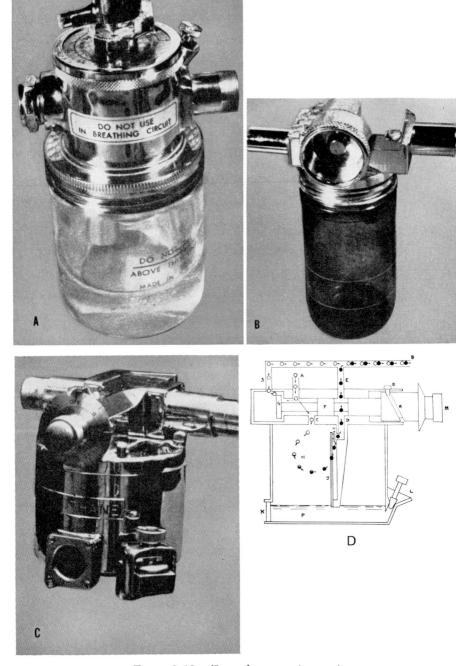

FIGURE 9–18.   (*Legend on opposite page*)

container of warm water or use of a heavy thermoconductive sheath for the vaporizer jar (Foregger Copper Kettle).

Because of its extreme potency, special vaporizers have been developed for metering halothane (Fig. 9–18). These are intended to increase its safety and also make its use more economical. Most of them are calibrated in percentage of halothane by volume in the anesthetic mixture.

Carbon Dioxide Absorption

In general, two types of filters are in use for removal of carbon dioxide. These are (1) the to-and-fro, and (2) the circle (Fig. 9–19).

These are so designated because of the direction gases flow within the system. In circle systems, exhaled gases pass from the patient through a soda lime canister to the rebreathing bag. They are then inhaled from the rebreathing bag by the patient, thus completing a circle. Valves within the system dictate the direction of flow. In to-and-fro systems the patient exhales through the soda lime canister into the rebreathing bag. On inhalation the gases are drawn back through the soda lime.

Removal of carbon dioxide generates considerable heat which in the to-and-fro system may become excessive. In the early developmental years the to-and-fro filter was the most popular, but it has gradually been supplanted by the more efficient circle filter. Today, in hospitals for humans, approximately 95% of inhalation anesthesia utilizing rebreathing is performed with the latter type.

With the to-and-fro system, it has been shown that absorption is most efficient when the tidal volume of the patient is equal to the air space in the canister filled with soda lime. Efficiency decreases when the air space is more or less than the tidal volume, thus small canisters should be used with small patients and *vice versa* (Fig. 9–20). It has been demonstrated that the canister size-tidal volume relationship is also important in the circle filter. However, in the latter absorption is unsatisfactory if the air space is less than the tidal volume, whereas, it continues to be effective if the air

---

FIGURE 9–18. Three types of halothane vaporizer: The Ohio-Heidbrink (*A*); the FNS (*B*); and the Fluotec (*C*). The Fluotec (*D*) is a temperature compensated drawover vaporizer. Gas enters port A and exits port *B* when no vaporization is desired. When plunger M-F-G is pulled forward and rotated clockwise port *C* is opened into vaporizing chamber *N*. Gas then flows over liquid *P* and makes its exit through port *H* and passage D-E to join the portion of the flow not diverted through the vaporizing chamber. Port *H* is temperature compensated by the bimetallic strip *J* to maintain constant vaporization. (Illustrations *A*, *B*, *C* from MacKay, I. M. and Kalow, W.: A Clinical and Laboratory Evaluation of Four Fluothane Vaporizers. Canadian Anaes. Soc. J., *5*, 248, 1958. Illustration *D* from Dripps, R. D., Eckenhoff, J. E., and Vandam, L. D.: *Introduction to Anesthesia*, W. B. Saunders Co., 1961.)

11

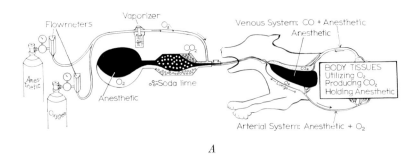

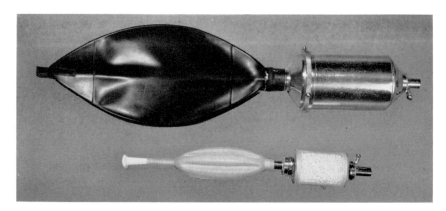

FIGURE 9–19.   Schematic drawings of (A) to-and-fro and (B) circle systems for closed administration of inhalation anesthetics.   Examples of this equipment are shown in Figures 9–13 and 9–15 respectively. (After American Medical Association: *Fundamentals of Anesthesia*, 3rd ed. W. B. Saunders Co., 1954.)

FIGURE 9–20.   A conventional size to-and-fro canister and rebreathing bag is shown (top) in comparison to one used for small dogs and cats (bottom).

space is greater than the tidal volume. For sustained absorption it is important to have the air space greater than the tidal volume in circle filters.

Neither unit will remove all the carbon dioxide for any length of time. For years the ill effects of hypercarbia were not appreciated, but now it is known that high carbon dioxide blood levels predispose to ventricular fibrillation. Since certain patients tolerate incomplete removal of carbon dioxide better than others, the objective is total removal of carbon dioxide from the system.

Soda lime, the agent which absorbs carbon dioxide, is not a specific chemical compound. It varies in fragility, porosity, moisture content, and carbon dioxide absorptive capacity, according to the manufacturer.

Soda lime is essentially a mixture of sodium and calcium hydroxide which furnishes free OH^- ions. The chemical reaction occurring in the canister is caused by carbon dioxide combining with water to form carbonic acid which is then neutralized by the base.

$$2CO_2 + 2H_2O \longrightarrow 2H_2CO_3 \longrightarrow 4H + 2CO_3$$
$$2NaOH \longrightarrow 2OH + 2Na$$
$$Ca(OH)_2 \longrightarrow 2OH + Ca$$
$$\downarrow$$
$$4H_2O + Na_2CO_3 + CaCO_3$$

Absorption of carbonic acid does not easily occur because it is a weak, poorly ionized substance. Because the distance between granules of soda lime is relatively great, carbon dioxide molecules can pass between the granules. In addition, some which do contact the soda lime are not converted to carbonic acid. Therefore, some carbon dioxide passes through soda lime and returns to the patient. The concentration of carbon dioxide in the system thus gradually increases as alkali on the surface of the granules is converted to carbonates. Adriani and Rovenstine (1941) have arbitrarily selected 0.5% carbon dioxide as the average point where patients will show signs of hypercarbia.

Soda lime must contain 15 to 20% moisture in order to be efficient. Additional moisture caused by humidification of gases in the system does not increase the efficiency.

Today, considerable attention is paid to the production of soda lime. Moisture content is controlled. Potassium hydroxide, which is more active chemically than sodium hydroxide, is added in small quantities to improve absorption. Silicates, which confer hardness but decrease efficiency, have been eliminated. The reaction, of sodium carbonate and calcium hydroxide to regenerate sodium hydroxide, keeps pace with carbon dioxide absorption in the soda limes commercially available.

It has been shown that there is no difference in efficiency when canisters are placed in the horizontal or vertical positions. Likewise, a center tube in the canister to diffuse gases through the soda lime makes no appreciable difference. The to-and-fro filter is dependent upon tidal volume which varies considerably. The circle filter offers more efficient absorption if a large capacity canister is used. Some canisters are now divided into two equal-sized compartments which are interchangeable. As one half becomes exhausted, the other half is shifted into position and the exhausted half replenished.

In the most efficient systems 1 gm. of soda lime will absorb 175 cc. of carbon dioxide. The ordinary single canister will absorb from 100 to 125 cc. of carbon dioxide/gm. of soda lime. The total hours of effective use of soda lime is roughly proportional to the amount used. Once exhausted, soda lime does not regenerate upon being aerated and, therefore, should be discarded.

Most soda limes contain an indicator, such as ethyl violet, which changes color as exhaustion occurs (usually this is from white or pink to violet). The color change is due to a shift in pH to the acidic side. Under ordinary conditions the average canister is effective for 5 to 8 hours of continuous anesthesia with the dog.

If soda lime inadvertently becomes exhausted during an operation, the patient will develop hypercapnea with resultant hyperpnea. The mucous membranes will remain bright pink with *no evidence of cyanosis.* Continued use of exhausted soda lime will result in acidosis and shock; death will rapidly intervene. It is imperative, therefore, that the condition of the soda lime be checked before each anesthetic period and occasionally during prolonged anesthesia.

Manometers

If open chest surgery is to be performed, a manometer is desirable. Connected to the rebreathing system, it serves to prevent harmful over-expansion of the lungs. Both spring-operated and water types are available, both usually being set at 15 to 18 cm. of water (Fig. 9–21). If excessive pressure is exerted on the rebreathing bag, or otherwise develops in the system, gas is automatically vented through the manometer when pressure exceeds the setting.

Gas Machine Operation

In operating a gas machine the following steps are performed:

1. The machine is checked to determine that everything is working properly, that the soda lime is not exhausted, and

that there is sufficient oxygen and anesthetic agent to complete the anesthetic period.

2. Endotracheal catheters of appropriate size are checked to insure that the cuff is patent.

3. The patient is anesthetized using a thiobarbiturate intravenously. (For an alternate type of induction see step 15).

4. An endotracheal catheter is inserted and the cuff inflated and clamped.

5. The adapter of the catheter is connected to the gas machine.

6. Oxygen is run into the system in sufficient quantity to inflate the rebreathing bag to approximately two-thirds capacity.

7. Oxygen flow is then adjusted to a rate estimated to meet the

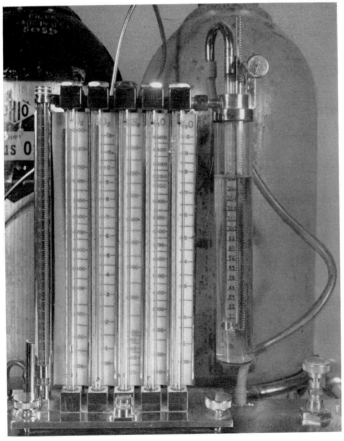

FIGURE 9–21. Sphygmomanometer (left), flowmeters (center), and water manometer (right) on a Foregger Iowa Model gas machine. The flowmeters are of the rotating bobbin type and must be perpendicular to function properly. Leveling screws and a level-bubble are built into the base of the flowmeter stand. A rachet adjusts the depth of insertion of the water manometer and thereby controls pressure within the system.

metabolic requirements of the animal. This varies from 50 to 250 cc./minute for most dogs.

8. Additional anesthetic is administered as needed, either by turning on the vaporizer in case a volatile liquid agent is used, or by turning the valve which introduces anesthetic gas into the system.

9. Once the proper depth of anesthesia is reached, administration of anesthetic is stopped and only oxygen flow to the patient is continued.

10. Additional anesthetic must be given periodically during the operative procedure as need arises.

11. If the chest is opened the anesthetist will have to "bag" the animal. This is accomplished by rhythmically compressing the rebreathing bag at a rate of 8 to 12 times a minute.

12. If anesthesia becomes too deep the system is flushed by opening the expiratory valve and expelling the anesthetic mixture from the rebreathing bag into the room. The valve is then closed and the rebreathing bag inflated with pure oxygen. This procedure is repeated until the animal shows evidence of recovery. If breathing has ceased, the anesthetist must "bag" the animal until spontaneous respiration resumes.

13. When anesthesia is to be terminated the same procedure is used, the gas in the system being expelled following which oxygen is introduced into the system.

14. As the patient shows signs of recovering from anesthesia, the adapter of the endotracheal catheter can be disconnected from the gas machine. After the patient has become accustomed to breathing room air, he can be returned to his cage to complete recovery. The catheter should be allowed to remain in position until the swallowing reflex returns. This is important, since occasionally a patient will not adapt to the sudden change from a high oxygen concentration to that of room air and hypoxia develops. In this case oxygen administration must be initiated again and the presence of a catheter is very desirable.

15. An alternate method of induction is by means of a mask connected to the machine, instead of a catheter. Preanesthetic sedation should be administered first. The animal is restrained by tapes to the operating table or is held by an assistant. The mask is held over the animal's face, a rapid flow of oxygen started, and the vaporizer turned on. In case an anesthetic gas is used the flow rate is adjusted to conform with the requirements for induction (see respective agents for per cent required for induction and maintenance). Once the animal is relaxed, it is usually easier to continue administration through an endotracheal catheter than to hold the mask.

Care of the Gas Machine

Most gas machines require little maintenance. Following each use the rebreathing bag should be washed, to remove any condensate which has collected in the bag, and hung to drain. The soda lime canister should be stoppered or otherwise protected from the air. Volatile liquid anesthetic agents should be returned to their original containers since most of them deteriorate on exposure to air and light. Valves on gas machines are usually of the needle type. They should be seated very loosely since excessive tightening will damage them.

Safety Precautions

Explosions and fires in the operating room are an occupational hazard with the anesthetist who uses volatile liquid or gaseous anesthetic agents.* An explosion will occasionally cause death of the patient. In man the ratio of explosions to anesthetic periods for the following three agents is listed by Collins (1952) as:

Ether	1:58,000
Ethylene	1:41,000
Cyclopropane	1:25,000

Veterinarians are particularly haphazard in their handling of explosive anesthetic agents. The fact that explosions do occur in veterinary hospitals is attested by the following newspaper article published in 1956.

3 INJURED IN HOSPITAL EXPLOSION
DR. _____ REPORTED IN FAIR CONDITION

Three men were injured, two seriously, when an ether bottle exploded in the operating room of a northside animal hospital yesterday morning.

Two of the men suffered multiple lacerations when particles of the exploded glass bottle scattered through the operating room of the _____ Small Animal Hospital.

The third man was treated at the hospital and released.

Another veterinarian said he was outside the operating room when he heard the explosion and the men started rushing by him.

Officers are uncertain what caused the blast. Dr. _____ was filling a pint glass jar with ether when the explosion occurred. _____ told deputies that they were operating on an animal and that Dr. _____ was forcing ether mixed with oxygen to the animal. The dog was not hurt.

The lights in the operating room were smashed and blood from the injured men was smeared on the walls. The ether bottle was made of heavy plated glass.

---

* A color film entitled "Fire and Explosion Hazards from Flammable Anesthetics" is available from Graphic Services, United States Department of Interior, Bureau of Mines Central Experiment Station, 4800 Forbes Avenue, Pittsburgh 13, Pennsylvania.

Only four commonly used inhalation anesthetic agents are non-inflammable and nonexplosive. These are nitrous oxide, chloroform, halothane, and methoxyflurane. In making anesthetic mixtures of any of the others the mixture passes into the explosive range. All except ethylene are more dense than air so that they have a tendency to pool along the floor. Ethylene, on the other hand, rises rather than falls.

Conditions for explosion develop when the following four factors are present:

1. A flammable substance.
2. Oxygen, either in air, in nitrous oxide, or in the pure form.
3. An explosive mixture of 1 and 2 above.
4. An ignition source.
   a. Open flame: cigarettes, cigars, pipes, or gas burners.
   b. Electric sparks: cauteries, electric switches, clippers, endo-scopic equipment, fans, surgical lamps, suction pumps, defective wiring.
   c. Static electricity: wool blankets, rubber goods, clothing, hair, plastics, tearing adhesive.

Static electricity is the most important ignition source. Electrical charges are developed on various surfaces by friction. This results in potential differences between surfaces and, when the proper distance separates the two, a spark jumps the gap.

Clothing of silk, wool, or plastic develops static electricity. Cotton clothing does not possess this property. Leather shoes should be worn; rubber-soled shoes insulate the wearer, allowing a charge to develop on the body. Rubber mats have the same effect and should never be used. Gases flowing through dry tubing develop a charge on the tubing; therefore, anesthetic gases should not be blasted through tubes of gas machines.

Other precautions which should be taken include the following:

1. Leaks in anesthetic equipment should be prevented.
2. Electrical switches and outlets should be at least 5 feet above the floor.
3. When possible, anesthetic gases should be vented outside the building.
4. Adequate circulation of air through the operating room should be provided to dissipate agents which escape.
5. Intercoupling of patient, operating table, gas machine, and anesthetist should be performed. This will dissipate charges of static electricity which may develop.
6. Humidity above 65% will discharge nearly all static charges;

therefore, dehumidification of operating areas should not be attempted.

7. In purchasing operating room equipment, it should be made certain that motors meet underwriter approval for use under explosive conditions and that conductive casters are used on all types of apparatus.

8. In construction of new hospitals installation of sparkproof electrical connections and conductive floors should be considered.*

* When planning new hospitals refer to Dornette, W. H. L.: *Hospital Planning for the Anesthesiologist.* Charles C Thomas, Springfield, Ill., 1958.

References

ADRIANI, J. and ROVENSTINE, E. A.: Experimental Studies on Carbon Dioxide Absorption for Anesthesia. Anesthesiology, *2*, 1, 1941.

BOOTH, N. H., RANKIN, A. D., and WILL, D. H.: Simplified Apparatus and Method for Administering Oxygen and Ether to the Dog. J.A.V.M.A., *137*, 114, 1960.

BROOKS, E. I., SAWABE, S., and SALEM, H.: Maintenance of Small Animal Anesthesia and Resuscitation. Small Animal Clinician, *2*, 37, 1962.

COLLINS, V. J.: *Principles and Practice of Anesthesiology.* Lea & Febiger, Philadelphia, 1952.

HARDENBERGH, J. G. and MANN, F. C.: The Auto-Inhalation Method of Anesthesia in Canine Surgery. J.A.V.M.A., *71*, 493, 1927.

SINGLETON, B.: Safe Small Animal Anesthesia. Bio-Chemic Review, *30*, 12, 1961.

STILES, S. W.: Induction of Ether Anesthesia in Cats. J.A.V.M.A., *134*, 275, 1959.

ZAUDER, H. L. and ORKIN, L. R.: Chamber for Anesthetization of Small Animals. Anesthesiology, *20*, 707, 1959.

THE BARBITURATES
AND
THIOBARBITURATES

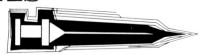

Chapter 10

BARBITURIC acid was first prepared by Conrad and Gutzeit in 1882. In 1903, Fischer and von Mering introduced a derivative, diethyl barbituric acid (veronal, barbital), for use as a hypnotic agent. Fischer is believed to have named the drug veronal from the Latin *vera* since he thought it to be the "true" hypnotic.

Chemical Structure

The barbiturates all contain a pyrimidine nucleus resulting from the condensation of malonic acid and urea (Fig. 10–1). Barbituric acid itself has no hypnotic activity. By substituting alkyl or aryl groups on the R_1 or R_2 positions (Fig. 10–2), various compounds with hypnotic activity are produced. Replacement of the oxygen atom in position X by a sulfur atom produces the ultrashort-acting thiobarbiturates.

Substituted R_1–R_2 derivatives of barbituric acid behave as weak acids and unite with fixed alkalies to form soluble salts. These salts hydrolyze in water to varying degrees and form alkaline solutions.

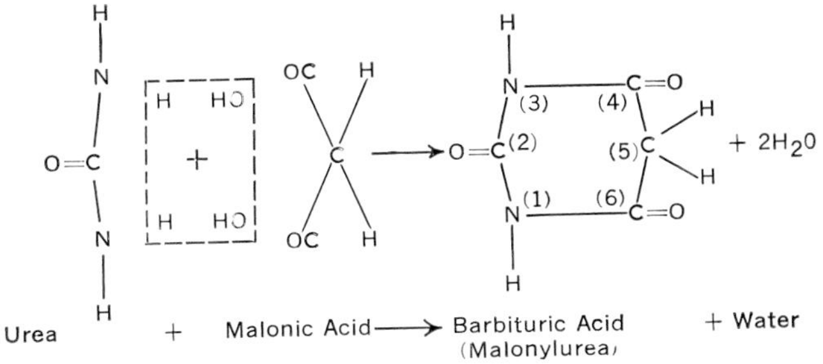

FIGURE 10–1. Formation of barbituric acid from urea and malonic acid.

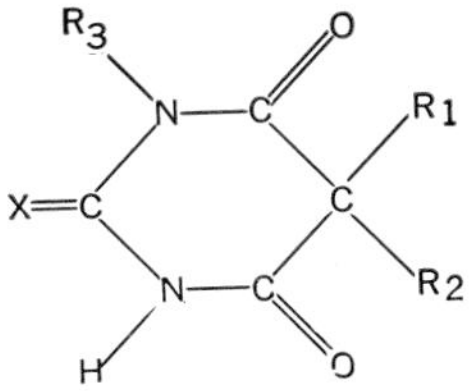

FIGURE 10–2. General formula of the barbiturates

Those commonly employed in veterinary medicine have a pH of 10 or above and for this reason may cause severe tissue damage and slough if injected perivascularly in any appreciable quantity.

General Pharmacology

The barbiturates are used both as hypnotics and general anesthetics. The principle effect of a barbiturate is depression of the central nervous system by interference with passage of impulses to the cerebral cortex. In hypnotic doses the barbiturates have little effect upon respiration, while in anesthetic doses respiration is depressed. Overdoses produce respiratory paralysis and death. With anesthetic doses there is depression of circulation both centrally and peripherally with a fall in blood pressure.

In hypnotic doses barbiturates have little effect on the basal metabolic rate. With anesthetic doses basal metabolism is depressed resulting in lowered body temperature.

Various investigators have studied the distribution of barbiturates in the body. Following injection of barbital sodium Dille *et al.* (1935) found liver, kidney, and heart muscle usually contained more barbiturate than skeletal muscle, intestine, or stomach. They stated that barbital distribution is probably controlled by blood supply to an organ and for this reason the concentration in all organs is never the same.

Maynert and Van Dyke (1950) studied barbiturate distribution using barbital labeled with N^{15}. They found that barbital is not destroyed or metabolized in the body. As much as 85% of both barbital and phenobarbital may be recovered from the urine over a period of several days following administration. The short-acting barbiturates, pentobarbital, amytal, and seconal, are destroyed principally by the liver. Their rapid destruction in the body accounts for their short action.

The placenta does not serve as a barrier to the passage of barbiturates from the mother to the fetus *in utero*.

Classification

The barbiturates have been classified into four groups according to duration of action (Tables 10–1 and 10–2). These are long, intermediate, short, and ultrashort. All of those used for clinical anesthesia fall in the short or ultrashort classification; whereas, those used for sedation or control of convulsions are of long or intermediate action.

Therapeutic Uses of Barbiturates in Small Animals

Barbiturates are used for three purposes in small animals:

1. *For Sedation and Hypnosis.* In this respect they have been supplanted, in most instances, by tranquilizers.
2. *As Anti-convulsants.* The ability of barbiturates to depress the motor cortex has been utilized to treat convulsions associated with poisoning, particularly strychnine, "running fits", distemper encephalitis, and overdosage of local anesthetics.
3. *For Anesthesia.* It is for this purpose that barbiturates are most frequently used in veterinary medicine.

Addiction to Barbiturates

While barbiturate addiction can be produced in animals, it is by its very nature self-limiting; however, in man, repeated oral use of barbiturates as soporifics or sedatives may become habit forming. For this reason, many states have enacted legislation to prohibit use of these drugs without a prescription. Veterinarians should be acquainted with applicable laws regarding their sale to prevent liability.

Barbiturates

Barbital Sodium, U.S.P.   (Barbitone, Veronal, Medinal)

The first barbiturate synthesized which proved to be of clinical value was barbital. Because of its prolonged depressive action it is

Table 10–1.—Names, Status, Chemical Structures, Duration of Action, and Excretion of the Barbiturates

Barbiturate	Status	Commercial Names or Synonyms	R_1	R_2	R_3	X	Duration of Action	Organ of Degredation and/or Excretion
Allylbarbituric Acid	N.F.	Sandoptal	allyl	isobutyl	H	O	Intermediate	III
Amobarbital	U.S.P.	Amytal	ethyl	isoamyl	H	O	Intermediate	III
Aprobarbital	N.F.	Alurate	allyl	isopropyl	H	O	Intermediate	II
Barbital	N.F.	Veronal, Barbitone	ethyl	ethyl	H	O	Long	I
Butabarbital†	N.N.R.	Butisol	ethyl	sec-butyl	H	O	Intermediate	—
Butallylonal†	N.F.	Pernoston	2-bromallyl	sec-butyl	H	O	Intermediate	II
Butethal	N.F.	Neonal	ethyl	n-butyl	H	O	Intermediate	II
Cyclobarbital	N.F.	Phanodorn	ethyl	cyclohexenyl	H	O	Short	II
Cyclopal	—	—	allyl	cyclopentenyl	H	O	Short	II
Diallylbarbituric Acid	N.F.	Dial	allyl	allyl	H	O	Long	II
Hexethal†	N.N.R.	Ortal	ethyl	n-hexyl	H	O	Intermediate	III
Hexobarbital‡	N.F.	Evipal, Hexo-barbitone	methyl	cyclohexenyl	CH₃	O	Ultrashort	IV
Kemithal‡	—	—	allyl	cyclohexenyl	H	S	Ultrashort	IV
Mephobarbital	N.F.	Mebaral	ethyl	phenyl	CH₃	O	Long	II
Pentobarbital	U.S.P.	Nembutal	ethyl	1-methylbutyl	H	O	Short	III
Phenobarbital	U.S.P.	Luminal, Pheno-barbitone	ethyl	phenyl	H	O	Long	I
Probarbital†	N.F.	Ipral	ethyl	isopropyl	H	O	Intermediate	III
Propallylonal	—	Nostal	isopropyl	2-bromallyl	H	O	Intermediate	III
Secobarbital†	U.S.P.	Seconal	allyl	1-methylbutyl	H	O	Short	III
Thiamylal‡	N.N.R.	Surital	allyl	1-methylbutyl	H	S	Ultrashort	IV
Thiopental‡	U.S.P.	Pentothal	ethyl	1-methylbutyl	H	S	Ultrashort	IV
Vinbarbital†	N.F.	Delvinal	ethyl	1-methyl-1-butenyl	H	O	Intermediate	II

† Employed principally as the sodium salt.
‡ Used for intravenous anesthesia, as sodium salt.
I Mainly excreted by kidney.
II Degraded by liver and excreted by kidney.
III Degraded by liver.
IV Absorbed by body fat, degraded by liver, and excreted by kidney.
(From Goodman, L. S. and Gilman, A.: *The Pharmacological Basis of Therapeutics.* 2nd ed. The Macmillan Co., 1958, with additions.)

(173)

Table 10-2.—Historical and Clinical Data of the Barbiturates and Thiobarbiturates

Agent (Generic Name)	Barbiturates				Thiobarbiturates			
	Pentobarbital	Secobarbital	Hexobarbital	Methohexital	Thiamylal	Thiopental	Thialbarbitone	Methitural
Trade Name	Nembutal Sodium® Registered by Abbott Laboratories	Seconal Sodium® Registered by Eli Lilly & Company	Evipal Sodium® Registered by Parke, Davis & Company	Brevane® Registered by Corn States Laboratories	Surital Sodium® Registered by Parke, Davis & Company	Pentothal Sodium® Registered by Abbott Laboratories	Kemithal Sodium® Registered by Fort Dodge Laboratories	Neraval Sodium® Registered by Schering Corporation
Chemical Name	Sodium 5-ethyl-5-(1-methylbutyl)-barbiturate	Sodium 5-allyl-5-(1-methylbutyl)-barbiturate	Sodium 1,5-dimethyl-5-(1-cyclo-hexenyl)-barbiturate	Sodium α-dl-1-methyl-5-allyl-5-(1-methyl-2-pentynyl)-barbiturate	Sodium 5-allyl-5-(1-methylbutyl)-2-thiobarbit-urate	Sodium 5-ethyl-5-(1-methylbutyl)-2-thiobarbit-urate	Sodium 5-allyl-5-(2-cyclohexenyl)-2-thiobarbit-urate	Sodium 5-(1-methylbutyl)-5-[2-(methyl-thio)-ethyl]-2-thiobarbit-urate
Formula	$C_{11}H_{17}N_2O_3$ Na	$C_{12}H_{17}N_2O_3$ Na	$C_{12}H_{15}N_2O_3$ Na	$C_{14}H_{17}N_2O_3$ Na	$C_{12}H_{17}N_2O_2$ SNa	$C_{11}H_{17}N_2O_2$ SNa	$C_{13}H_{15}O_2N_2$ SNa	$C_{12}H_{20}N_2O_2$ S$_2$Na
Discovery of Compound	1930 by Volwiler	1930 by Shonle	1932 by Krepp & Taub	1955 by Doran	1929 by Dox	1929 by Taburn & Volwiler	1938 by Carrington	1954 by Zima, Von Werder & Hotovy
Discovery of Anesthetic or Relaxant Properties	1930 by Volwiler & Tabern	1931 by Swanson	1932 by Weese & Scharpff	1955 by Gibson	1933 by Gruhzit	1933 by Tatum	1946 by Carrington & Raventos	—
Type of Compound	5-substituted barbiturate	5-substituted barbiturate	N-substituted barbiturate	N-5-substi-tuted barbiturate	5-substituted thiobarbit-urate	5-substituted thiobarbit-urate	5-substituted thiobarbit-urate	5-substituted thiobarbit-urate
Molecular Weight	248.26	260.27	258.25	284.0	276.33	264.23	286.3	288.44
Buffer Employed	None	None	None	Sodium carbonate	6% Sodium carbonate	6% Sodium carbonate	None	5% Sodium carbonate

(174)

Preservative or Stabilizing Agent Used	None	Phenol, 0.25% and polyethylene glycol 200, 50%	None	None	None	None	None	None
Thermostability	Precipitates on heating	Precipitates on heating	Free acid melts at 146° C.	Deteriorates when boiled	Precipitates when boiled	Precipitates when boiled	Thermolabile	Precipitates on autoclaving
Chemostability	Solution stable indefinitely	Solution stable up to 18 months in sealed container, decomposes on exposure to air	Solution stable for 48 hours if tightly stoppered	Solution stable at room temperature for 6 months	Solution stable for 48-72 hours if tightly stoppered	Solution stable for 48-72 hours if tightly stoppered	Solution stable 7 days if refrigerated, indefinitely if frozen	Solution stable for 24-48 hours if tightly stoppered
Onset of Action Duration of Action	30-60 seconds 1-2 hours	30-60 seconds 1-2 hours	30-60 seconds 15-30 minutes	10-30 seconds 5-15 minutes	20-30 seconds 10-15 minutes	20-30 seconds 10-15 minutes	20-30 seconds 15-45 minutes	10-30 seconds 10-15 minutes
Route and/or Organ of Detoxification or Elimination	Detoxified by the liver	Detoxified by the liver	Detoxified by the liver	Detoxified by the liver	Absorbed by fat and detoxified by the liver	Absorbed by fat and detoxified by the liver	Absorbed by fat and detoxified by the liver	Absorbed by fat and detoxified by the liver
Usual Mode of Administration	Intravenous, intrathoracic, intraperitoneal	Intravenous	Intravenous	Intravenous	Intravenous	Intravenous	Intravenous, intrathoracic, intraperitoneal	Intravenous
Specific Pharmacologic Antagonist	None (Oxygen administration and artificial respiration recommended in respiratory arrest.)				Methetharimide may be specific for thiobarbiturates (Oxygen administration and artificial respiration are recommended in respiratory arrest.)			
pH of Solution	6%-pH 10.0-10.3	5%-pH 9.8-10.1	2.5%-pH 3.5-10.5	5%-pH 10.4-11.4	2.5%-pH 10.5-11	2.5%-pH 10.5-11	10%-pH 10.6	2.5%-pH 10.58, 5%-10.62

(175)

(From data compiled by Dr. W. H. L. Dornette and published by the Ohio Chemical and Surgical Equipment Company, with additions.)

used primarily as a sedative and hypnotic (Fig. 10–3). The duration of action is slightly shorter than that of phenobarbital. Use of this drug in the dog is not recommended since the anesthetic dose (0.09 mg./lb.), approaches the minimum lethal dose (0.11 mg./lb.) (Sharaf, 1947). The oral sedative dose of barbital sodium for the dog is 150 to 1000 mg. (2.5 to 15 gr.) daily, depending upon the size of the animal and indications for its use (Jones, 1957). The dose for the cat is 100 to 300 mg. Barbital sodium has been replaced in clinical use by phenobarbital sodium.

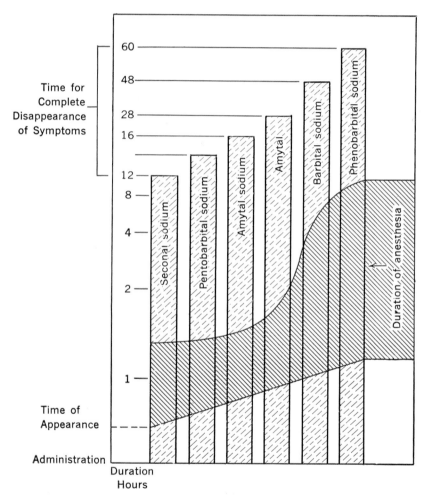

FIGURE 10–3. Time of appearance, duration of anesthesia, and time needed for complete disappearance of symptoms after oral administration of equivalent single anesthetic doses in animals. (Jones, L. M.: *Veterinary Pharmacology and Therapeutics,* 1957, courtesy of Iowa State University Press.)

Phenobarbital Sodium, U.S.P. (Phenobarbitone, Luminal)

Phenobarbital was synthesized in 1912 in Germany and marketed under the tradename Luminal. It is a long-acting barbiturate and advantage has been taken of its prolonged action in treating various convulsive disorders. In control of convulsions due to distemper encephalitis, it appears to be as effective as any of the newer drugs and considerably cheaper. Because it is excreted slowly in the urine, it has a tendency to be cumulative. An oral "loading dose" should be administered first, followed by a daily maintenance dose. In the average dog (10 kg.) this would be 1 gr. initially followed by $\frac{1}{4}$ gr. three times a day. Loss of motor coordination results from overdose and when this occurs the dose should be reduced. In convulsions due to strychnine poisoning, if it is felt that anesthesia should be maintained for a long period of time, phenobarbital solution may be given intravenously "to effect" in the same manner as one would administer pentobarbital sodium.

Mephobarbital, N.N.R. (Mebaral)

Chemically mephobarbital is N-methylphenobarbital. Butler et al. (1952) studied its metabolism and found that in the dog it is almost completely converted to phenobarbital. This conversion appears to occur principally in the liver and little is excreted unchanged in the urine. Jones (1957) has pointed out that the use of mephobarbital is questionable since it is (1) expensive, (2) poorly absorbed from the gastrointestinal tract and therefore must be given in large doses, and (3) is converted to phenobarbital much more rapidly than phenobarbital is eliminated, thus tends to become cumulative.

In clinical practice mephobarbital is used principally for its depressant action on the motor areas of the brain. In the dog it has been used in the treatment of distemper encephalitis and epileptic convulsions.

Amobarbital Sodium, U.S.P. (Amytal)

Amobarbital, introduced in 1928, was the first intravenous barbiturate to be used to any extent in animals and man. Relatively large doses are needed for anesthesia, and it produces a profound sleep predisposing to pneumonia. Excitement during the recovery stage is common. Amobarbital is not used for anesthesia; it has found use, however, as a sedative and anticonvulsant. The fatal oral dose in the dog is 57 mg./lb. (125 mg./kg.) of body weight (Swanson and Shonle, 1931). The oral dose for sedation of most species is 2 to 5 mg./lb. of body weight.

12

Pentobarbital Sodium, U.S.P.　(Nembutal)

Pentobarbital sodium came into general use as an anesthetic agent for dogs and cats in the early '30s. It slowly supplanted ether and ACE mixture, administered by open mask methods, as the anesthetic of choice. By 1940 its use was widespread and today it is the most commonly used small animal anesthetic in the United States.

Pentobarbital sodium occurs as a white powder or crystalline granules. It is freely soluble in water or alcohol. It forms a clear colorless solution which is marketed under a number of trade names.

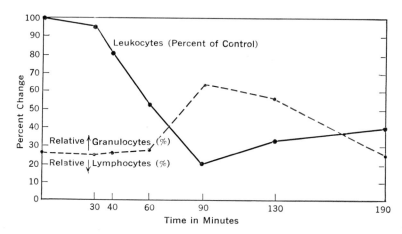

FIGURE 10–4. The relative per cent change in white cell counts with intravenous pentobarbital sodium anesthesia in 12 dogs as compared to control levels in unanesthetized dogs. The relative per cent distribution of lymphocytes and granulocytes is shown on the same scale. (From Graca, J. G. and Garst, E. L.: Early Blood Changes in Dogs Following Intravenous Pentobarbital Anesthesia. Anesthesiology, *18*, 461, 1957.)

Aqueous solutions have an alkaline pH and may precipitate on standing, but the drug can be redissolved by addition of alkali such as sodium hydroxide. Commercial solutions for anesthesia contain 64 mg. (1 gr.) of pentobarbital sodium per milliliter of solution. The calculated dose for dogs and cats is 13 mg. ($\frac{1}{5}$ gr.) per pound of body weight or 1.0 ml./5 lb. of body weight; however, it should be emphasized that pentobarbital is given "to effect."

Following a single intravenous dose of pentobarbital there is early depression of blood pressure. The heart rate decreases for 40 to 60 minutes and then stabilizes or increases. Respiration is initially depressed and gradually increases with time.

Light pentobarbital anesthesia has little influence on renal hemodynamics. Deep anesthesia will depress renal function, both blood and urine flow, by circulatory depression and also by reflex renal vasoconstriction. Pentobarbital also sharply inhibits water diuresis by stimulating release of antidiuretic hormone (Blake, 1957).

A striking and constant leukopenia is found in dogs, which reaches its height in approximately 90 minutes (Graca and Garst, 1957). Leukocyte counts drop to 20% of control values (Fig. 10–4). After 90 minutes there is a gradual rise in cell numbers so that at 190 minutes the mean value is 39% of the control. While the absolute differential white count decreases, there is a relative lymphocytosis which reaches its peak at 90 minutes and then returns to normal.

The red cells decrease also, the lowest count being reached 30 minutes following injection with a reading of 84.6% of control values. The count returns to normal in 130 minutes. Hemoglobin and hematocrit values show corresponding changes. Hausner et al. (1938) have shown radiographically that pentobarbital, amytal, and thiopental produce dilation of the spleen which presumably accounts for the decrease in erythrocytes. Maximum dilation usually occurs 20 to 30 minutes after injection of the anesthetic. Sedimentation rate and coagulation time are both increased, while prothrombin time is decreased. Oddly, oral administration of pentobarbital sodium in sedative doses does not affect the blood constitutents in the same fashion.

In some animals the effect produced by pentobarbital anesthesia is difficult to differentiate from shock produced in other ways and may actually terminate with death of the animal. Size of the dose and method of its administration are the major factors in variation of response to pentobarbital. Also, individual variations undoubtedly exist. Roughly one of four animals given a dose of 30 mg./kg. develops side effects which may mimic some phases of experimental shock (Mylon et al., 1943).

On intraperitoneal administration the peak concentration in the blood is reached more slowly than with intravenous injection, and the portion of drug absorbed into the portal system will be subjected to early destruction in the liver. When a 2.5% aqueous solution is given intraperitoneally in a dose of 30 mg./kg. of body weight, the anesthesia produced usually is not accompanied by impaired renal function and effective renal plasma flow occurs. Arterial blood pressure is elevated in dogs so anesthetized, with a mean of 146.7 mm. Hg (Corcoran and Page, 1943).

Pentobarbital freely crosses the placental barrier and enters the fetus. For this reason its use for cesarean section results in high mortality in the newborn. These animals are born viable, but usually do not recover from anesthesia, are unable to nurse, and die within the first 24 to 48 hours postoperatively.

Dogs given pentobarbital containing N^{15} orally, excrete about 60% of the total dose of N^{15} in the urine during the first 24 hours

(Van Dyke *et al.*, 1947). Over 92% of the N^{15} is excreted as metabolic products derived from the drug, and only 3% is in the form of pentobarbital.

Injection of glucose in dogs awakening from pentobarbital anesthesia will cause return of the anesthetic state in 25% of the animals, no response in 25%, and in the remaining 50% a doubtful response (Lamson *et al.*, 1951). This phenomenon termed a "glucose reaction" has undoubtedly killed many dogs unwittingly treated for postoperative shock with intravenous glucose. A species variation in susceptibility to this effect has been demonstrated; guinea pigs, chickens, pigeons, rabbits, and hamsters are very susceptible, dogs are intermediate, and mice, rats, goldfish, and tadpoles are refractory or negative. Intermediates in the glycolysis of glucose and in the Kreb's cycle have been shown to have the same effect. The "glucose reaction" presumably occurs with all barbiturates and thiobarbiturates but not with inhalation or other anesthetics.

Epinephrine given intravenously to dogs or mice also causes a return of sleep on awakening from hexobarbital or chloral hydrate anesthesia. Norepinephrine is less effective in producing this effect (Lamson *et al.*, 1952). This phenomenon presumably is due to increased glucose levels in the blood and should be remembered when the use of epinephrine is considered in barbiturate-anesthetized dogs.

The duration of surgical anesthesia with pentobarbital varies widely with individual animals, averaging about 30 minutes. Complete recovery usually occurs in 6 to 18 hours. Occasional animals, particularly cats, may not rouse for as long as 24 to 72 hours.

Animals awakening from pentobarbital anesthesia tend to exhibit the same signs as when being anesthetized, except in reverse order. These include crying, shivering, involuntary running movements, thrashing, increased respiratory movements followed by recovery of the right reflex, and later, ability to stand with a staggering gait (Table 7-2, p. 115). Because recovery is slow, without preanesthetic agents these actions may become so exaggerated that the animal injures itself through contact with the cage or causes wound disruption. Greyhounds are notable for this effect. Show animals have been known to break canine teeth, much to the embarrassment of the veterinarian. Administration of meperidine or a tranquilizer is *always* indicated in these cases.

Pentobarbital in excessive dosage is often given intravenously for euthanasia. Appendix C (page 410) contains directions for preparing such a solution.

Secobarbital Sodium, U.S.P.   (Seconal)

Secobarbital sodium is a barbiturate of short duration. It has been used in man as a central nervous system depressant for any degree desired, from light depression to hypnosis, by varying the dose.

As all other barbiturates, it depresses respiration and circulation. It is detoxified in the liver.

While secobarbital has been used alone as an anesthetic agent in dogs and cats, it is now used chiefly in combination with mephenesin, a muscle relaxant (see Chapter 12, pg. 231). A sterile solution containing 50 mg. ($\frac{3}{4}$ gr.) of secobarbital sodium and 30 mg. ($\frac{5}{12}$ gr.) of mephenesin/ml. is available commercially.* Advantages claimed for this mixture are quick onset of anesthesia, short duration, and smooth rapid return of consciousness. The average intravenous dose is 1 ml./6.6 lb. of body weight and the duration of surgical anesthesia is approximately 1 hour (Harris and Hyder, 1953).

Because it has the least effect of all barbiturates on the EEG, secobarbital is sometimes used for anesthesia of dogs during electroencephalography.

Table 10–3.—Effects of Certain Barbiturates Injected Intravenously in Dogs

	Number of Dogs	Dose (mg./kg.)	Duration of Anesthesia* (min.)	Down Time* (min.)	Return to Normal* (min.)	Average Respiratory Rate
Pentobarbital sodium	8	25	200	'252	358	11
Hexobarbital sodium	12	40	69	183	340	19
Thiopental sodium	12	26	50	69	137	15

* Anesthesia   = absence of pad reflex.
  Down time   = from onset of anesthesia until animal stood.
  Return to normal = from onset of anesthesia until the dog could climb stairs without ataxia.
(After Hunt, W. H., Fosbinder, R. J., and Barlow, O. W.: Anesthetic Effects of Some New Barbituric Acid Derivatives Administered to Dogs. J. Am. Pharm. Assoc. (Scient. Ed.), 37, 1, 1948.)

Hexobarbital Sodium, N. F. (Evipal)

Hexobarbital sodium was introduced in 1932, and was considered the best ultrashort-acting barbiturate for intravenous anesthesia until the advent of thiopental sodium. It produces anesthesia of brief duration (15 to 60 minutes) depending upon the amount given. For short-lasting anesthesia in the dog and cat, 10 mg./lb. of 5% solution is injected intravenously. A comparison of the effects of hexobarbital in high dosage with pentobarbital and thiopental is shown in Table 10–3.

* See Myothesia, Appendix A, p. 403.

Weaver *et al.* (1958) reported trials of hexobarbital for anesthesia in dogs. They found it to be unsatisfactory because induction was not smooth and recovery was characterized by a marked increase in excitability. A dose of 35.4 mg./kg. was found to produce maximum relaxation.

Methohexital Sodium   (Brevane)

Methohexital sodium is an ultrashort-acting barbiturate, which is unique in that it contains no sulfur atom and hence is not a thiobarbiturate. Its short duration is due to rapid metabolism in the tissues. Blood concentrations necessary to produce anesthesia are approximately one-half those required with thiopental or thiamylal.

According to the manufacturer a double dose rapidly administered intravenously causes temporary apnea. The lethal dose is said to be approximately 2.5 times greater than the median anesthetic dose. Animals which die show respiratory failure followed by cardiac failure.

Methohexital sodium is supplied as 500 mg. of dry powder in rubber-stoppered vials. It is diluted with water for injection or normal saline to form a 2.5% solution. Solutions are said to be stable for as long as 6 months at room temperature.

The dose for the dog or cat is 1 ml./5 lb. of body weight of 2.5% solution. Half of the estimated dose is injected intravenously at a rapid rate following which administration is continued to effect. Surgical anesthesia for 5 to 15 minutes is obtained by an initial injection. More prolonged anesthesia can be maintained by intermittent administration or continuous drip. Recovery is quick and may be accompanied by muscular tremors and violent excitement which detract from the usefulness of the drug. Dogs are usually ambulatory 30 minutes after administration ceases.

Thiobarbiturates

Thiopental Sodium, U.S.P.   (Pentothal)

Thiopental was the first thiobarbiturate to gain popularity as an anesthetic agent for small animals. It is the thio analog of pentobarbital sodium, and only differs in that the number two carbon has a sulfur atom attached to it instead of an oxygen atom. Thiopental sodium is a yellow crystalline powder which is unstable in aqueous solution or when exposed to atmospheric air. For this reason it is dispensed in sealed containers as a powder buffered with sodium carbonate. It is usually mixed with sterile water or saline to form a 6.4% solution (1 gr./ml.). Thiopental solutions should be stored in a refrigerator at 5 to 6° C. (41 to 42° F.) to retard deterioration. As solutions age they become turbid and crystals precipitate. This results in progressive loss of activity but does not increase toxicity of the drug. Since the potency is decreased, larger quantities of solution must be used to produce the desired effect (Robinson, 1947).

Taylor et al. (1952) studied the metabolism of thiopental and found it to be exceedingly complex. Following injection with thiopental containing radioactive sulfur (S^{35}), monkeys produce at least 12 different metabolic products which are excreted in the urine. About 86% is found in the urine within 4 days after intravenous injection; small amounts are also found in the tissues and feces.

The initial toxic effect produced by thiopental is a marked depression of the respiratory centers, both rate and amplitude being affected. The pulse rate is slowed and blood pressure is depressed. Approximately 16 times more thiopental is needed to stop the heart than is needed to paralyze respiration (Wiedling, 1948).

Booker et al. (1952) determined that there is a prominent hyperglycemia, increase in lactic acid and amino acids of the blood, and decrease in liver glycogen during prolonged thiopental anesthesia. Insulin was shown to prevent the decrease of liver glycogen or favor increased storage of liver glycogen. Furthermore, increased glycogen storage in the liver seemed to favor destruction of thiopental, as evidenced by the fact that increased amounts of thiopental were necessary to maintain surgical anesthesia when insulin was administered. Animals on a high protein diet or high carbohydrate diet were also found to require more thiopental for surgical anesthesia than animals maintained on a "normal diet". They stated, ". . . the evidence supports the view that the nutritional state, good protein intake and good liver glycogen storage, are indispensable factors in determining the ability of the organism to dispose of Pentothal."

Repeated doses of thiopental have a cumulative effect as shown in Figure 10–5. Prolonged periods of anesthesia may result from this effect if numerous doses are administered.

Brodie et al. (1952) found that thiopental has an ultrashort action not because it is rapidly metabolized, but because it is rapidly localized in body fat. As concentrations in the plasma, muscle, and liver fall, the thiopental level in fat continues to rise (Fig. 10–6).

Anderson and Magee (1956) have shown the same effect occurs after a fatty meal. A high chylomicron level in the blood will produce a significant reduction in sleeping time. They believe that because thiopental is in more intimate contact with chylomicrons and a smaller diffusion distance is present, blood fat is much more potent than depot fat in reducing thiopental sleeping time.

Thiamylal Sodium, N.N.R.   (Surital)

Thiamylal sodium is the thio analog of the barbiturate, seconal sodium. It differs from thiopental sodium in that the ethyl radical of the latter (on R_1) is replaced by an allyl radical. According to

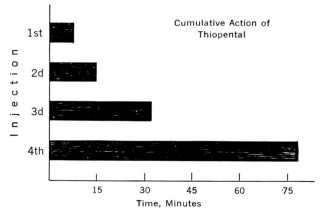

FIGURE 10–5.   The average duration of anesthesia after successive hourly intravenous injections of equal doses of thiopental to dogs. (From data of Wyngaarden, J. B., Woods, L. A., Ridley, R., and Seevers, M. H.:   Anesthetic Properties of Sodium-5-allyl-5 (1-methylbutyl)-2-thiobarbiturate (Surital) and Certain Other Thiobarbiturates in Dogs. J. Pharm. & Exper. Therap., *95*, 322, 1949.)

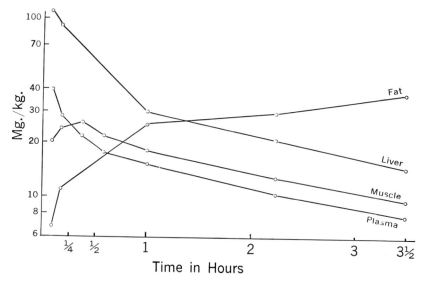

FIGURE 10–6.   Concentrations of thiopental in various tissues of a dog after the intravenous administration of 25 mg./kg. (From Brodie, B. B., Bernstein, E., and Mark, L. C.:   The Role of Body Fat in Limiting the Duration of Action of Thiopental. J. Pharm. & Exper. Therap., *105*, 421, 1952.)

Swanson (1951) it was first synthesized by Shonle and his associates. Thiamylal sodium is marketed as a mixture with sodium carbonate, the mixture being prepared by adding thiamylal sodium and sodium carbonate to just enough sodium hydroxide solution to dissolve the salts. The pH is adjusted to between 10.7 and 10.9. The solution is made to volume with water, filtered, sterilized, and lyophilized. The finished product consists of pale yellow, hygroscopic, agglutinated masses of crystals with no pronounced odor. On addition of distilled water, it readily dissolves forming a clear yellow solution

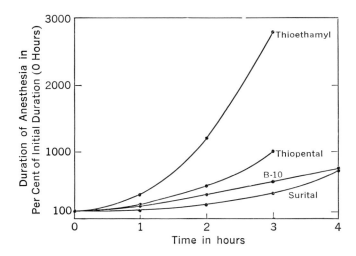

Figure 10–7. Cumulative action of hourly injections of four thiobarbiturates. Time values on the abscissa represent the hour on which injections were administered. (From Wyngaarden, J. B., Woods, L. A., Ridley, R., and Seevers, M. H.: Anesthetic Properties of Sodium-5-allyl-5-(1-methyl butyl)-2-thiobarbiturate (Surital) and Certain Other Thiobarbiturates in Dogs. J. Pharm. & Exper. Therap. 95, 326, 1949.)

with a pH of 10.3 (in 2.5% solution). Solutions have a pungent odor which has been described as that of sulfur or garlic. Reduction in pH of the solution results in precipitation of the drug; a few drops of alkali will redissolve precipitated material. According to Helrich (1950) normal saline is the preferred diluent. He states that solutions of thiamylal and saline have been kept for as long as 14 days without loss of potency or change in appearance.

Wyngaarden *et al.* (1947) compared the action of thiamylal and some other thiobarbiturates in dogs and found that the anesthetic potency of thiamylal was 1.5 compared to 1 for thiopental. Thiamylal was found to be less cumulative than thiopental as shown in Figure 10–7.

Swanson (1951) found no tolerance developed to thiamylal from repeated administration every other day for 4 weeks. There was slowing of the pulse rate with reduction in blood pressure. No inhibition of the vagus in dogs was observed following anesthetic doses as occurs with some other barbiturates. Thiamylal may be less cardiotoxic than thiopental according to Woods *et al.* (1947) who studied their action in both heart-lung preparations and intact dogs.

Depression of respiration is pronounced on rapid intravenous injection. When dogs are given excessive doses of thiamylal or thiopental by continuous injection, the respiratory rate and amplitude progressively decrease but blood pressure does not drop significantly until respiratory arrest occurs. Then it drops precipitously (Woods *et al.*, 1949). Dogs artificially respired will tolerate $1\frac{1}{2}$ to $3\frac{1}{2}$ times the dose of thiamylal tolerated with spontaneous respiration. Artificially ventilated animals show a very gradual decline in blood pressure to low levels. Anoxia secondary to respiratory failure is the cause of death.

Shideman *et al.* (1947) studied the role of the liver in degradation of the thiobarbiturates. By producing liver damage with carbon tetrachloride, they demonstrated that it plays an important role in detoxification of thiopental and thiamylal. This fact was confirmed in a second experiment which reduced liver blood flow by production of an Eck fistula.

Reutner and Gruhzit (1948) repeatedly injected groups of dogs with 15, 17.5, 20, 22.5, and 25 mg./kg. of thiamylal, some dogs receiving as many as 18 injections over a period of 49 days. Red, white, and differential blood cell counts and hemoglobin values remained unchanged. Urine specimens were free of sugar and albumin throughout the test period. Likewise, the total blood non-protein nitrogen, blood sugar, and bromsulfalein liver function tests remained normal.

Thiamylal is usually prepared as a 4% solution by adding 25 ml. of sterile water or saline to 1 gm. of powder. A dose of 17.5 mg./kg. ($\frac{1}{8}$ gr./lb.) intravenously will produce surgical anesthesia in dogs for approximately 15 minutes, with complete recovery in about 3 hours. If anesthesia of longer duration is desired repeated increments can be administered. It has been used with a wide variety of preanesthetic agents and muscle relaxants with excellent results.

Because of its low toxicity thiamylal is used in very young, aged, and poor-risk patients. It has won universal acclaim for its safety and is probably the most widely used thiobarbiturate in small animal practice.

Thialbarbitone Sodium (Kemithal)

Thialbarbitone sodium is a pale yellow, water-soluble powder. A 10% solution has a pH of 10.6. Solutions are stable for approximately one week when refrigerated.

According to Edds and Trace (1954) equiactive doses of thialbarbitone and thiopental produce anesthesia of similar onset and duration. They state that thialbarbitone produces less respiratory depression and less laryngospasm than does thiopental. Thialbarbitone has been administered intravenously to dogs and cats and intraperitoneally, intrathoracically, and rectally to cats.

Thialbarbitone is supplied in rubber-stoppered vials containing 1 gm. of dry powder. Ten ml. of sterile distilled water is added to make a 10% solution. The dose schedule for dogs is as follows:

Under 10 pounds	0.30 ml/lb.
10 to 30 pounds	0.25 ml./lb.
30 to 50 pounds	0.20 ml./lb.
Over 50 pounds	0.15 ml./lb.

Thialbarbitone stimulates salivation and for this reason preanesthetic atropine is indicated.

According to Carrington and Raventos (1946) thialbarbitone sodium is safer, produces less respiratory depression, and less fall in blood pressure than does thiopental.

Clinical studies indicate that good muscle relaxation is obtained. A respiratory lag develops on induction following which respirations become deep and regular. Some advantages claimed for thialbarbitone are (1) no excitement on induction, (2) the anesthetic can be given much more rapidly than pentobarbital sodium, (3) anesthesia of 15 to 45 minutes duration, and (4) rapid recovery with little excitement.

Arañez and Forteza (1955) administered toxic doses of thialbarbitone ranging from 41 to 46 mg./lb. to dogs. During the stage of deep anesthesia the pulse was weak and rapid, respirations were slow and shallow, and shivering was observed in all dogs. Urination and defecation occurred in some, along with cyanosis of the mucous membranes. Pulse rates were increased and respiratory rates lowered. The recovery period varied from 18 to 36 hours. The minimum lethal dose was found to be 46.9 mg./lb. of body weight. Respiratory arrest followed by cardiac arrest was observed in those animals which died.

Arañez and Tacal (1957) reported the use of thialbarbitone as an anesthetic for cats. When given intravenously, induction was rapid and generally without excitement. The length of surgical anesthesia varied from 15 to 72 minutes when 20 to 30 mg./lb. of body weight were administered. Slight respiratory depression, contraction of the pupils, complete muscular relaxation, congestion of the mucous membranes, tachycardia, and occasional ptyalism were noted. The recovery period ranged from 37 to 269 minutes and generally was smooth.

Doses of 31 to 32 mg./lb. of body weight are toxic to cats and the minimum lethal dose is 33 mg./lb. (Arañez and Tacal, 1957).

Methitural Sodium (Neraval)

Methitural sodium is an ultrashort-acting thiobarbiturate. It differs from other thiobarbiturates in that on the number five position, it has a second sulfur atom in a methylthioethyl radical. This radical, which is also present in methionine, probably accounts for the very rapid action of the anesthetic. The potency of methitural is approximately two-thirds that of thiopental in the dog, cat, and monkey and one-half that of thiopental in the rat. In general, the

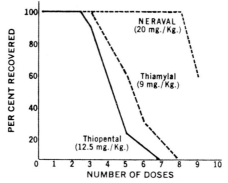

FIGURE 10-8. Repeated administration of comparable anesthetic doses of methitural sodium (Neraval), thiopental sodium, and thiamylal sodium to dogs at 1 hour intervals. (Courtesy of Schering Corp., from data of Irwin, S., Stagg, R. D., Dunbar, E. and Govier, W. M.: Methitural, A New Intravenous Anesthetic: Comparison with Thiopental in the Cat, Dog and Monkey. J. Pharm. & Exper. Therap., *116*, 317, 1956.)

effects of methitural are the same as those of thiopental and thiamylal with the exception that anesthesia is not so prolonged. The various reflexes of the dog, cat, and monkey disappear in the same order for both methitural and thiopental.

Methitural is very rapidly absorbed by fat, and is degraded by the liver more quickly than is thiopental. The speed of these two factors accounts for its very rapid action as compared with other thiobarbiturates. No methitural is excreted unchanged in the urine of the dog. The cumulative action is considerably less than thiopental or thiamylal. This was demonstrated by Irwin *et al.* (1956) who repeatedly administered equivalent anesthetic doses of these agents to three groups of dogs at hourly intervals (Fig. 10-8).

After three doses of thiopental or four doses of thiamylal some animals began to exhibit incomplete recovery. Nine doses of methitural were required to produce the same effect, demonstrating that there is a lessened cumulative effect of methitural as compared with the other two thiobarbiturates.

Methitural is supplied in rubber-stoppered vials containing 1 gm. of methitural sodium plus 50 mg. of anhydrous sodium carbonate as a stabilizing buffer. A 5% aqueous solution has a pH of 10.62. The intravenous dose for the dog is 45 mg./kg. It is recommended that a 4.5% solution be prepared by dissolving the contents of a 1-gram vial in 22.5 ml. of sterile distilled water or normal saline. The resulting solution contains 45 mg./ml. and the intravenous dose for the dog is 1 ml./kg.

The entire dose should be injected in about 30 seconds, otherwise poor anesthesia results. Occasionally slight muscle twitching may be observed during induction as a result of myoneural junction stimulation. Salivation also may occur and is best prevented by preanesthetic atropine.

The intravenous dose for cats is 35 mg./kg. Intraperitoneally the dose for the cat is 85 to 100 mg./kg.; an irregular response is common.

The period of surgical anesthesia is very brief, usually not more than 10 minutes. Recovery from methitural anesthesia is quite rapid and generally without excitement. Most animals will be walking 1 hour after induction.

Clinical trials of methitural sodium have been reported by Lieberman (1958) who used 1 ml./4 lbs. of 5% solution. With preanesthetic demerol or morphine-atropine the dose was reduced to 1 ml./5 lbs. and deep anesthesia for 15 to 20 minutes was produced.

This product has not met with universal acclaim, probably because of its very short duration.

Combinations of Barbiturates

In an effort to produce an anesthetic agent intermediate in duration between the thiobarbiturates and pentobarbital, combinations of these have been developed. Two of these are Combuthal* and Pento-short*; both are mixtures of thiopental and pentobarbital. Each gram of powder contains 750 mg. of thiopental sodium and 250 mg. of pentobarbital sodium.

Depending upon the dose and rate of administration, surgical anesthesia is produced for an average of 25 to 45 minutes. The recovery period as judged by ability of the patient to stand is 1 to 3 hours and is relatively free of excitement. Advantages claimed for the mixtures are smoothness of induction, excellent anesthesia, and a smooth rapid recovery. Solutions for injection are prepared by adding 30 ml. of sterile water, normal saline or Ringer's solu-

* See Appendix A, p. 402 for manufacturer.

tion to 1 gm. of dry powder. This produces a solution containing 30 mg. ($\frac{1}{2}$ gr.) per ml. In animals weighing over 30 pounds it is suggested that only 15 ml. of diluent be used so that each ml. contains 60 mg. (1 gr.). Solutions should be stored in a refrigerator and used within 48 hours; however, clinical reports indicate that potency is maintained for as long as 10 to 14 days. Cloudy solutions or those containing recrystallized drugs should be discarded.

In clinical practice it appears that little is gained by use of mixtures such as those above.

Intravenous Injection

Barbiturates are administered by a number of routes depending upon the anesthetist, the patient, and the effect desired. For anesthesia the intravenous route is preferable since the anesthetic can be given "to effect". Because of wide variation in patient response this type of dose control is very desirable. With intrathoracic, intraperitoneal, and intramuscular administration, control is difficult since a precalculated dose must be given. The oral route is slow and unpredictable, and therefore is used chiefly when sedation is sought.

For intravenous anesthesia the cephalic vein on the anterior aspect of the forelimb is most commonly used. In dogs second choice is generally the saphenous vein on the lateral surface of the hind limb just proximal to the hock. In cats the femoral vein on the inner surface of the thigh is second choice. Other veins less frequently used are the jugular and the marginal vein of the ear. In dogs already anesthetized the lingual veins on the ventral surface of the tongue are easily accessible. There is a tendency for these to bleed rather profusely, however, following venipuncture.

Care should be taken in selection of needles and syringes for administration. In large breeds 18 or 20 gauge needles are used, since a considerable quantity of anesthetic must be injected rapidly to carry the patient through the excitement stage. In smaller animals 22 to 24 gauge needles aid in venipuncture and help slow the rate of injection. There is a careless tendency to use large syringes on very small animals. This is dangerous because the dose cannot be accurately controlled. A syringe of size commensurate with the dose should always be employed; use of large syringes with small doses is an invitation to disaster.

In very small animals (less than 5 pounds) it is advisable to dilute the anesthetic with sterile water. By making a 50% dilution more accurate dose control is achieved.

When intravenous injection is to be made, hair over the vein should be removed with clippers or scissors and the skin prepared by swabbing with a suitable antiseptic. The latter procedure, in addition to cleaning the area, tends to distend the vein.

In the dog if injection is to be made into the cephalic vein of the right foreleg, the assistant stands by the animal's left side with his left arm circling the neck and his right arm extended over the dog's back. The right hand grasps the right foreleg just below the elbow (Fig. 10–9A). The right index finger is extended over the dorsal surface of the limb, the thumb is held around the ventral surface of the leg and, by compressing thumb and forefinger, the vein is occluded causing it to distend with blood. The wrist is turned slightly so that the skin covering the dorsal aspect of the foreleg and the cephalic vein is rotated outward. The anesthetist grasps the paw of the right foot with his left hand and, if the vein is not easily seen, by rapidly squeezing the paw several times pumps blood from the paw to distend the vein. If the carpus is flexed acutely the vein is stretched tightly over the underlying muscles and rolling is prevented. Good technique demands that the needle used for injection be threaded up the vein so that the hub is at the site of venipuncture. The leg and syringe are both held in the left hand during injection so they will move as a unit if the animal moves. This prevents accidental retraction of the needle from the vein.

Persons experienced with pentobarbital administration usually estimate the weight of the animal and draw an excess of solution into a syringe. The first one-third to one-half of the dose is rapidly injected while the anesthetist watches the animal's facial expression closely. As injection is made the animal will often lick his lips as though tasting the drug. Frequently dogs move the head from side to side as the anesthetic effect begins. These movements are seen early in the course of administration and indicate more drug must be given. The eyes begin to lose their alert expression and the animal then relaxes. At this point it is usually best to lay the patient on his side without restraint so that the rate and depth of respiration can be observed.

As injection is continued, the operator can, with his thumb and forefinger placed behind the canine teeth, open the animal's jaw. If in a light state of anesthesia, the patient will further open the jaw, curl the tongue, and simulate a yawn. At this point the corneal and pedal reflexes are still present and the animal is not in a state of surgical anesthesia. Administration of anesthetic should be continued cautiously and in small amounts, with careful attention paid to the respiration and reflexes. Surgical anesthesia is reached when the pedal reflex is abolished. At this point further administration of drug is dangerous.

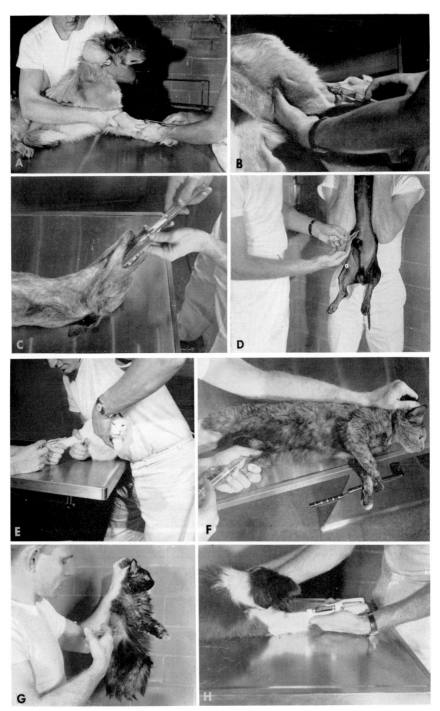

FIGURE 10–9. Methods of parenteral administration of barbiturates.
(A) Cephalic vein, dog. (B) Saphenous vein, dog. (C) Sublingual vein, dog. (D) Intraperitoneal injection, dog. (E) Cephalic vein, cat. (F) Femoral vein, cat. (G) Intra-thoracic injection, cat. (H) Method of taping syringe to limb for intermittent injections.

One should constantly bear in mind that anesthesia is most safely accomplished when administration of the final portion is done quite slowly. In many practices it is routine procedure to anesthetize the animal lightly, following which the syringe containing the agent is taped to the limb (Fig. 10–9H). A short piece of tape is applied parallel to the barrel and plunger of the syringe to prevent venous back pressure from pushing the plunger out of the barrel. At this point the animal is clipped, scrubbed, and prepared for surgery following which final administration of anesthetic is made. The syringe is left in position throughout the operation so that small increments can easily be given as needed.

Intraperitoneal Injection

Intraperitoneal injection has been employed extensively in the past, but has the disadvantage that the dose cannot be as accurately controlled as it can by intravenous administration. Usually with this method the animal is restrained by an assistant, who holds it in a vertical position against his body with the abdomen facing the anesthetist. An area just lateral to the umbilicus is clipped and a suitable antiseptic applied. The needle is then thrust through the abdominal wall and the injection made (Fig. 10–9D). The dose for intraperitoneal administration is calculated in the same manner as the intravenous. The peak concentration in the blood is reached more slowly and drug absorbed into the portal system is subject to early destruction in the liver (Corcoran and Page, 1943).

Intramuscular Injection

Under unusual circumstances, such as when wild animals are anesthetized, intramuscular or subcutaneous injection of barbiturates may be indicated. Because of their high alkalinity, there is a tendency for tissue necrosis to develop following this procedure.

Bleicher (1958) has advocated intramuscular pentobarbital sodium for basal and general anesthesia in laboratory dogs. The solution is injected in the rectus femoris muscle, care being taken to avoid the sciatic nerve. Up to 8 ml. of undiluted pentobarbital has been injected in one site. For basal anesthesia prior to ether 20 mg./kg. of body weight is used, for moderate anesthesia 30 mg./kg., and for surgical anesthesia of 1 to 2 hours 40 mg./kg. is administered. Induction requires about 15 minutes and anesthesia reaches its height about 30 minutes following injection. While this procedure is not generally acceptable in small animal practice, in certain situations it may prove expedient.

Intrathoracic Injection

Because of difficulty in restraining cats for intravenous injection, some individuals prefer to anesthetize them by injecting a barbiturate intrathoracically. The technique was first described by Sternfels (1955) who used 4% thiamylal and injected 1 ml./5 lb. of body weight. He stated that the injection should be made posterior and dorsal to the heart at the level of the 8th rib using a 25 gauge $\frac{1}{2}$-inch needle (Fig. 10–9G). With thiamylal, anesthesia develops in 4 to 6 minutes and lasts 15 to 45 minutes. No excitement occurs on induction or recovery.

Niemeyer (1958) advocated the use of pentobarbital intrathoracically and indicated that the site of injection is not too important. He preferred a low thoracic approach, 1 cm. below and 1 cm. behind the flexed elbow joint, and used the same dose as for intravenous anesthesia. He stated, "No cats have been lost as a direct result of this method, nor have we had any pulmonary complications following injections. The only objection to this method is occasional sneezing while the animal is going under the anesthetic. This is due to deep injection . . . This deep injection can be avoided by using careful technique."

On the other hand Holzworth (1958) strongly opposed intrathoracic administration of anesthetic to cats, stating there is bound to be some risk to the heart, pericardium, and lung and that barbiturate is irritating to the serosal surfaces. The latter fact can be confirmed on necropsy of animals destroyed with intrathoracic barbiturates. Enold (1962) found pleural thickening, bronchitis, and coagulative necrosis of the lung on examination of experimentally injected cats.

Administration of Thiobarbiturates

In general, thiobarbiturates are administered intravenously in the same manner as barbiturates. Thiobarbiturates produce more respiratory depression on induction than barbiturates; often one-third of the calculated dose will cause the patient to collapse and respiration to stop. This transient apnea is alarming to those not aware of this reaction. When it occurs, injection of anesthetic should be suspended until spontaneous rhythmic respirations resume. This usually occurs as soon as the blood carbon dioxide level rises and stimulates the respiratory center. Injection is then continued using the same signs to determine the depth of anesthesia as are used with barbiturates.

Intrathoracic injection of thiamylal in cats has been advocated by Sternfels (1955), whereas, intraperitoneal and intramuscular injections of the same strength do not produce sufficient anesthesia for surgical procedures. This is probably due to slower absorption.

Barbiturate Slough

Occasionally an animal may struggle during induction of barbiturate anesthesia and some of the drug may be administered perivascularly. This should be avoided because of the possibility of a tissue slough developing. Experienced anesthetists prevent this by threading the needle up the vein. This makes it unlikely that the needle will come out of the vein if the syringe is jarred or the animal moves. Sloughs due to anesthesia require from 2 to 4 weeks to heal and leave an unsightly scar. Nothing can infuriate an owner more than development of a slough in his animal.

If it is suspected that barbiturate solution has been injected perivascularly, the area should be infiltrated with 1 or 2 ml. of 2% procaine solution. According to Elder and Harrison (1944) there are two reasons for procaine to be effective in this condition. First, procaine is a vasodilator and prevents vasospasm in the area; it thus aids in dilution and absorption of the barbiturate. Second, procaine is broken down by an alkaline medium and in this reaction the alkali (barbiturate) is neutralized.

References

ANDERSON, E. G. and MAGEE, D. F.: A Study of the Mechanism of the Effect of Dietary Fat in Decreasing Thiopental Sleeping Time. J. Pharm. & Exper. Therap., *117*, 281, 1956.

ARAÑEZ, J. B. and FORTEZA, T. F.: Kemithal Sodium as a General Anesthetic for Dogs. J.A.V.M.A., *127*, 411, 1955.

ARAÑEZ, J. B. and TACAL, J. V., JR.: Kemithal Sodium as a General Anaesthetic for Cats. Indian Vet. J., *34*, 7, 1957.

BLAKE, W. D.: Some Effects of Pentobarbital and Anesthesia on Renal Hemodynamics, Water and Electrolyte Excretion in the Dog. Am. J. Physiol., *191*, 393, 1957.

BLEICHER, N.: Intramuscular Nembutal in Canine Anesthesia. Vet. Med., *53*, 372, 1958.

BOOKER, W. M., MALONEY, A. H., TUREMAN, J. R., and RATLIFF, C.: Some Metabolic Factors Influencing the Course of Thiopental Anesthesia in Dogs. Am. J. Physiol., *170*, 168, 1952.

BRODIE, B. B., BERNSTEIN, E., and MARK, L. C.: The Role of Body Fat in Limiting the Duration of Action of Thiopental. J. Pharm. & Exper. Therap., *105*, 421, 1952.

BUTLER, T. C., MAHAFFEE, D., and MAHAFFEE, C.: The Role of the Liver in the Metabolic Disposition of Methobarbital. J. Pharm. & Exper. Therap., *106*, 364, 1952.

CARRINGTON, H. C. and RAVENTOS, J.: Kemithal: A New Intravenous Anaesthetic. Brit. J. Pharmacol., *1*, 215, 1946.

CORCORAN, A. C., and PAGE, I. H.: Effects of Anesthetic Dosage of Pentobarbital Sodium on Renal Function and Blood Pressure in Dogs. Am. J. Physiol., *140*, 234, 1943.

DILLE, J. M., LINEGAR, C. R., and KOPPANYI, T.: Studies on Barbiturates. XII. Factors Governing the Distribution of Barbiturates. J. Pharm. & Exper. Therap., *55*, 46, 1935.

EDDS, G. T. and TRACE, J. C.:   A New General Anesthetic for Small Animals. Vet.
    Med., *49*, 81, 1954.
ELDER, C. K. and HARRISON, E. M.:   Pentothal Sodium Slough. Prevention by Pro-
    caine Hydrochloride. J.A.M.A., *125*, 116, 1944.
ENOLD, G. L.:   Pathologic Effects of Intrathoracic Barbiturate Anesthesia in Cats.
    J.A.V.M.A., *140*, 795, 1962.
GRACA, J. G. and GARST, E. L.:   Early Blood Changes in Dogs Following Intravenous
    Pentobarbital Anesthesia. Anesthesiology, *18*, 461, 1957.
HARRIS, J. R. and HYDER, N.:   The Use of Secobarbital Sodium and Mephenesin as an
    Anesthetic for Dogs. J.A.V.M.A., *123*, 297, 1953.
HAUSNER, E., ESSEX, H. E., and MANN, F. C.:   Roentgenologic Observations of the
    Spleen of the Dog under Ether, Sodium Amytal, Pentobarbital Sodium and Pen-
    tothal Sodium Anesthesia. Am. J. Physiol., *121*, 387, 1938.
HELRICH, M., PAPPER, E. M., and ROVENSTINE, E. A.: Surital Sodium: A New Anesthetic
    Agent for Intravenous Use. Preliminary Clinical Evaluation. Anesthesiology, *11*,
    33, 1950.
HOLZWORTH, J.:   Intrathoracic Administration of General Anesthesia.   Modern Vet.
    Practice, *39*, 48, 1958.
IRWIN, S., STAGG, R. D., DUNBAR, E., and GOVIER, W. M.:   Methitural, a New In-
    travenous Anesthetic: Comparison with Thiopental in the Cat, Dog and Monkey.
    J. Pharm. & Exper. Therap., *116*, 317, 1956.
JONES, L. M.:   *Veterinary Pharmacology and Therapeutics.* 2d ed.   The Iowa State Col-
    lege Press, Ames, Iowa, 1957.
LAMSON, P. D., GREIG, M. E., and HOBDY, C. J.: Modification of Barbiturate Anesthesia
    by Glucose, Intermediary Metabolites, and Certain Other Substances. J. Pharm. &
    Exper. Therap., *103*, 460, 1951.
LAMSON, P. D., GREIG, M. E., and WILLIAMS, L.:   Potentiation by Epinephrine of the
    Anesthetic Effect in Chloral and Barbiturate Anesthesia.   J. Pharm. & Exper.
    Therap., *106*, 219, 1952.
LIEBERMAN, L. L.:   An Ultrashort-Acting Anesthetic. Vet. Med., *53*, 601, 1958.
MAYNERT, E. W. and VAN DYKE, H. B.:   The Absence of Localization of Barbital in
    Divisions of the Central Nervous System. J. Pharm. & Exper. Therap., *98*, 184, 1950.
MYLON, E., WINTERNITZ, M. C., and DE SUTO-NAGY, G. J.:   Studies on Therapy in
    Traumatic Shock. Am. J. Physiol., *139*, 313, 1943.
NIEMEYER, K. H.:   Intrathoracic Anesthesia. Modern Vet. Practice., *39*, 12, 1958.
REUTNER, T. F. and GRUHZIT, O. M.:   Surital Sodium a New Anesthetic and Hypnotic:
    Studies in Dogs. J.A.V.M.A., *113*, 357, 1948.
ROBINSON, M. H.:   Deterioration of Solutions of Pentothal Sodium. Anesthesiology, *8*,
    166, 1947.
SHARAF, A. E. A.:   Medical (Soluble Veronal) Hypnosis Anaesthesia and Toxicity in
    Dogs. Brit. Vet. J., *103*, 358, 1947.
SHIDEMAN, F. E., KELLY, A. R., and ADAMS, B. J.:   The Role of the Liver in the Detoxi-
    cation of Thiopental (Pentothal) and Two Other Barbiturates. J. Pharm. & Exper.
    Therap., *91*, 331, 1947.
STERNFELS, M.:   Intrathoracic Anesthesia in Cats. Vet. Med., *50*, 365, 1955.
SWANSON, E. E.:   Sodium 5-Allyl-5-(1-Methylbutyl)-2-Thiobarbiturate, A Short
    Acting Anaesthetic. J. Pharmacy and Pharmacol., *3*, 112, 1951.
SWANSON, E. E. and SHONLE, H. A.:   The Oral, Rectal and Intravenous Administration
    of Sodium Iso-Amyl-Ethyl-Barbiturate (Sodium Amytal). J. Pharm. & Exper.
    Therap., *41*, 289, 1931.
TAYLOR, J. D., RICHARDS, R. K., and TABERN, D. L.:   Metabolism of S[35] Thiopental
    (Pentothal). J. Pharm. & Exper. Therap., *104*, 93, 1952.
VAN DYKE, H. B., SCUDI, J. V., and TABERN, D. L.:   The Excretion of N[15] in the Urine
    of Dogs after the Administration of Labeled Pentobarbital. J. Pharm. & Exper.
    Therap., *90*, 364, 1947.
WEAVER, L. C., BURCH, G. R., ABREU, B. E., and RICHARDS, A. B.:   A Study of the
    Anesthetic Properties of Combinations of Hexobarbital Sodium and Thialbarbitone
    Sodium in Dogs. Am. J. Vet. Res., *19*, 940, 1958.
WIEDLING, S.:   A Simple Method for Direct Comparison of the Depressant Effect of the
    Barbiturates on the Respiration and Circulation. Nature (London), *162*, 1003, 1948.

Woods, L. A., Wyngaarden, J. B., Rennick, B., and Seevers, M. H.: The Cardiovascular Effects of Sodium Pentothal and Sodium 5-Allyl-5-(1-Methylbutyl)-2-Thiobarbiturate in the Dog. Fed. Proc., 6, 387, 1947.

Woods, L. A., Wyngaarden, J. B., Rennick, B., and Seevers, M. H.: Cardiovascular Toxicity of Thiobarbiturates: Comparison of Thiopental and 5-Allyl-5(1-Methylbutyl)-2-Thiobarbiturate (Surital) in Dogs. J. Pharm. & Exper. Therap., 95, 328, 1949.

Wyngaarden, J. B., Woods, L. A., and Seevers, M. H.: The Cumulative Action of Certain Thiobarbiturates in Dogs. Fed. Proc., 6, 388, 1947.

OTHER METHODS OF PRODUCING GENERAL ANESTHESIA

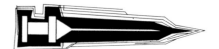

Chapter 11

Chloral Hydrate
Chlorobutanol (Chloretone)
Chloralose
Urethane (Ethyl Carbamate)
Paraldehyde
Magnesium Sulfate

Tribromoethanol Solution (Avertin)
Hydroxydione Sodium (Viadril)
Hypothermia
Induction of Hypothermia in the Dog
Cardiopulmonary Bypass Techniques
Electronarcosis

WHILE the anesthetic agents previously described are those most commonly employed, a number of miscellaneous agents and techniques may be used for general anesthesia under special circumstances. Several drugs are used for anesthesia of laboratory animals which do not find application in routine clinical use. Among them are chloral hydrate, chlorobutanol, chloralose, urethane, paraldehyde, and magnesium sulfate. Tribromoethanol has been used in a number of wild species, while hydroxydione, a steroid anesthetic, is more a curiosity than a clinical tool. Some of the procedures hereafter described, such as hypothermia and electronarcosis, are still in the developmental stage and may in the future find more widespread application in the clinic.

Chloral Hydrate, U.S.P.

Liebrich, who introduced chloral hydrate as a hypnotic in 1869, thought that because it released chloroform *in vitro* it would do the same *in vivo*. This has subsequently been proven a misconception. The use of chloral hydrate in small animals was abandoned long ago in the United States. However, in France and some other countries it has been used until recently.

Chloral hydrate occurs as colorless translucent crystals which volatilize on exposure to air with an aromatic, penetrating odor. It has a bitter, caustic taste. One gram of the crystals will dissolve in 0.25 ml. of water. It may be administered orally, or solutions may be injected intravenously or intraperitoneally. It is irritant to the gastric mucosa and may cause vomiting if not diluted in water, but is readily absorbed from the gastrointestinal tract. A small amount of chloral hydrate is excreted unchanged in the urine. The greater portion is reduced to trichlorethyl alcohol, a less potent hypnotic, and this is in turn conjugated with glycuronic acid to form urochloralic (trichlorethylglycuronic) acid which has no hynotic property. The latter is excreted in the urine. In animals with liver damage, chloral hydrate may be found in larger quantities and urochloralic acid in smaller quantities in the urine.

Chloral hydrate depresses the cerebrum with loss of reflex excitability. In subanesthetic doses, motor and sensory nerves are not affected. Chloral hydrate is a good hypnotic, but a poor anesthetic since it produces deep sleep which lasts for several hours. It has very weak analgesic action. In hypnotic doses, the medullary centers are not affected. Anesthetic doses of chloral hydrate depress the vasomotor center severely, resulting in a fall in blood pressure. Hypnotic doses depress respiration and anesthetic doses markedly depress the respiratory center. Death from chloral hydrate administration is caused by progressive depression of the respiratory center. The margin of safety is such that it is not a satisfactory surgical anesthetic.

When given to dogs in a 30% solution intravenously, at a rate of 0.3 gm./kg. of body weight, anesthesia lasting 60 to 85 minutes is produced (Mahmoud and Kamel, 1953). Salivation, defecation, micturition and vomition may occur. The muscles are relaxed and the reflexes absent, the pedal reflex being the last to disappear. The pupils are contracted, respiratory rate diminished, pulse weak and temperature depressed.

Chlorobutanol, U.S.P. (Chloretone)

Chlorobutanol occurs as colorless crystals which are sparingly soluble in water and readily soluble in alcohol. It has been administered orally or intravenously for anesthesia in laboratory animals. The MLD for dogs is 238 mg./kg. orally. It formerly was used as a sedative and hypnotic, but currently is used chiefly as a preservative for various solutions, particularly those for parenteral administration.

Chloralose

Chloralose is prepared by heating anhydrous glucose and trichloroacetaldehyde (anhydrous chloral) in a water bath. Both alpha and beta chloralose are formed, the alpha form being the active fraction. It has been used in studies of the baroreceptor reflexes since it produces a higher blood pressure and more active reflexes than other agents (Brown and Hilton, 1956).

Chloralose is usually prepared as a 1.0% aqueous solution. Heat is necessary to dissolve the drug but solutions should not be boiled. The intravenous anesthetic dose for dogs of alpha chloralose is approximately 0.11 gm./kg. For adult cats it is 36 mg./lb. (King and Unna, 1954).

Urethane, N. F. (Ethyl Carbamate)

Urethane is prepared by heating urea with alcohol under pressure or by warming urea nitrate with alcohol and sodium nitrite. The drug is marketed in the crystalline state. One gram dissolves in 0.5 ml. of water, the aqueous solution being neutral. It is most often used as an anesthetic in laboratory animals and fish. The lethal intravenous dose for rabbits is 2.0 gm./kg. The dose for dogs and cats is 0.6 to 2.0 gm. Up to 500 mg./kg. may be used as a hypnotic dose. Mice given urethane develop an exceptionally high incidence of lung tumors, regardless of the route of administration. Tumors also develop in treated rats and rabbits. There are no known instances where lung tumors have developed in humans from urethane. However, until further work is done, there is definite justification for concern over the health of individuals in prolonged contact with urethane or its solutions (Wood, 1956).

Paraldehyde, U.S.P.

Paraldehyde is a polymer of acetaldehyde. In hypnotic doses, it has a wide margin of safety because it depresses only the cerebrum and not the medullary centers. When given to dogs at a rate of 2 ml./kg./minute intravenously, a 9% aqueous solution may cause hemoglobinuria. The LD_{50} for dogs is 3.5 gm./kg.

Magnesium Sulfate

Dilute aqueous solutions of magnesium sulfate can be used to produce surgical anesthesia in small animals; however, all parts of the central nervous system are depressed and the result is often fatal respiratory arrest. For this reason, and since it is relatively inexpensive, the drug is used principally for euthanasia, a saturated solution being administered intravenously. Its effect, however, is not as desirable as that achieved with the barbiturates, animals sometimes showing a period of excitement prior to collapse.

Magnesium anesthesia can be counteracted by intravenous injection of a soluble calcium salt such as calcium gluconate or calcium chloride. Animals so treated will show an immediate and almost total recovery. Combined neostigmine (0.35–0.63 mg./kg.) and pentylenetetrazol (10 mg./kg.) intravenously will produce the same result in rabbits (Borglin and Lindsten, 1949).

About 70% of injected magnesium sulfate is excreted by the kidneys in 48 hours.

Tribromoethanol Solution, U.S.P. (Avertin)

Tribromoethanol is a white crystalline powder, slightly soluble in water. Therefore, it is dissolved in amylene hydrate to form a solution containing 100 gm. of tribromoethylene in each 100 ml. of solution. For administration, this stock solution is dissolved in warm distilled water (40° C.) to make the desired strength of solution (usually 2.5 or 3%).

Because it is easily decomposed by light and high temperatures, the solution must be tested prior to use by addition of one drop of Congo red to 5 ml. of solution. A purple color develops at a pH below 5 indicating decomposition to dibromoacetic aldehyde and hydrobromic acid. If these are present the solution should be discarded.

Tribromoethanol solution may be given either orally or rectally, neither method giving accurate dose control. For dogs the dose is 400–600 mg./kg. and for cats 300 mg./kg.

The solution is rapidly absorbed; the onset of narcosis is evident in 2 or 3 minutes and the maximum effect is attained in approximately 15 minutes. The duration is maximal for about 2 hours.

Both blood pressure and respirations are reduced with tribromoethanol anesthesia. Death is due to respiratory failure.

Tribromoethanol is conjugated with glucuronic acid in the liver and excreted in the urine as tribromoethyl glucuronide. For this reason the drug is contraindicated in hepatic or kidney disease. It is also to be avoided where toxemia, septicemia, or dehydration are present. Amylene hydrate, the solvent, is eliminated unchanged in urine and from the lungs. Delayed toxic effects resembling those seen with chloroform have been reported, including renal and hepatic damage.

Rectal administration in cats is accomplished by inserting a rubber tube through the anus approximately 6 inches into the colon. The solution is then injected and the hindquarters elevated until narcosis develops. It is not necessary to empty the colon prior to injection and enemas are contraindicated (Wright and Hall, 1961).

When given rectally to healthy cats tribromoethanol has a mortality rate of approximately 2% (Wright, 1952). Sodium thiosulfate is an antidote and should be given at the rate of 40 ml. of 25% solution per rectum for each 1 ml. of the drug. Other resuscitative measures such as artificial respiration are, of course, also indicated.

Hydroxydione Sodium (Viadril)

Hydroxydione is a steroid hypnotic and basal anesthetic agent. It occurs as a crystalline solid and forms an aqueous solution with a pH of 7.8 to 10.2. When administered orally or intravenously it will produce surgical anesthesia in mice, rats, rabbits, dogs, and monkeys (P'An *et al.*, 1955). One hundred mg./kg. intravenously produces surgical anesthesia for an average of 1 hour in dogs. It has a high therapeutic index for mice as shown in Table 11–1. There is a relatively mild degree of respiratory and cardiac depression as compared with thiopental. No hormonal effects have been demonstrated with this agent despite its steroid structure.

Table 11–1.—Comparative Anesthetic Effect of Hydroxydione and Thiopental Sodium in Mice, Rats, and Rabbits

Compound	Animal Species	Sex of Animal	Route of Administration	AD_{50}	LD_{50}	T.I.*
Hydroxydione				mg./kg.	mg./kg.	
	Mice	Male	I.V.	21.5	250.0	11.6
	Rats	Male	I.V.	24.5	190.0	7.8
	Mice	Male	Oral	100.0	1200.0	12.0
	Rats	Male	Oral	155.0	700.0	4.5
	Rabbits	Male	I.V.	15.0	95.0	6.3
Thiopental sodium	Mice	Male	I.V.	17.5	80.0	4.6
	Mice	Male	Oral	100.0	208.0	2.1
	Rats	Male	I.V.	24.0	61.0	2.5
	Rats	Male	Oral	75.0	117.0	1.6

* T.I. = Therapeutic index = LD_{50}/AD_{50}

(From P'An, S.Y., Gardocki, J. F., Hutcheon, D. E., Rudel, H., Kodet, M. J., and Laubach, G. D.: General Anesthetic and Other Pharmacological Properties of a Soluble Steroid, 21-Hydroxypregnanedione Sodium Succinate. J. Pharm. & Exper. Therap., *115*, 432, 1955.)

Hydroxydione is rapidly inactivated in the liver, but the anesthetic activity is not prolonged by liver damage (P'An *et al.*, 1955).

Two and one-half to 5% solutions may be used. Because of its highly irritant nature hydroxydione tends to produce phlebitis when given intravenously and should never be injected perivascularly.

To date this drug has not been used to any extent clinically in small animals and remains largely a pharmacological curiosity.

Hypothermia

As the body temperature of a warm-blooded animal falls, there is a reduction in metabolism and, therefore, a diminished need for oxygen. Bigelow *et al.* (1950) found that oxygen uptake in dogs is reduced by approximately 50% at 30 °C. and 65% at 25 °C. Thus the heart, brain, liver, or other vital organ can survive at a low temperature for a considerably increased period of time when deprived of all or a portion of its blood supply. Hypothermia may be artifically produced in the entire body, or in only a portion such as the heart or head. While it has been tried in many situations, it has found its greatest usefulness in surgery of the heart and central nervous system.

It would seem at first glance that the colder an animal was made to become the less oxygen would be required by a given organ. This has been suggested by Lynn *et al.* (1954) who postulated that at 10°

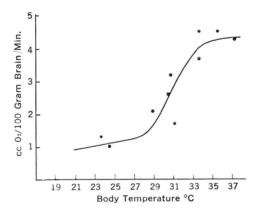

FIGURE 11–1.   Relation of oxygen uptake by the brain to temperature. (From Bering, E. A., Jr., Taren, J. A., McMurray, J. D., and Bernhard, W. F.: Surg. Gynec. & Obstet., *102*, 134, 1956.)

C. the oxygen uptake would be zero. It has been shown, however, that there is a variation in reduced oxygen consumption for different organs. For example, the work done by the heart at 26 to 27° C. is little less than that at normal temperature, and while the general oxygen uptake by the body at this temperature is reduced to 40% of normal, that of the heart is still 50%. Bering *et al.* (1956), working with monkeys, found little change in cerebral oxygen uptake until a temperature of 31° C. is reached. At this point it falls sharply and through the next 4° there is a drop of about 25%. Below 27° C. oxygen consumption continues to fall but at a much slower rate. The relationship of oxygen consumption to temperature was shown to be S-shaped rather than linear (Fig. 11–1).

Several species of warm-blooded animals have been subjected to drastic hypothermia. It has been found possible to cool small laboratory animals to 0° C., and even lower, followed by recovery. Andjus and Lovelock (1955) reported 80 to 100% recovery in rats after cooling to temperatures just above the freezing point with cardiac and respiratory arrest for 1 hour. Smith (1956) kept golden hamsters "on ice" with circulatory arrest for up to 7 hours. These animals even survived super-cooling to –5 or –6° C. When the circulation has been maintained with a pump-oxygenator, dogs have survived cooling to 1.5° C. (Gollan *et al.*, 1955). Niazi and Lewis (1957) anesthetized 6 adult monkeys with thiopental and reduced the body temperature to between 4 and 9° C. Cardiac standstill occurred when the body temperature reached 14 to 11° C. and lasted for periods of 42 minutes to 2 hours. Five of the monkeys survived and appeared normal.

In order to induce the hypothermic state as quickly as possible, it is necessary to control shivering. Claude Bernard in 1876 indicated that shivering increased metabolism and was an important mechanism in protection against cold. Shivering is induced by an increased temperature gradient between cold receptors in the skin and centers in the hypothalamus (Davis and Mayer, 1955). Even without visible shivering there is general hypertonicity of the skeletal muscles, which results in increased metabolic, heart, and respiratory rates. Shivering can be prevented by deep anesthesia, or light anesthesia with curarization or tranquilization (promazine, chlorpromazine). The latter drugs are thought to exert their effect through a peripheral action on muscle fibers and on the hypothalamic temperature control center.

Three methods of whole-body cooling have been utilized: (1) surface, (2) body cavity, and (3) extracorporeal. Surface cooling is usually accomplished by direct immersion of the unprotected body in ice water or by placing the body on a mattress through which ice water is circulated. Hyperventilation is maintained throughout the procedure to keep the blood pH on the alkaline side of normal. This has been shown to reduce cardiac arrhythmias and fibrillation. Below 28° C. (82.4° F.) no anesthetic is needed and the patient is maintained on artificial ventilation alone. Active cooling is stopped when approximately two-thirds of the desired temperature fall has been accomplished. Otherwise, the temperature will continue to drop once the desired degree of hypothermia has been reached.

Body cavity cooling is accomplished by pouring cold saline solution into the open thoracic cavity (Blades and Pierpont, 1954). This method has the disadvantage of being slow and requiring large volumes of saline solution. In addition, cold saline solution comes into direct contact with the heart and cardiac irregularities are common. Intragastric cooling, performed by running cold water into a balloon inserted in the stomach, has been used in animals and man (Khalil and MacKeith, 1954). This method also is slow since the total surface area of the balloon is small.

Extracorporeal cooling can be accomplished by running blood from a cannulated artery through tubing immersed in a cooling medium and returning it to the venous system (Boerema *et al.*, 1951). A pump is required to force the blood through the system. Lucas (1956) has suggested that a jar filled with a mixture of carbon dioxide snow, saline, and alcohol be used as the coolant. Thrombosis is prevented by administration of heparin.

Extracorporeal cooling has been used to lower the brain temperature below that of the general body temperature. Kimoto *et al.* (1956) developed this method in dogs, cannulating the carotid artery with polyethylene tubing so that the blood could pass through a cooling coil and return to the distal artery. With this technique the brain temperature is lowered to 14° C. while body temperature remains at 31 or 32° C.

Extracorporeal cooling carries with it the dangers of hemolysis and interference with the blood coagulation mechanism. It also presents the hazard of thrombosis. The most obvious advantage is that it provides the best control over body temperature and rewarming can be carried out quickly and efficiently.

With other methods warming is accomplished by covering the patient with blankets and by application of heat. Patients are sometimes heated rapidly by the use of warm water baths or diathermy; the latter, however, is somewhat dangerous and its use is not suggested.

Since hypothermic anesthesia is a form of general anesthesia, it has all the risks involved in this procedure. In addition, it has its own hazards which may be grouped under (1) the circulatory system, (2) the skin and internal organs, and (3) the metabolism.

Blood pressure falls during hypothermia due to decreased cardiac output and vasodilation. Occasional severe drops in blood pressure may occur. The fall in heart rate seen with hypothermia is due to depression of the SA node and bundle of His. These conduction changes are manifested by a prolongation of the PR interval, spreading of the QRS complex, and lengthening of the ST interval. In dogs a cardiac crisis occurs between 23 and 15° C. This is characterized by cessation of sinus rhythm, intense bradycardia, ventricular extrasystoles, and ventricular fibrillation. Atropine does not relieve the bradycardia. Ventricular fibrillation has been shown to occur most often when the temperature of the heart muscle is below 28° C. and when the heart is manipulated. It occurs less frequently in young animals than in adults. Hypercarbia with acidemia, hyperkalemia, and myocardial hypoxia appear to cause fibrillation also.

The incidence of spontaneous ventricular fibrillation has been shown to vary with the anesthetic used to initiate hypothermia. Pentobarbital results in a higher incidence than does thiopental or ether (Covino et al., 1954). Cyclopropane also produces a high rate of arrhythmias (Steinhaus et al., 1959).

Several drugs have been used in an effort to prevent fibrillation. Among these are procaine, neostigmine, and acetylcholine. Covino and Hegnauer (1956) reported that 2-diethylaminoethyl-isonicotinimide (Ambonestyl) reduced the incidence of ventricular fibrillation during ventriculotomy in acidotic dogs at 25 to 23° C. from 80 to 30%. Combined with hyperventilation, fibrillation was completely prevented.

An important blood change during hypothermia is alteration in coagulation. In addition, there is a decrease in platelets, hemoconcentration, reduction in eosinophil and leukocyte counts, with a fall in the mean corpuscular hemoglobin concentration.

Knocker (1955) has shown that hypothermia causes severe damage to the liver, kidneys, and adrenal glands in dogs when temperatures of around 25° C. are maintained for hours. Short periods of cooling, however, do not appear to cause demonstrable damage.

Hypothermia has been used for surgery of the heart and great vessels, brain and spinal cord, in some other surgical procedures, in treatment of shock, and to prevent brain damage following a severe hypoxic episode. The chief factor limiting its use in heart surgery is that the maximum time of circulatory arrest at 28° C. cannot be over 10 minutes, because of hypoxic brain damage. For this reason older patients and those with cardiac defects requiring extensive repair should be managed with some form of heart-lung bypass. The greatest application for hypothermia in man is in neurosurgery. Here it is often combined with induced hypotension. While hypothermia has been used in dogs for removal of heartworms and repair of cardiac anomalies, its use is not widespread. This is probably due to the fact that considerable equipment and trained personnel are required to perform the technique safely and efficiently.

Induction of Hypothermia in the Dog

To produce hypothermia in the dog 1 mg./lb. of promazine is given intravenously as a preanesthetic agent. Thiamylal is injected for general anesthesia following which an endotracheal catheter is inserted and halothane is used for maintenance. A slow intravenous drip of 5% dextrose is started, and 2 mg./kg. of gallamine is given in the drip tubing to abolish respirations. Artificial respiration is then started.

The animal is positioned on its back in a sink, bathtub, or other container, with its head and feet above the proposed water level (Fig. 11–2). An electronic thermometer is placed in the esophagus and needle electrodes of an ECG machine inserted in the feet. From this point constant monitoring of the ECG on an oscilloscope is desirable since cardiac fibrillation may occur at any time during the cooling period and requires immediate corrective measures.

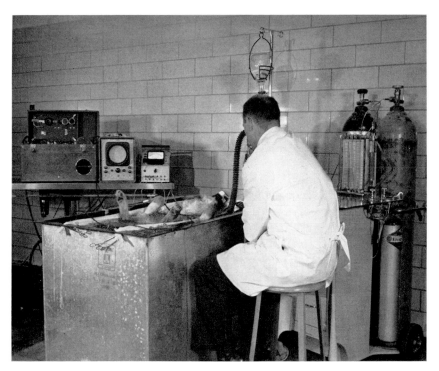

FIGURE 11–2. Induction of hypothermia in a dog. An electrocardiograph with coupled oscilloscope (left) monitors the heart. A multichannel thermometer, with probes in the patient's esophagus and rectum, determines temperature of the patient's body and the water bath. Oxygen and halothane are administered by means of the gas machine at right.

Ice water is used for rapid cooling. It should be constantly agitated by hand or with a pump. The dog should be removed from the bath before the desired body temperature is reached, since it will continue to decline after removal from the water. Generally an intraesophageal temperature of 85° F. (30° C.) is optimum since cardiac fibrillation commonly occurs at temperatures below 82° F. (28° C.).

After removal from the water the dog should be dried with towels and placed on a heating pad during the operative period. Rewarming can then be started as soon as closure of the surgical wound is begun. While seldom necessary, for quick rewarming the animal can be placed in a warm water bath. As anesthesia is discontinued and shivering commences, the body temperature quickly begins to rise. If the operation is short, rewarming in a water bath may be necessary along with administration of atropine and edrophonium to reverse the paralysis produced by gallamine.

Cardiopulmonary Bypass Techniques

As previously mentioned, in order to do lengthy intracardiac surgery various bypass techniques have been developed. The advantage is that the surgeon is able to visualize directly the operative field within the bloodless heart. Hypothermia alone does not allow this procedure for more than 10 minutes. Cardiopulmonary bypass may be performed in conjunction with hypothermia or without the latter; however, the use of extracorporeal circulation with hypothermia reduces the work load of the heart and enables periods of cardioplegia for as long as 60 minutes (Sealy *et al.*, 1961).

Heart-lung preparations consist essentially of two pieces of equipment, an oxygenator which is a substitute for the patient's lungs, and a pump (or pumps) which substitute for the heart. The simplest oxygenators are those in which oxygen is bubbled directly through the blood and are available as disposable units (Fig. 11–3). Other more complicated oxygenators involving semipermeable membranes, screens over which the blood streams, and rotating disks are also in use. Two types of pumps are commonly employed, one in which the action is intermittent, the other in which blood is forced through an elastic tube by the action of rollers or fingers. To initiate this technique, a thoracotomy is performed and the patient heparinized by intravenous administration of 1.5 mg./kg. of heparin. The oxygenator and tubing are primed with 5% dextrose solution or 5% dextrose in 0.2% sodium chloride solution (Cooley *et al.*, 1962). The latter is more isotonic, minimizing hemolysis and the tendency toward hyponatremia which occurs postoperatively when 5% dextrose is used. Catheters are inserted in the anterior and posterior vena cava and blood is withdrawn, run through the oxygenator, and pumped into the aorta via the femoral artery (Fig. 11–4). In dogs flow rates seldom exceed 75 mg./kg./minute. The aorta is clamped distal to the sinus of Valsalva to prevent retrograde flow. As the heart is opened, blood is removed from it by suction and returned to the system through a separate inlet. During the bypass procedure, blood in the oxygenator is warmed by infrared lamps if normothermia is to be maintained.

When the cardiac surgery is completed, the aortic clamp is removed, blood in the oxygenator is pumped into the patient, the cannulae are removed, and the chest incision closed. Utilizing a heart-lung bypass, the accepted upper limit of ischemia of the dog's heart at normothermia is 20 minutes (Wesowski *et al.*, 1952).

Two techniques have been devised to give a completely flaccid heart during surgery. With mild hypothermia (28° C.) and bypass apparatus, the heart can be arrested by injection of a solution of potassium citrate (0.8%), magnesium sulfate (2.47%), and prostigmine (0.001%). To accomplish this the aorta is mobilized and

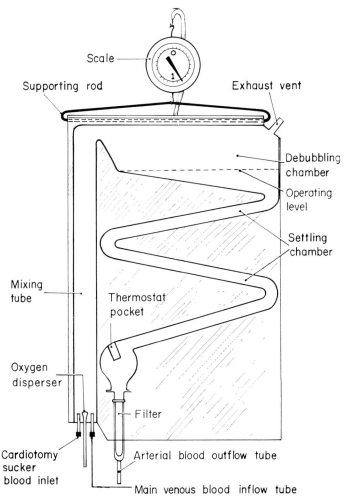

FIGURE 11–3. Schematic drawing of a plastic sheet oxygenator suspended from a spring scale. Venous blood from the patient enters the bottom of the mixing tube where it is oxygenated. It then flows through the debubbling chamber and into the settling chamber, from which it is pumped to the patient. The scale makes it possible to maintain a constant blood volume in the unit. Heat loss is controlled by directing infrared heat lamps on the settling chamber. (From Gott, V. L., Sellers, R. D., DeWall, R. A., Varco, R. L., and Lillehei, C. W.: A Disposable Unitized Plastic Sheet Oxygenator for Open Heart Surgery. Dis. Chest., *32*, 615, 1957.)

clamped about 2 inches distal to the heart and the solution injected proximal to the clamp so that it enters the coronary arteries. With this technique the heart will withstand 30 to 60 minutes of ischemia. When the operation is complete the clamp is removed from the aorta, blood from the heart-lung machine flushes out the solution, and the

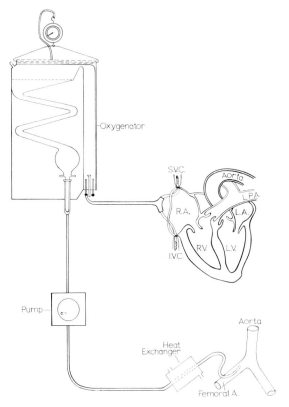

FIGURE 11–4. Schematic diagram of cardiopulmonary bypass apparatus. Venous blood is collected by gravity from the superior and inferior vena cava (S.V.C., I.V.C.), oxygenated, and pumped into the femoral artery. A heat exchanger may be used to maintain or lower the temperature of the blood as desired. (R.A. = right atrium, R.V. = right ventricle, L.A. = left atrium, L.V. = left ventricle.)

heart beat resumes.   Paradoxically, use of potassium citrate at normothermia is harmful.

Recent work indicates that ventricular fibrillation, while undesirable, is not as serious as was formerly assumed. Thus deep hypothermia alone (7° C.) has been used to cause cardioplegia. Many hearts on rewarming will spontaneously resume a normal beat and those which fibrillate can be successfully managed with massage and electrical defibrillation. Since effective heart action stops at temperatures below 25° C., no attempt at electrical defibrillation should be made until the heart temperature rises to 28° C.

Protamine sulfate is given intravenously to neutralize the anticoagulant effect of heparin. It is available in 1% solution. The dose is 1 to 2 times the amount of heparin previously administered. Occasionally, protamine may cause a dangerous hypotension.

Hexadimethrine bromide may also be used to neutralize heparin after cardiac surgery. It is available in an isotonic aqueous solution containing 10 mg./ml. The recommended dose is 1 mg. for each 100 U.S.P. units of heparin.* The required quantity of solution should be diluted with isotonic saline or 5% dextrose solution to give a final concentration of 1 mg./ml. of solution. The dose should be given intravenously over a period of 10 to 15 minutes.

Electronarcosis

Passage of electricity through the brain to produce anesthesia has been investigated for many years. In the veterinary field, clinical trials were conducted by Sir Frederic Hobday in England as early as 1932. Despite considerable research, much remains to be learned about this technique before it can be applied generally for small animal anesthesia. It may be of greatest use in situations where prolonged anesthesia is required.

Direct, pulsating direct, and alternating current have been used to produce electronarcosis. Early workers were bothered by respiratory depression, convulsions, and fatalities. Recently, alternating current of 700 cycles, 35 to 50 milliamperes, and approximately 40 volts has been employed (Hardy et al., 1961). Others have used combined direct and alternating current, modified to produce a rectangular wave of 1.0 to 1.4 milliseconds duration, with a frequency of 100 waves per second (Smith et al., 1961a). Most instruments deliver the current through electrodes applied to the head (Fig. 11–5). Continuous electrode contact is important to maintain anesthesia. Individual variation among dogs requires that the current be adjusted for each according to the response observed.

Electrical anesthesia is characterized by convulsions on induction unless a muscle relaxant is first administered. An exception to this is the method of Smith et al. (1961a), which employs direct current for induction and then both direct and alternating current. Profuse salivation develops on induction and continues throughout. This can be counteracted by use of atropine. Endotracheal intubation should always be performed. Hyperthermia, probably due to disturbance of the thermoregulatory center in the hypothalamus, is commonly seen. The EEG immediately following anesthesia is de-

---

* U.S.P. XV requires heparin to have a potency of not less than 110 units/mg.

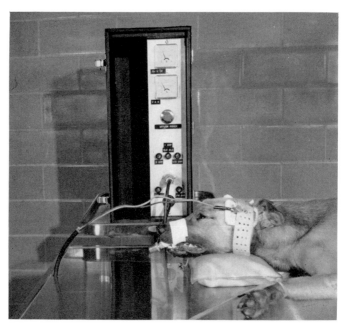

FIGURE 11–5.—Electronarcosis. An electrode is placed on either side of the head and held with a latex strap. Contact is enhanced by use of plastic foam pads soaked with ECG electrode solution. An endotracheal catheter is inserted to maintain a patent airway. (Courtesy of Dr. R. A. Herin, Colorado State University, Fort Collins, Colorado.)

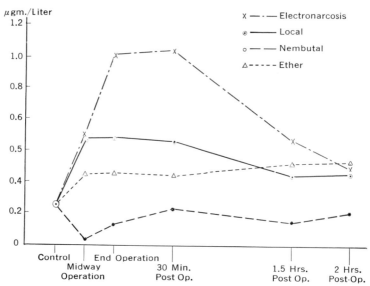

FIGURE 11–6.   Epinephrine secretion in response to a standard laparotomy: A comparison of different agents for anesthesia. The points on each curve represent the average values from seven dogs. Electronarcosis and laparotomy produced the greatest rise in epinephrine secretion, with response to procaine and to ether next in order, respectively. Nembutal depressed the epinephrine level of plasma despite the associated surgery. (From Hardy, J. D., Carter, T. and Turner, M. D.:   Catechol Amine Metabolism. Ann. Surg., 150, 669, 1959.)

(212)

creased in amplitude and increased in frequency, but returns to normal within 30 minutes. No brain lesions have been found following electronarcosis but skin burns from the electrodes have been reported (Smith *et al.*, 1961*b*).

Electrical anesthesia appears to produce severe stress as evidenced by an increased plasma level of hydroxycorticoids, epinephrine, and norepinephrine (Fig. 11–6). The blood pressure rises sharply and then gradually falls to near normal levels (Fig. 11–7). The clotting

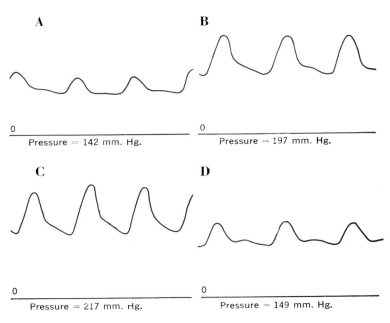

A

B

0   0

Pressure = 142 mm. Hg.   Pressure = 197 mm. Hg.

C

D

0   0

Pressure = 217 mm. Hg.   Pressure = 149 mm. Hg.

FIGURE 11–7. Mean femoral artery blood pressure in a dog under electronarcosis: (A) preinduction, (B) induction, (C) beginning surgical anesthesia, and (D) 15 minutes after onset of surgical anesthesia. (Courtesy of Dr. R. A. Herin, Colorado State University, Fort Collins, Colorado.)

time, sedimentation rate, hemoglobin, hematocrit, total and differential white blood cell counts do not differ from preinduction values (Herin, 1962). There is little effect on blood oxygen; blood carbon dioxide content and pH are lowered, while blood glucose rises. It has been suggested that electrical anesthesia, which produces an uninhibited response of the adrenal medullary and cortical systems, may be more desirable than an anesthetic, such as pentobarbital, which depresses this response (McNeil and Hardy, 1959).

It is difficult to assess the depth of electrical anesthesia in dogs. Muscle relaxation varies from adequate to poor. Pain induced by surgery may cause body movements in animals which appear unconscious. The photomotor reflex is probably the best means of determining the depth of anesthesia if a large dose of atropine has not been used (See Chapter 12, p. 219).

Analgesia persists for several minutes following removal of the current, and the animal often appears hypnotized. A slight stimulus may then cause arousal, following which the animal resumes all normal activities.

Advantages of electronarcosis are economy, immediate recovery of the patient when the current is turned off, and apparent lack of deleterious tissue reactions. In the future it may be widely utilized in clinical anesthesiology.

References

ANDJUS, R. K. and LOVELOCK, J. E.: Reanimation of Rats from Body Temperatures Between 0 and 1° C by Microwave Diathermy. J. Physiol., *128*, 541, 1955.

BERING, E. A., JR., TAREN, J. A., McMURREY, J. D., and BERNHARD, W. F.: Studies on Hypothermia in Monkeys. II. The Effect of Hypothermia on the General Physiology and Cerebral Metabolism of Monkeys in the Hypothermic State. Surg., Gynec. & Obstet., *102*, 134, 1956.

BIGELOW, W. G., LINDSAY, W. K., HARRISON, R. C., GORDON, R. A., and GREENWOOD, W. F.: Oxygen Transport and Utilization in Dogs at Low Body Temperatures. Amer. J. Physiol., *160*, 125, 1950.

BLADES, B. and PIERPONT, H. C.: A Simple Method for Inducing Hypothermia. Ann. Surg., *140*, 557, 1954.

BOEREMA, I., WILDSCHUT, A., SCHMIDT, W. J. H., and BROEKHUYSEN, L.: Experimental Researches into Hypothermia as an Aid in the Surgery of the Heart. Arch. chir. neerl., *3*, 25, 1951.

BORGLIN, N. E. and LINDSTEN, T.: On the Combined Effect of Neostigmine and Pentamethylenetetrazol or Beta-Phenylisopropylamine on Magnesium Anaesthesia. Acta. Pharmacol., *5*, 309, 1949.

BROWN, R. V. and HILTON, J. G.: The Effectiveness of the Baroreceptor Reflexes under Different Anesthetics. J. Pharm. & Exper. Therap., *118*, 198, 1956.

COOLEY, D. A., BEALL, A. C., JR., and GRONDIN, P.: Open Heart Surgery by a Simplified Technique: Using Disposable Oxygenators, 5 per cent Dextrose Solution Prime, and Normothermia. Paper presented at the Foundation Cardiologique Princesse Liliane International Cardiology Symposium, Brussels, Belgium, 1962.

COVINO, B. G., CHARLESON, D. A., and D'AMATO, H. E.: Ventricular Fibrillation in the Hypothermic Dog. Am. J. Physiol., *178*, 148, 1954.

COVINO, B. G. and HEGNAUER, A. H.: Hypothermic Ventricular Fibrillation and Its Control. Surgery, *40*, 475, 1956.

DAVIS, T. R. A. and MAYER, J.: Nature of the Physiological Stimulus for Shivering. Amer. J. Physiol., *181*, 669, 1955.

GOLLAN, F., TYSINGER, D. S., JR., GRACE, J. T., KORY, R. C., and MENEELY, G. R.: Hypothermia of 1.5° C in Dogs Followed by Survival. Amer. J. Physiol., *181*, 297, 1955.

HARDY, J. D., TURNER, M. D., and McNEIL, C. D.: Electrical Anesthesia. III. Development of a Method and Laboratory Observations. J. Surg. Res., *1*, 152, 1961.

HERIN, R. A.: Electrical Anesthesia in the Dog. J.A.V.M.A, *142*, 865, 1963.

KHALIL, H. H. and MacKEITH, R. C.: A Simple Method of Raising and Lowering Body Temperature. Brit. Med., J. *4*, 734, 1954.

KIMOTO, S., SUGIE, S., and ASANO, K.: Open Heart Surgery under Direct Vision with the Aid of Brain-Cooling by Irrigation. Surgery, *39*, 592, 1956.

KING, E. E. and UNNA, K. R.: The Action of Mephenesin and Other Interneuron Depressants on the Brain Stem. J. Pharm. & Exper. Therap., *111*, 293, 1954.

KNOCKER, P.: Effects of Experimental Hypothermia on Vital Organs. Lancet, *2*, 837, 1955.

LUCAS, B. G. B.: Discussion on the Application of Hypothermia to Surgical Procedures. Proc. R. Soc. Med., *49*, 345, 1956.

LYNN, R. B., MELROSE, D. G., CHURCHILL-DAVIDSON, H. C., and McMILLAN, I. K. R.: Hypothermia: Further Observations on Surface Cooling. Ann. R. Coll. Surg. Engl., *14*, 267, 1954.

MAHMOUD, A. H. and KAMEL, S. H.: Chloral Hydrate, Anaesthesia and Toxicity in Dogs. Brit. Vet. J., *109*, 437, 1953.

McNEIL, C. D. and HARDY, J. D.: Electrical Anesthesia: Some Metabolic Observations and Comparisons. Surgical Forum, *9*, 394, 1959.

NIAZI, S. A. and LEWIS, F. J.: Profound Hypothermia in the Monkey with Recovery After Long Periods of Cardiac Standstill. J. Applied Physiol., *10*, 137, 1957.

P'AN, S. Y., GARDOCKI, J. F., HUTCHEON, D. E., RUDEL, H., KODET, M. J., and LAUBACH, G. D.: General Anesthetic and Other Pharmacological Properties of a Soluble Steroid, 21-Hydroxypregnanedione Sodium Succinate. J. Pharm. & Exper. Therap., *115*, 432, 1955.

SEALY, W. C., YOUNG, W. G., JR., LESAGE, A. M., and BROWN, I. W., JR.: Observations on Heart Action During Hypothermia Induced and Controlled by a Pump Oxygenator. Ann. Surg., *153*, 797, 1961.

SMITH, A. U.: Resuscitation of Hypothermic, Supercooled and Frozen Mammals. Proc. R. Soc. Med., *49*, 357, 1956.

SMITH, R. H., GOODWIN, C., FOWLER, E., SMITH, G. W., and VOLPITTO, P. P.: Electronarcosis Produced by a Combination of Direct and Alternating Current. A Preliminary Study. Anesthesiology, *22*, 163, 1961.

SMITH, R. H., GRAMLING, Z. W., SMITH, G. W., and VOLPITTO, P. P.: Electronarcosis by Combination of Direct and Alternating Current. 2. Effects on Dog Brain as Shown by EEG and Microscopic Study. Anesthesiology, *22*, 970, 1961.

STEINHAUS, J. E., SIEBECKER, K. L., and KIMMEY, J. R.: Comparative Effects of Anesthetic Agents on Cardiac Irritability During Hypothermia. J.A.M.A., *169*, 76, 1959.

WESOWSKI, S. A., FISHER, J. H., FENNESSEY, J. F., CUBILES, R., and WELCH, C. S.: Recovery of the Dog's Heart After Varying Periods of Acute Ischemia. Surgical Forum, *3*, 270, 1952.

WOOD, E. M.: Urethane as a Carcinogen. Progressive Fish Culturist, *18*, 135, 1956.

WRIGHT, J. G.: *Veterinary Anaesthesia*. Alexander Eger, Inc., Chicago, 1952.

WRIGHT, J. G. and HALL, L. W.: *Veterinary Anaesthesia and Analgesia*. 5th ed. The Williams & Wilkins Company, Baltimore, 1961.

THE MUSCLE RELAXANTS AND OTHER ADJUVANTS TO ANESTHESIA

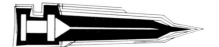

Chapter 12

The Muscle Relaxants

A number of drugs can be used in conjunction with anesthetic agents to produce more complete muscle relaxation. On occasion their use alone may be indicated; for example, they may be used to relax the patient for endotracheal intubation. Considerable information is available concerning these drugs and a knowledge of it is necessary for their intelligent use.

There are three ways in which muscle relaxation can be effected. First, by administration of drugs acting centrally, such as the intravenous or inhalant anesthetics. These depress the central nervous system and this is reflected in the activity of the ventral horn cells of the spinal cord, a decreased activity causing lowered muscle tone. However, certain disadvantages are found when profound muscular relaxation is produced in this manner. Depression of the vasomotor and respiratory centers may result in severe hypotension and hypoxia.

Local anesthetics will produce muscle relaxation peripherally if injected directly into a muscle or around the nerve which supplies it. Transmission of impulses which maintain muscular tone is thus abolished. Certain disadvantages pertain here also; namely, restraint may be a problem with this type of anesthesia and, with epidural or spinal anesthesia, hypotension may result due to paralysis of sympathetic nerves.

A third means of producing muscle relaxation is with drugs known as *muscle relaxants*. All muscle relaxants produce their effect on the neuromuscular junction with the exception of mephenesin which acts upon synapses in the spinal cord.

Since curare was first used to produce muscle relaxation, the term *curariform* has been applied to the action of this group of drugs. Actually from the pharmacological standpoint they are divided into four categories:

1. Depolarizing Agents
    a. Decamethonium (Syncurine, C-10)
    b. Succinylcholine (Anectine, Suxamethonium)
2. Nondepolarizing Agents
    a. d-Tubocurarine chloride
    b. Dimethyl tubocurarine (Metubine, Mecostrin)
    c. *Chondodendron tomentosum* Extract, purified, N.N.R. (Intocostrin)
    d. Gallamine (Flaxedil)
    e. Benzoquinonium (Mytolon)
3. Dual Blocking Agents
    a. Hexabiscarbacholine (Imbretil)
4. Miscellaneous
    a. Mephenesin (Myanesin, Tolserol)

When a motor nerve impulse arrives at the terminal nerve fibers, acetylcholine is liberated. The acetylcholine reacts with a protein receptor substance on the specialized end-plate region of the muscle fiber. It thus produces a change in permeability of the membrane in the end-plate region to all ions, causing a variation in the resting potential of the end-plate known as the "end-plate potential". As the end-plate potential reaches a critical level it fires, producing an electrical wave propagated along the sarcolemma which is known as the "muscle action potential". Once the action is produced, acetylcholine is then hydrolized to acetic acid and choline by an enzyme, cholinesterase, which is found in the end-plate region.

Transmission of the nerve impulse may be interfered with in several ways:

1. By anything which interferes with release of acetylcholine. Procaine, magnesium ions, or deficiency of calcium ions will slow or stop production of acetylcholine at the nerve terminal.

2. Delay in breakdown of acetylcholine at the end-plate region will cause persistent depolarization of the membrane and transmission of subsequent impulses is impossible. Delay of breakdown can be caused by anticholinesterase drugs among which are neostigmine.

3. Agents which produce depolarization and continue to persist at the end-plate will stop transmission of impulses at the neuromuscular junction. Among drugs which act in this manner are decamethonium (C-10) and succinylcholine (Suxamethonium); these are not hydrolyzed by cholinesterase. The persistent nature of the block by these drugs has been explained on the basis that it is a total depolarization and also that a decreased sensitivity to acetylcholine exists at the end-plate. Regardless of cause, these drugs produce an initial depolarization of the end-plate region and are termed *depolarizing agents*.

4. A fourth type of block is produced by drugs, such as d-tubocurarine, which have affinity for the protein molecules of the motor end-plate receptors. These drugs combine loosely with the end-plate receptors and prevent excitation of the muscles by acetylcholine. This block is referred to as "competitive inhibition" since these drugs compete with acetylcholine for the end-plate receptor sites. In addition to d-tubocurarine many other drugs competively inhibit the action of acetylcholine and the term *nondepolarization block* is used to describe the action of these agents.

A peculiar effect seen after the administration of depolarizing drugs is termed *dual block*. Depolarization of the muscle fibers occurs first and gradually the type of block changes until it exhibits the characteristics of a nondepolarizing block.

In all species of animals relaxant drugs produce approximately the same sequence of muscle relaxation (Fig. 12–1). The facial muscles, the jaw and tail are affected first, usually within 30 to 60 seconds following intravenous injection of the agent. This is followed by paralysis of the neck and limb muscles and then the swallowing and phonatory muscles. The abdominal musculature is affected next, followed by the intercostal muscles. The diaphragm is last to become paralyzed and when this occurs, unless artificial respiration is performed, the animal will die of respiratory failure. The recovery pattern is in the reverse order.

Early workers attempted to give a dose which would just paralyze the abdominal musculature without paralyzing the diaphragm. It was found, however, that this procedure reduced the respiratory minute volume to the point that artificial respiration was necessary. Therefore, at the present time the dose of relaxant is not determined on this basis; rather, enough is given to paralyze all respiratory muscles and artificial respiration is administered. An exception is the production of limb relaxation in which case a small dose of relaxant may be administered without interfering with respiration.

Because muscle relaxants produce a progressive paralysis which in high doses affects the respiratory muscles, their use without a means for artificial respiration is dangerous and foolhardy. *Oxygen should always be available when these drugs are used.*

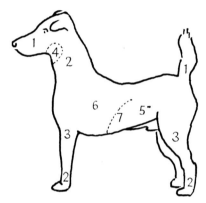

FIGURE 12–1. Sequence of muscle paralysis.
1. The muscles of expression, the jaw muscles and tail muscles.
2. The neck muscles and distal limb muscles.
3. The proximal limb muscles.
4. The swallowing and phonatory muscles.
5. The muscles of the abdominal wall.
6. The intercostal muscles.
7. The diaphragm.

(From Wright, J. G. and Hall, L. W.: *Veterinary Anaesthesia and Analgesia.* 5th ed The Williams & Wilkins Co., 1961.)

None of the muscle relaxants produce analgesia; thus, though an animal may be completely immobilized it feels all painful stimuli. For this reason, analgesics or anesthetics should always be administered concurrently. When a relaxant is used with light general anesthesia, it is difficult to distinguish, by the usual voluntary muscle reflexes, between true unconsciousness and consciousness masked by immobilization (Croft, 1961). The photomotor reflex (contraction of the pupil of the eye on stimulation with a bright light) can be used as a differential test provided not more than 0.032 mg./kg. of atropine has been given as premedication. For best results the eyes should be covered for a short period prior to stimulation.

Table 12–1 summarizes the activity and actions of these drugs in various species.

Table 12-1.—Drugs Affecting the Neuromuscular Junction

Drug	Animal[1]	Neuromuscular Blocking Potency mg (cation)/kg	LD_{50} mg (cation)/kg	Antagonist or Antidote	Other Effects
Decamethonium halide (C-10; Eulissin; Syncurine)	Man	0.02–0.025		Hexa- or pentamethonium.	Cardiovascular.
	Cat	0.015–0.018		Hexa- or pentamethonium, stilbazolinium salts.	
	Monkey	0.125		Hexa- or pentamethonium.	
	Mouse	0.35	0.4–0.5		
	Rabbit	0.04–0.09		Hexa- or pentamethonium.	Anticholinesterase; muscarinic.
	Rat	1.25	1.5		
	Chick	0.025			
	Frog[2]	5.5–6.2	>123	Hexa- or pentamethonium.	Contracture.
Gallamine triethiodide (Flaxedil)	Man	0.45–0.6		Neostigmine, tensilon.	Histamine release; parasympathetic.
	Cat	0.3–1.1			
	Dog	0.25	0.5	Tensilon.	
	Mouse	1.2	1.9–2.7		
	Rabbit	0.2–0.3	0.4	Neostigmine.	
	Rat		3.3		Histamine release.
	Frog[2]	6 and 36			

Drug	Species				
Benzoquinonium chloride (Mytolon chloride; Win 2747)	Man	0.06–0.24			Bradycardia, salivation, bronchorrhea.
	Cat[4]	9.5	11.7		
	Dog	0.1		Neostigmine.	
	Mouse[3]	0.5	1.4 (0.5 i.v.)		
	Rabbit	0.025	0.04	Neostigmine.	
	Rat		1.1		
Succinylcholine (Suxamethonium halide; Succinoylcholine; Scoline; Brevedil M; Celocurine; Anectine; Lysthenon; Curacit)	Man	0.1–0.3		Plasma cholinesterase.	Anticholinesterase; nicotinic; initial stimulation of muscular contraction.
	Cat	0.05–0.1			Nicotinic; initial stimulation of muscular contraction.
	Dog	0.1	0.15	Plasma cholinesterase.	Anticholinesterase.
	Mouse	0.05–0.1	0.25		
	Rabbit	0.1	0.5		
	Sparrow	5.0	10.0		Contracture.
	Frog[2]	2.5			Nicotinic; contracture.
d-Tubocurarine chloride (Tubarine)	Man	0.08–0.19		Neostigmine, tensilon.	Cardiovascular; histamine release.
	Cat	0.12–0.23			Histamine release; ganglion blocking.
	Dog	0.08–0.15	0.38	Tensilon.	Ganglion blocking.
	Monkey	0.06			

Table 12-1.—Drugs Affecting the Neuromuscular Junction (Continued)

Drug	Animal[1]	Neuromuscular Blocking Potency mg (cation)/kg	LD_{50} mg (cation)/kg	Antagonist or Antidote	Other Effects
d-Tubocurarine chloride (Tubarine)	Mouse	0.06-0.09	0.11-0.15		
	Rabbit	0.09-0.15	0.165	Neostigmine.	Ganglion blocking.
	Rat	0.04-0.06	0.08		Histamine release.
	Chick	0.13			
	Frog[2]	1.4, 4.1 and 7.5	>20.0	Acetylcholine.	
	Man	0.027		Tensilon, neostigmine.	
	Cat	0.02			Ganglion blocking; histamine release.
Dimethyl ether of d-tubocurarine iodide (Dimethine; Metubine)	Mouse	0.08-0.1	0.16		
	Rabbit	0.01-0.015	0.02	Neostigmine.	
	Rat	0.009	0.025-0.03	Neostigmine.	Histamine release.
	Frog[2]	0.94	14.4		

[1] Unless otherwise indicated, drug administered by intravenous injection. [2] Ventral lymph sac injection. [3] Subcutaneous injection. [4] Oral administration. (From Spector, W. S.: *Handbook of Biological Data.* W. B. Saunders Co., 1956.)

Agents Producing Depolarization Block

Depolarization block differs from nondepolarization block as follows:

1. Paralysis is preceded by transient stimulation of the muscle fibers thought to be caused by initial depolarization. This muscle twitching may be visible in animals.
2. Antagonists to the nondepolarizing agents tend to potentiate the depolarizing drugs, hence, may prolong their action.
3. In nerve-muscle preparations it can be shown that after partial paralysis due to a nondepolarizing drug there is rapid loss of induced tetanus, whereas after paralysis caused by depolarizing agents induced tetanus is maintained.
4. The depolarizing agents probably never produce a pure neuro-muscular block. In dogs they cause both depolarization and nondepolarization. In contrast the nondepolarizing relaxants always have a pure nondepolarizing action.
5. The depolarizing relaxants have been shown to affect the red muscle fibers more than the white in the cat, rat, and mouse; the nondepolarizing agents have an opposite effect.

Wright and Hall (1961) have pointed out that in veterinary anesthesia little clinical difference exists between a depolarizing and nondepolarizing action, the main difference between the two types being that the former agents produce an initial muscle contraction.

Decamethonium (Syncurine; C-10)

Decamethonium is a white odorless crystalline solid which forms aqueous solutions with a pH of about 5.5. It has the simplest chemical structure of the common blocking agents. In general, the drug is relatively inert and very stable in solution. Three milligrams of decamethonium are roughly equivalent in action to 15 to 20 mg. of d-tubocurarine.

When injected intravenously into unanesthetized animals decamethonium bromide is 1 to 1½ times as active as d-tubocurarine chloride in the rabbit, twice as active in the dog, and about one-fourth as active in the mouse. In the cat it is 7 to 10 times as potent.

When injected slowly, intravenously, into the rabbit and dog, decamethonium paralyzes the muscles of the hind legs followed by those of the head and neck and the front legs. On rapid intravenous injection of curarizing doses the paralysis appears to occur simultaneously in all these muscles. The paralysis produced in the rabbit and dog is shorter than that produced by an equivalent dose of d-tubocurarine chloride, but in the cat appears to last longer. Decamethonium has the advantage over d-tubocurarine chloride in a relative sparing action on the respiration, equipotent doses causing less depression.

In curarizing doses decamethonium causes no significant blood pressure drop in the dog or cat. When a dose large enough to depress the respiration is given, a typical asphyxial rise in blood pressure develops. Eighty to 90% can be recovered in the urine indicating little is metabolized in the body (Kalow, 1959). Prostigmine and edrophonium are *not* antidotes; no antidote is available.

This drug is probably more toxic than d-tubocurarine chloride in the rabbit, dog, cat, and man. Since it displays a weak curarizing action in the mouse compared to the other species, it is less toxic for mice than d-tubocurarine (Castillo *et al.*, 1949).

Irwin *et al.* (1957) have indicated a minimum of 0.2 mg./kg. is required to produce apnea in thiopental-anesthetized dogs. Subsequent doses of 0.02 mg./kg. will maintain apnea.

Succinylcholine (Anectine; Suxamethonium)

Succinylcholine is a white odorless solid marketed as an aqueous solution with a pH of 3.2 to 3.5. Warm solutions at a pH of 7.4 hydrolyze appreciably.

Succinylcholine is prepared as a chloride or an iodide anhydrous salt; the chloride is $1\frac{1}{2}$ times as potent as the iodide. Because it is similar chemically to two molecules of acetylcholine, it is sometimes referred to as diacetylcholine. Opened vials of solution gradually lose potency.

Succinylcholine produces depolarization of the motor end-plate. The muscles of the eyes are affected first followed by the muscles of the throat, peripheral muscles, intercostal muscles, and lastly the diaphragmatic musculature. A general uncoordinated muscular twitching accompanies the depolarizing action. In man this produces pain, not during the main action of the drug but in the recovery period, the pain outlasting the period during which the drug is known to be present in the body.

Of the muscle relaxants only succinylcholine has a rapid rate of destruction, due to hydrolysis in the serum where no membranes have to be passed in order to reach the hydrolyzing enzyme. Less than 2% of an injected dose of succinylcholine appears in the urine. Plasma cholinesterase (pseudocholinesterase) hydrolyzes succinylcholine quickly to form succinylmonocholine and choline. Succinylmonocholine then is broken down into choline and succinic acid. Acetylcholinesterase (true cholinesterase of erythrocytes) cannot hydrolyze succinylcholine. According to Hall *et al.* (1953) plasma cholinesterase activity in the dog shows a wide range of variation depending upon the breed.

The liver is probably the site of synthesis of true (red cell, brain, muscle) and pseudo (plasma) cholinesterase production. In liver disease the plasma cholinesterase level is decreased and on administration of succinylcholine apnea and respiratory depression are prolonged. Procaine is hydrolyzed by a nonspecific cholinesterase, and thus may compete with succinylcholine for the same enzyme. Procaine has been shown to intensify the myoneural action of succinylcholine if injected after the relaxant. The action is antagonized if procaine is injected before administration of succinylcholine.

Succinylcholine is free from the usual complications of muscle relaxants such as hypotension, tachycardia, histamine release, bronchospasm, urticaria, and cumulative effects. Lack of cumulative effect permits almost instantaneous change in the degree of muscle relaxation. Because it is rapidly hydrolyzed, it produces no residual respiratory paralysis. The chief disadvantage is that the effective dose and duration of effect are inconsistent between individuals. In dogs prolonged apnea may follow administration of three or more doses (Hall, 1959).

Minimal doses may produce muscular tremors in dogs, particularly in the head and front limbs. On intravenous injection approaching the respiratory failure level, parasympathomimetic action is observed (intestinal hypermotility, micturition, and salivation). Sialism is an indication of subsequent respiratory paralysis. Salivation can be corrected by administration of atropine and its use is advisable. Many dogs will exhibit depression after recovery, lasting in some instances as long as 18 hours.

When given intravenously, effective doses produce muscular relaxation within 15 seconds. The mean effective dose of succinylcholine *chloride* intravenously for *unanesthetized* dogs is 18 to 26 mcg./lb. of body weight; it is suggested that 22 mcg./lb. be the initial dosage and further amounts be given to effect (Knill, 1956). In dogs anesthetized with thiopental-trichloroethylene, the minimum relaxing dose of succinylcholine *iodide* is 0.067 mg./kg. of body weight (Table 12–2). The use of succinylcholine in thoracic surgery is of particular value because paralysis of the diaphragm can easily be produced. The usual dose of succinylcholine *iodide* for this purpose is about 0.15 mg./kg. of body weight. The intraperitoneal and subcutaneous routes of administration are very ineffective probably due to the rate of absorption; consequently, these are not suitable for clinical use.

Neostigmine, other anticholinesterases, and edrophonium do not antagonize succinylcholine but rather prolong its action. No specific pharmacological antagonist is available. However, in patients show-

15

ing little recovery, infusion of fresh plasma or whole blood will restore plasma cholinesterase activity and thus hydrolyze the drug.

Succinylcholine is contraindicated in dogs suffering from respiratory or liver disease.

Equipment and methods for using succinylcholine in capture and restraint of wild animals are described in Chapter 14 under *The Cap-Chur Gun*, p. 300.

Table 12–2.—Effect of Succinylcholine Iodide on Neuromuscular Transmission, Ventilation, and Blood Pressure on Intravenous Injection in the Dog

Experiment (No.)	Celocurin (mg./kg.)	Max. degree of relaxation[1] (%)	Duration of effect (min.)	Ventilation[2] (%)	Duration of respiratory arrest	Variation in blood pressure (mm. Hg)
I	0.022	25	2–3	100	0	− 1
II	0.045	50	5–7	75	0	+ 4
III	0.060	50	6–11.5	50	0	+ 8
IV	0.066	>50	11–14	50	0	+15
V	0.085	>50	8–11	0	45 sec.	− 8
VI	0.11	>50	18–21	0	10 min.	− 6
VII	0.22	>50	23–27	0	10 min.	− 9

[1] The degree of relaxation denotes the ratio of the amplitude of the normal muscle to that of the "curarized" muscle. A degree of relaxation of 50% usually suffices for clinical purposes.

[2] Ventilation denotes the difference between expiratory and inspiratory pressure in the trachea as a percentage of the basic value of the difference.

(From Hansson, C. H.: Succinylcholine Iodide as a Muscular Relaxant in Veterinary Surgery. J.A.V.M.A., *128*, 288, 1956.)

Agents Producing Nondepolarization Block

Agents which act by nondepolarization (competitive blockers, or "true curarizing drugs") produce the following effects:

1. Transmission of the motor nerve impulse across the myoneural junction is prevented and thus voluntary striated muscle is paralyzed.
2. On direct stimulation both the nerve and muscle fiber remain excitable throughout the block.
3. Acetylcholine is produced in normal quantities at the end-plate region during the block by stimulation of the motor nerve.
4. Anticholinesterases (neostigmine, edrophonium) are antagonistic to these blocking agents.

Drugs of clinical importance in this group are:

1. The curare alkaloids, including d-tubocurarine, the dimethyl ether of d-tubocurarine (Metubine, Mecostrin), and Intocostrin.
2. Synthetic compounds such as gallamine (Flaxedil) and benzoquinonium (Mytolon).

d-Tubocurarine Chloride, U.S.P.

d-Tubocurarine chloride is a white or yellowish-white crystalline solid which forms aqueous solutions with a pH of approximately 3. Tubocurarine is obtained from the plant, *Chondodendron tomentosum*, and standardized by biological assay. It is sold for medical use dissolved in sterile isotonic solution, each ml. containing the equivalent of 2.7 mg. of anhydrous tubocurarine chloride or 3.0 mg.

Table 12–3.—Species Variation of d-*Tubocurarine (A Typical Non-depolarizing Muscle Relaxant) and Decamethonium (A Typical Depolarizing Muscle Relaxant)*

The mg./kg. Paralyzing Dose

	Cat	Man	Baboon	Rabbit	Monkey	Mouse	Rat	Frog
d-Tubocurarine	0.3	0.25	—	0.20	0.09	0.12	0.08	5.5
Decamethonium	0.03	0.05	0.14	0.15	0.25	0.70	2.5	11.0

(From Paton, W. D. M., and Zaimis, E.: Brit. J. Pharmacol., *4*, 381, 1949.)

of the pentahydrate. The biopotency of the anhydrous salt is 6.8 units/mg. in the rabbit head-drop assay. The drug is quite stable and aqueous solutions can be stored for long periods or even autoclaved without serious decomposition.

A wide species variation in response to d-tubocurarine has been observed (Table 12–3). Commercial solutions of curare are too concentrated for safe administration to small animals. For this reason they are diluted with physiological saline so that each ml. contains 2 units. Curare, like pentobarbital, should be given "to effect" and a full 2 minutes should be taken for the injection. Rapid injection may produce bradycardia, tachycardia, or even cardiac collapse.

The use of curare with a general anesthetic such as pentobarbital or thiopental permits the use of less anesthetic and good muscular relaxation is still obtained.

When administration with thiopental is desired, the anesthetic is diluted so that each ml. contains $\frac{1}{2}$ gr. (32 mg.) and the dose is calculated at $\frac{1}{6}$ to $\frac{1}{8}$ gr./lb. Tubocurarine is mixed with the anesthetic at a rate of 1 ml. (3 mg.) for each 40 lbs. of body weight. Injection is made intravenously over a 3- to 5-minute period.

Using dogs, Pickett (1951) tried combinations of curare with ether, pentobarbital, and thiopental. All injections of curare were made intravenously and prostigmine 1:2,000 was used as an antidote. It was found that $\frac{1}{4}$ unit/lb. of body weight administered without an anesthetic produced little effect while $\frac{1}{2}$ unit was occasionally capable of causing respiratory paralysis. Depression necessitating artificial respiration was frequently produced by $\frac{3}{4}$ unit/lb. In dogs anesthetized with pentobarbital or thiopental, $\frac{3}{8}$ unit/lb. seemed to be the optimum dose. Brinker (1951) used 4% thiamylal solution containing $\frac{3}{8}$ unit of d-tubocurarine chloride/ml. and reported the delivery of viable puppies by cesarean section.

Wright and Hall (1961) state that the effective dose for dogs is 0.2 mg./lb. and that at this level a fall in blood pressure due to blocking of autonomic ganglia and histamine release occurs. Its use in this species, therefore, is at best somewhat risky. Similar hypotension occurs on intravenous administration to cats.

Pickett reported that when used with ether in $\frac{1}{8}$ or $\frac{1}{4}$ unit doses/lb. of body weight, respiration became shallow and labored. Because some fatalities occurred despite administration of prostigmine, he believed that curare was definitely contraindicated with ether anesthesia. According to Booth (1963) curare is not contraindicated with ether but, because the latter has a curariform action, only one-third the dose of curare should be used.

About two-thirds of injected d-tubocurarine is destroyed in the body, since only one-third is excreted in the urine and practically none in the feces.

Prostigmine methylsulfate (1:2,000), given in 0.5 to 2 ml. doses, is a limited antagonist for curare and is effective only against minimal paralytic doses. It is ineffective against larger doses of curare and may actually prolong curarization.

Dimethyl Tubocurarine, N.F.

The iodide of dimethyl tubocurarine, *Metubine*, is an odorless, pale yellow, crystalline powder. It is slightly soluble in water forming aqueous solutions with a pH of about 6.1. It is prepared from d-tubocurarine by substitution of two hydroxyl groups with OCH_3 groups. The substitution is accompanied by an increase in potency. The chloride of dimethyl tubocurarine is called *Mecostrin*.

In dogs dimethyl tubocurarine is two to three times more potent than d-tubocurarine chloride. It is similar in action to d-tubocurarine, but the duration of neuromuscular block is slightly shorter. It is claimed to have less effect on autonomic ganglia and to produce less histamine release. According to Wright and Hall (1961), equipotent doses of dimethyl tubocurarine and d-tubocurarine produce comparable depression of blood pressure.

Chondodendron Tomentosum Extract, Purified, N.N.R.
(Intocostrin)

Purified *Chondodendron tomentosum* extract is available in biologically standardized aqueous solution for intramuscular or intravenous use. Each milliliter provides 20 units of curare activity or is equivalent in potency to 3 mg. of d-tubocurarine chloride. The action produced by this drug is essentially the same as that of d-tubocurarine chloride. The liver and kidneys are involved in its detoxification and for this reason it is contraindicated in hepatic and renal disease.

Gallamine Triethiodide (Flaxedil)

Gallamine triethiodide is a white, odorless, crystalline solid which is soluble in water. The commercially available solution has a pH of about 3.2; it is marketed in 10 ml. multiple-dose vials, each ml. containing 20 mg. It has three quaternary ammonium groups which form salts with acids and dissolve to produce weak acid solutions. In general gallamine is non-reactive and stable in solution. Seven milligrams of gallamine are approximately equivalent in action to 1 mg. of d-tubocurarine chloride.

Gallamine produces a nondepolarization block at the neuromuscular junction. In addition it produces some vagal block and tachycardia occurs quickly after intravenous injection in the dog. It does not produce histamine release in the dog and for this reason is the nondepolarizing relaxant of choice in this species. There is no indication that in clinical doses there is any action on the central nervous system, liver, or kidneys. In cats a transient fall in blood pressure occurs on intravenous injection and this has been attributed by Wright and Hall (1961) to its inhibitory effect on cholinesterase produced by the liver.

Gallamine is not detoxified in the body and is excreted unchanged in the urine. Thirty to 100% of the total dose injected into cats can be recovered from the urine within 2 hours (Mushin *et al.*, 1949). For this reason it is contraindicated in animals suffering from renal failure but may be used in animals with compensated chronic nephritis.

For complete paralysis in dogs 0.5 mg./lb. should be given intravenously. Apnea will last for 15 to 20 minutes. Similar doses in cats produce 10 to 20 minutes of apnea. No adverse side effects occur in either species though, as previously mentioned, a transient hypotension may occur in the cat.

Gallamine has been used extensively as an immobilizing agent for wild animals and, when edrophonium is used as an antidote, has proved to be very effective (See Chapter 14, p. 307).

Benzoquinonium Chloride (Mytolon)

Benzoquinonium is a nondepolarizing relaxant. In addition to its neuromuscular blocking action it stimulates the vagus causing a marked increase in salivary and bronchial secretions with a tendency for bradycardia. These side effects can be prevented with atropine or scopolamine.

In dogs the average dose producing complete arrest of nerve impulse transmission in nerve-muscle preparations is 0.11 mg./kg. The dose required for respiratory arrest is only slightly larger than the one causing arrest of nerve transmission.

About 80% of administered benzoquinonium can be recovered in the urine. Its use is contraindicated in acute or chronic respiratory disease or in disturbances of cardiac conductivity.

Artifically ventilated dogs may tolerate more than 200 times the paralyzing dose of benzoquinonium (Hoppe, 1950). Neostigmine is an effective antagonist.

Dual Blocking Agents

Hexabiscarbacholine (Imbretil)

Hexabiscarbacholine, a long-acting muscle relaxant, was synthesized in Austria and first tested pharmacologically by Klupp *et al*, in 1953. It is a white, crystalline, slightly hydroscopic powder, soluble in water and alcohol but almost insoluble in ether, chloroform, or benzene. An aqueous solution is clear, colorless, and has a pH of 7.45.

Hexabiscarbacholine is said to have a "dual-block" action, the initial phase or depolarizing block lasting a few minutes, followed by a persistent paralysis of the curare type. Reversal of effects has been reported with neostigmine and other anticholinesterase drugs. Ngai (1959) reported 10 mcg./kg. intravenously in anesthetized cats produced generalized muscular fasciculations followed by 10 to 30 minutes of complete paralysis. Twenty to 30 mcg./kg. was necessary to produce apnea.

Cardiac activity, blood pressure, and intestinal function are not influenced by therapeutic doses. Large doses (20 to 30 times the muscle relaxing dose) cause a slight transient rise in blood pressure in animals. The drug action is cumulative and tachyphylaxis does not occur with repeated injections. Hexabiscarbacholine is unaffected by cholinesterase and is probably excreted unaltered in the urine. In dogs approximately 50% is eliminated within 2 hours after a single intravenous dose and 75% within 6 to 8 hours. Excretion is almost complete in 48 hours.

Repeated injections cause an increasingly prolonged action, being approximately four times as effective as the initial dose. Both hypertension and hypotension may be seen. There is little evidence of histamine release following its injection.

The chief advantage is its ability to produce profound abdominal relaxation almost equivalent to that obtained with spinal anesthesia. The greatest disadvantage is the lack of a reliable antagonist. Neostigmine methylsulphate is probably effective in most species but potentiates the action of hexabiscarbacholine in cats (Ngai, 1959).

Miscellaneous Relaxants

Mephenesin (Myanesin; Tolserol)

Mephenesin is a colorless crystalline solid, sparingly soluble in water but very soluble in alcohol and propylene glycol. It is a neutral substance and the pH of its solution is practically the same as that of the pure solvent. Solutions are stable and unaffected by light, heat, cold, and air.

The mechanism of action is quite different from curare, since neuronal conduction and neuromuscular transmission are not depressed with conventional doses. Its effect is apparently due to depression of reflexes in the spinal cord, the site of action being the internuncial cells. Mephenesin has been shown experimentally to be an efficient strychnine antagonist.

Mephenesin is probably degraded in the liver. In dogs less than 2% of the drug can be recovered from the urine.

Rabbits injected intravenously with 30 to 50 mg./kg. develop flaccid paralysis without loss of consciousness. Muscle power is regained 5 to 10 minutes after injection. The mean lethal dose for mice after intraperitoneal injection is 610 ± 10 mg./kg.; the mean paralyzing dose is 178 ± 8 mg./kg. Excitement, tremors, or convulsions are not seen at any time.

Intravenous injection of 30 mg. in rabbits or cats does not cause change in blood pressure or respiration. Larger doses cause a fall in blood pressure accompanied by decreased rate and increased depth of respiratory movements. Toxic doses cause death by respiratory paralysis. Simultaneous injection of an ineffective dose of mephenesin and an ineffective dose of hexobarbital causes deep narcosis without excitement on induction and with complete muscular relaxation.

Mephenesin has been added to barbiturate solutions (Myotal*, Myothesia†) to produce more profound muscular relaxation during anesthesia. It has not met with universal acceptance, however.

* The Warren-Teed Products Company. Each ml. contains 64 mg. of pentobarbital sodium and 32 mg. of mephenesin.

† The S. E. Massengill Company. Each ml. contains 50 mg. of secobarbital sodium and 30 mg. of mephenesin.

Anticurariform Agents

Antagonists to the muscle relaxants are at the present time limited to those effective against the antidepolarizing drugs. There seems to be little to choose from between edrophonium (Tensilon) and neostigmine (Prostigmine), both of which are anticholinesterases. The neuromuscular action of these drugs is probably due to their inhibitory effect on acetylcholine hydrolysis, thus intensifying acetylcholine effects.

The time elapsing between intravenous injection of edrophonium (30 to 60 seconds) is shorter than for neostigmine (120 to 240 seconds). Temporary improvement of neuromuscular activity followed by recurarization may occur with edrophonium and occasionally also with neostigmine. For this reason seemingly recovered patients should never be left unobserved.

Complications and side effects caused by neostigmine and edrophonium are due chiefly to an excess of acetylcholine acting on the postganglionic parasympathetic fibers. These are more pronounced with neostigmine than edrophonium and include salivation, bronchial secretion, intestinal hypermotility, and bradycardia.

The use of antagonists should seldom be necessary if proper care is exerted in administration of muscle relaxants. When respiratory exchange is inadequate, it is recommended that artificial respiration be administered until spontaneous respiration resumes (Foldes, 1957). If an antagonist is needed, the initial dose should be small and atropine given concurrently to prevent side effects.

Table 12–4 gives the approximate dose schedule for neostigmine and edrophonium.

Ganglionic Blocking Agents

Ganglionic blocking agents have been used in veterinary practice for two purposes: (1) to produce general paralysis in animals difficult to restrain or capture, and (2) to produce hypotension during surgery.

In the first category nicotine is the only agent currently employed

Nicotine

Nicotine, an alkaloid, is obtained from several species of tobacco. In the purified form it is an odorless clear liquid with a specific gravity of 1.009. It darkens on exposure to light or atmospheric oxygen, assuming the characteristic odor of tobacco, and volatilizes at room temperature. It is miscible with water, soluble in most organic solvents, and forms salts with most acids (sulfate, salicylate, tartrate, lactate).

Table 12-4.—Recommended Dose of Antagonists for Nondepolarizing Muscle Relaxants

| Agent | Initial Dose | | Onset of Action in Minutes | Repeat Dose of Antagonist* | Minutes Between Doses |
	Antagonist	Atropine			
Neostigmine (Prostigmine)	0.03–0.10 mg./10 lbs.	0.02 mg./lb.	2–4	0.015–0.05 mg./10 lbs.	5–8
Edrophonium (Tensilon)	0.5–1.0 mg./10 lbs.	0.02 mg./lb.	0.5–1	0.25 mg./10 lbs.	2–4

* If initial dose does not produce desired effect.
(After Foldes, F. F.: Muscle Relaxants in Anesthesiology. Charles C Thomas, 1957.)

Nicotine has been considered a parasympathomimetic agent with curariform activity. It is biphasic in action, producing a short period of stimulation followed by paralysis of all autonomic gangila. Extremely small doses may produce sympathetic stimulation and with increased doses both divisions of the autonomic system may respond. There is wide species and individual variation, thus making it difficult to predict a specific reaction to nonlethal doses. Dogs, cats, and monkeys frequently vomit following administration, whereas ruminants do not. A marked excitement is sometimes seen in deer and goats prior to paralysis; this is not seen in cattle and horses. The therapeutic index of nicotine is 2 for most species; therefore, *it should be considered a dangerous drug and used with discretion.* The pure alkaloid can be absorbed through the intact skin.

Only a portion of injected nicotine is eliminated in the urine, the percentage varying with the amount injected. Urinary excretion is complete in 16 hours in dogs.

Toxic doses affect the central nervous system and myoneural junctions resulting in postural incoordination and paralysis. Death is due to paralysis of the respiratory muscles. The spinal centers may be stimulated sufficiently to cause convulsions which, in turn, contribute to asphyxial death.

There is no known antidote for lethal doses of nicotine though autonomic drugs have been used to treat the parasympathomimetic symptoms such as excessive salivation and increased peristalsis. In these instances the autonomic drugs appear only to hasten death. If convulsions are produced, pentobarbital sodium, cortisone, and amphetamine may be of some value (————, 1959). The lethal dose of nicotine for dogs is 10 mg./kg. orally or 3 mg./kg. intravenously.

Acute tolerance to nicotine occurs in many species; thus animals reinjected shortly after initial injection may show little response. However, the original threshold is regained within approximately 24 hours.

Equipment and methods for administration of nicotine to both wild and domestic animals are described in Chapter 14 under *The Cap-Chur Gun*, p. 300.

Hypotensive Agents

Control of blood loss during surgery has always presented a problem. A number of solutions have been advanced, including deliberate withdrawal of blood and subsequent reinfusion. The development of sympathetic blocking agents has led to their trial in deliberate induction of hypotension. They have been found particularly valuable in brain surgery of man. Among the agents which have been used are quaternary ammonium compounds, such as pentamethonium and hexamethonium, and thiophanium derivatives such as trimethaphan (Arfonad). Outwardly it would appear that this technique is shock producing. Paradoxically, however, it has been pointed out by Boba and Converse (1957) that there is good evidence to indicate lowered blood pressure with prevention of vasoconstriction, such as occurs with these agents, prevents or prolongs the onset of irreversible shock.

Pentamethonium Bromide and Hexamethonium Bromide

Penta- and hexamethonium compounds are used in human medicine and surgery to lower blood pressure and reduce gastric secretion. They are also used to produce temporary hypotension during surgical operations. They block impulses through the ganglia of both the sympathetic and parasympathetic nervous systems. Blood pressure is reduced by release of autonomic tone and not by direct action on the vascular system. This results in abolition of the normal pressor reflexes.

Clark and Weiss (1952) have described the use of these drugs in veterinary practice. When dogs anesthetized with pentobarbital were given a dose of 20 mg./100 lb. the mean arterial blood pressure dropped suddenly following which it rose and stabilized at a new level 15 to 45 mm. Hg below the original pressure. Repeated injections caused a further drop which was not proportional to the amount of drug administered. Considerable variation in susceptibility was noticed.

The recommended initial dose for dogs is 20 mg./100 lb. of the methonium compounds. Because blood pressure readings are not conveniently made in the dog, the effect is judged by the feel of the pulse, auscultation of the heart, and the amount of hemorrhage in the surgical field. With a mean blood pressure below 60 mm. Hg the femoral pulse in the dog can hardly be felt. In man the desired systolic pressure maintained is 55 mm. Hg.

The methonium drugs should be used with caution in dogs with chronic nephritis since they are excreted in the urine and their action may be excessively prolonged in animals with impaired kidney function. In this situation a pressor agent can be administered following surgery since sympathomimetics reverse the action of these drugs.

Tetraethylammonium Chloride or Bromide (TEA)

Among the quaternary ammonium compounds with nicotinic properties, the tetraethylammonium ion (TEA) is unusual in that its action is almost entirely confined to autonomic ganglia and it is solely depressant in its effect on these structures. It blocks transmission in both sympathetic and parasympathetic ganglia. It may be used either as the chloride or bromide.

Over a range of 0.1 to 10 mg./kg. intravenous tetraethylammonium bromide produces a fall in arterial blood pressure in the cat and dog anesthetized with pentobarbital. The least effective dose varies from 0.05 to 0.4 mg./kg., 1.0 mg./kg. producing as little as 10% or as large as 55% reduction in arterial pressure (Acheson and Moe, 1946). Occasionally pressor responses are obtained with large doses. Duration of depression is several minutes. Side effects are absent except with the largest doses.

In dogs under pentobarbital anesthesia, tetraethylammonium chloride produces a widely variable response in 5 to 10 mg./kg. doses. Even in the same animal depressor or pressor responses may occur on different days (Page, 1949).

Concentrations higher than those necessary for ganglionic blockade produce skeletal muscle fasciculation; large doses may cause curariform paralysis. Since the discovery of more effective hypotensive agents the use of TEA has been largely abandoned.

Trimethaphan (Arfonad)

Trimethaphan is a thiophanium derivative which has the characteristic ganglionic blocking and hypotensive effects of tetraethylammonium bromide. Intravenous doses ranging from 0.015 to 0.25 mg./kg. show an average of 30 times the potency and twice the duration of circulatory depressor effects of TEA in the dog, cat, and monkey. About 20 times the intravenous dose is required intramuscularly in the dog and cat to cause an equal vasodepression. Oral administration produces erratic results.

There is wide species variation in the acute toxicity of the thiophanium compounds. On intravenous injection trimethaphan is 2 to 4 times as toxic as TEA in mice, rats, and rabbits, and 75 times as toxic in dogs (Randall et al. 1949). In all species except the dog toxic doses of TEA and trimethaphan produce death by respiratory failure. In the dog death appears due to hemorrhagic shock, apparently from profound fall in blood pressure, with hemorrhage into the gastrointestinal tract and petechia in the internal organs. This state of hemorrhagic shock in dogs appears to be accompanied by release of histamine and heparin since administration of antihistamine and antiheparin agents modifies the lethal effect. A prolonged clotting time is also found in dogs after intravenous doses of trimethaphan ranging from 0.25 to 1.0 mg./kg. Because of these effects the drug is probably contraindicated in the dog; they have not been demonstrated in other species.

Neostigmine in large doses and ephedrine in doses of 1 mg./kg. intravenously will abolish the depressor and ganglionic blocking effects of both TEA and trimethaphan.

References

ACHESON, G. H. and MOE, G. K.: The Action of Tetraethylammonium Ion on the Mammalian Circulation. J. Pharm. & Exper. Therap., *87*, 221, 1946.

BOBA, A. and CONVERSE, J. G.: Ganglionic Blockade and Its Protective Action in Hemorrhage: A Review. Anesthesiology, *18*, 559, 1957.

BOOTH, N. H.: Personal Communication. Colorado State University, Fort Collins, Colorado, 1963.

BRINKER, W. O.: Use of Surital Sodium and Curare in Small-Animal Surgery. N. Amer. Vet., *32*, 832, 1951.

CASTILLO, J. C., PHILLIPS, A. P., and DE BEER, E. J.: The Curariform Action of Decamethylene-1, 10-Bis-Trimethylammonium Bromide. J. Pharm. & Exper. Therap., *97*, 150, 1949.

CLARK, R. and WEISS, K. E.: The Possible Applications of the New Hypotensive (Methonium) Drugs in Veterinary Practice. J. South Africa Vet. Med. Assoc., *23*, 15, 1952.

CROFT, P. G.: The Photomotor Reflex as an Indicator of Consciousness in the Immobilized Dog. J. Small Anim. Pract., *2*, 206, 1961.

FOLDES, F. F.: *Muscle Relaxants in Anesthesiology.* Charles C Thomas, Springfield, Ill., 1957.

HALL, L. W.: Accidents and Emergencies in Anesthesia. Modern Vet. Practice, *40*, 28 (August 1), 1959.

HALL, L. W., LEHMAN, H., and SILK, E.: Response in Dogs to Relaxants Derived from Succinic Acid and Choline. Brit. Med. J., *1*, 134, 1953.

HOPPE, J. O.: A Pharmacological Investigation of 2, 5-Bis-(3-Diethyl-aminopropyl-amino) Benzoquinone-Bis-Benzylchloride (Win 2747): A New Curarimetic Drug. J. Pharm. & Exper. Therap., *100*, 333, 1950.

IRWIN, R. L., DRAPER, W. B., and WHITEHEAD, R. W.: Urine Secretion During Diffusion Respiration after Apnea from Neuromuscular Block. Anesthesiology, *18*, 594, 1957.

KLUPP, H., KRAUPP, O., STORMANN, H., and STUMPF, C.: Uber die Pharmakologischen Eigenschaften Einiger Polymethlen-Decarbaminsaure-Bischolinester. Arch. internat. pharmacodyn., *96*, 161, 1953.

KALOW, W.: The Distribution, Destruction and Elimination of Muscle Relaxants. Anesthesiology, *20*, 505, 1959.

KNILL, L. M.: Pharmacodynamics of Succinylcholine Chloride in the Dog. Master's Thesis, Colorado State University, Fort Collins, Colorado, 1956.

MUSCHIN, W. W., WIEN, R., MASON, D. F. J., and LANGSTON, G. T.: Curare-like Actions of Tri-(Diethylaminoethoxy)-Benzene Triethyliodide. Lancet, *1*, 726, 1949.

NGAI, S. H.: Study of a New Relaxant-Imbretil-in the Cat. Fed. Proc., *18*, 427, 1959.

PAGE, I.: Mechanism of the Vascular Action of Tetraethylammonium Chloride. Am. J. Physiol., *158*, 402, 1949.

PICKETT, D.: Curare in Canine Surgery. J.A.V.M.A., *119*, 346, 1951.

RANDALL, L. O., PETERSON, W. G., and LEHMAN, G.: The Ganglionic Blocking Action of Thiophanium Derivatives. J. Pharm. & Exper. Therap., *97*, 48, 1949.

WRIGHT, J. G. and HALL, L. W.: *Veterinary Anesthesia and Analgesia.* 5th ed. The Williams & Wilkins Co., Baltimore, 1961.

————: Catalogue and Instructions for Use of Short and Long Range Syringe Projector and Cap-Chur Equipment. Palmer Chemical and Equipment Company, Inc., Atlanta, Georgia, 1959.

TOPICAL, INFILTRATION, FIELD BLOCK AND CONDUCTION ANESTHESIA

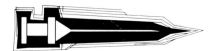

Chapter 13

Physiology of Nerve Conduction and Mechanism of Anesthetic Action

Nerve impulses are transient waves of electrical excitation which travel the length of a nerve fiber. A fiber may be likened to an insulated wire, containing a core of low resistance cytoplasm surrounded by an insulating membrane of high resistance. The tissue fluid surrounding the membrane is a low resistance media. In a resting state, the inner surface of the membrane is negatively charged while the outer surface is positively charged. Early physiologists determined that tissue fluids had a high concentration of sodium ions, while body cells contained a high concentration of potassium ions. It was also noted that a nerve impulse traveling along the nerve

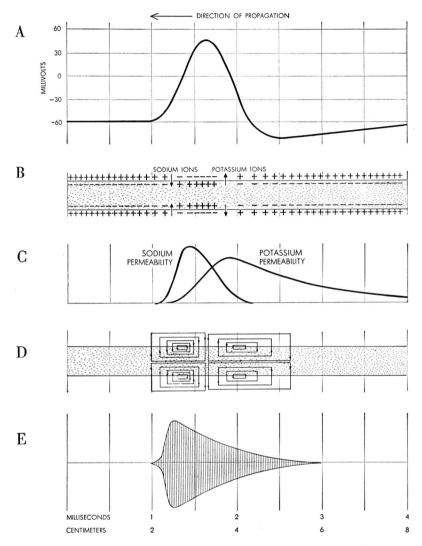

FIGURE 13–1.   Nerve impulse travels along a nerve fiber as a self-propagating wave of electrical activity.   The potential across the outer membrane of the fiber reverses and then returns to normal again (A).   These changes are caused by rises in ionic permeability (C), which permit rapid movement of sodium ions into the fiber, followed by an egress of potassium ions (B).   The altered potential across the disturbed part of the membrane causes electrical currents to flow in the external medium and within the fiber (D).   These depolarize the membrane ahead of the advancing impulse, triggering permeability changes and thus producing a wave of increased conductance (E).   (Keynes, R. D.:   The Nerve Impulse and the Squid.   Scientific American, *199*, 83 (Dec.), 1958).

could be demonstrated as a very brief period of electrical negativity on the outer surface of the nerve fiber membrane (Fig. 13–1). With these facts in mind, Bernstein, in 1902, proposed that selective permeability of the nerve membrane to potassium and impermeability to sodium accounted for the resting potential. A dynamic equilibrium is established in which a negative charge inside the membrane opposes the tendency of the positively charged potassium ions to escape. As an impulse traverses the fiber, the membrane momentarily loses its selective resistance to the electro-chemical pressure of the sodium ions outside. When sodium enters through the membrane, potassium escapes with a resultant fall in membrane potential. The electric current generated by the exchange of ions spreads the loss of selectivity of the membrane to the adjacent section, and the impulse travels along the fiber by self-depolarization regeneration.

Local anesthetic agents will prevent passage of the nerve impulse in (1) sensory nerve endings, (2) ganglionic synapses, (3) myoneural junctions, and (4) nerve trunks. Clinically, the important sites of action are sensory nerve endings and nerve trunks. The smallest nerve fibers are paralyzed first because of the greater surface area per unit of volume. In mixed nerves the sequence of anesthesia is autonomic, sensory, and motor. The order of anesthesia as determined by loss of sensation and action potential has been shown (Heinbecker et al., 1932, 1934) to be:

1. Unmyelinated nerves (vasoconstriction and vasodilation).
2. Smallest thinly myelinated nerves (temperature).
3. Small thinly myelinated nerves (pain).
4. Large thickly myelinated nerves (touch).
5. Largest thickly myelinated nerves (joint and pressure sense).

Return of sensation and action potential is in the reverse order.

In general, local anesthetics are acid salts of basic substances. The salt forms are water soluble; whereas, the substances themselves are water insoluble or lipoid soluble. Normal tissue fluids, which are slightly alkaline, hydrolyze the salt and liberate the base which is then absorbed by nerve tissue.

The exact mechanism of action is still controversial, though it is probably a surface action. The free base which contains positively charged ions is strongly absorbed by the negatively charged nerve fibers and nerve endings. This in turn brings about a decrease in nerve membrane permeability or electrical conductivity.

In concentrations used clinically, local anesthetics affect chiefly nerve cells. Higher concentrations may depress all living cells and lead to local tissue necrosis. The duration of anesthesia is roughly proportional to the concentration of the solution employed. Infected tissue, with an accumulation of pus, contains acid and is much more difficult to anesthetize than normal tissue.

Vasoconstrictors

In 1903 H. Braun discovered that when epinephrine hydrochloride was added to local anesthetic solutions a marked prolongation of anesthesia was produced. This prolongation occurs with all injectable local anesthetics presently in use. The effect of epinephrine is to produce a marked vasoconstriction; hence, the anesthetic is removed from the site of injection much more slowly. This results in longer anesthetic action and decreases the toxicity of the anesthetic, since it can be detoxified over a longer period of time. The maximum safe concentration of epinephrine with a local anesthetic agent is 1:50,000; greater concentration may cause local tissue necrosis. An exception to this rule is in epidural anesthesia where concentrations up to 1:10,000 may be safely used. Other vasoconstrictors employed less frequently are phenylephrine hydrochloride and cobefrin hydrochloride. They do not have any real advantage over epinephrine (Tainter et al., 1938).

Vasoconstrictors are contraindicated in extremities because the ischemia produced may cause gangrene.

Hyaluronidase

Hyaluronidase is a mucolytic enzyme which hydrolyzes hyaluronic acid, the ground substance preventing diffusion of foreign materials in the tissues. When hyaluronidase is added to solutions of local anesthetics it promotes diffusion and absorption. In therapeutic doses it is non-toxic, the ratio of toxic to therapeutic dose being 200:1 (Seifter, 1950).

For infiltration anesthesia, hyaluronidase is used in a concentration of 100 to 150 TRU (turbidity reducing units) per 100 ml. of anesthetic solution. The efficiency of a local anesthetic is increased since the area affected is enlarged. Outwardly it would seem to be of particular value in nerve blocks, in that the anesthetic would not have to be deposited so accurately. However, Moore (1950) and Eckenhoff and Kirby (1951) found that hyaluronidase did not increase the incidence of successful blocks. On the other hand, the duration of anesthesia is decreased and the toxicity increased due to more rapid absorption. This can be counteracted by addition of epinephrine to the solution. The effects produced by various combinations of procaine, epinephrine, and hyaluronidase are shown in Tables 13–1 and 13–2. Hyaluronidase does not increase the efficiency of solutions used for epidural or spinal anesthesia. Because of its cost it is seldom used with local anesthetic agents in small animals.

Table 13–1.—Spreading Effect of Hyaluronidase on Procaine Injected Subcutaneously

Number of Subjects	Solution Injected	Average Area of Skin Anesthesia
		(sq. cm.)
28	Procaine 1% (3 ml.)	8.8
25	Procaine 1% + hyaluronidase (1.6 mg. %)	15.7
13	Procaine 1% + hyaluronidase + epinephrine (1 to 100,000)	17.5

(Kirby, C. K., Eckenhoff, J. E., and Looby, J. P.: The Use of Hyaluronidase with Local Anesthetic Agents in Surgery and Dentistry. Ann. N. Y. Acad. Sci., 52, 1166, 1950.)

Table 13–2.—Effect of Hyaluronidase and Epinephrine on Duration of Anesthesia

Number of Subjects	Solution Injected	Average Duration of Anesthesia to Pinprick
		(min.)
28	Procaine (1%)	32
25	Procaine + hyaluronidase (3.2 mg.%)	23
13	Procaine + epinephrine (1 to 100,000)	188
13	Procaine + hyaluronidase + epinephrine	180

(Kirby, C. K., Eckenhoff, J. E., and Looby, J. P.: The Use of Hyaluronidase with Local Anesthetic Agents in Surgery and Dentistry. Ann. N. Y. Acad. Sci., 52, 1166, 1950.)

Toxicity of Local Anesthetics

Speaking of the use of local anesthetic agents in humans, Adriani (1956) has said:

"Few potentially hazardous drugs are used as thoughtlessly, as indiscriminately, and with less knowledge of their applied pharmacology, as are the local anesthetics. The number of fatalities and near catastrophies from the misuse of these drugs is difficult to estimate because statistics are not accurate. The number of fatalities and various types of untoward responses is higher than one surmises."

Fortunately, the problem of toxicity from local anesthetics is not as great in animals, with the exception of primates, as it is in man. This is perhaps due to the fact that smaller quantities of anesthetic solution are used and that domestic animals have a less well-developed nervous system. Deaths in small animals from injection of local anesthetics are uncommon and usually confined to very small or young animals.

Toxic symptoms produced by all local anesthetic agents are similar though toxic and lethal doses vary widely (Tables 13–3 and 13–4). Untoward responses are of two types, local and systemic. Local damage consists of transient or permanent injury to the tissues. The accepted drugs currently in use do not produce this difficulty. Systemic reactions occur when local anesthetics are absorbed into the general circulation in toxic levels. While all are ultimately absorbed, under ordinary circumstances a toxic level is not attained and no systemic effects occur.

Table 13–3.—The Intravenous Toxicity of a Series of Local Anesthetic Agents to Mice, Guinea Pigs, and Rabbits (Results Are Expressed as LD_{50}, in Terms of Mg. of Base/Kg. of Body Weight)

Agent	Mice	No. of animals	Guinea pigs	No. of animals	Rabbits	No. of animals
Procaine	78 ± 5	60	56 ± 4	25	41 ± 2	25
Neothesin	32 ± 4	40	16 ± 2	30	18 ± 6	35
Hexylcaine	24 ± 2	60	17 ± 2	25	14 ± 2	20
Cocaine	25 ± 4	40	13 ± 2	20	11 ± 1	15
Butacaine	19 ± 2	40	10 ± 2	25	10 ± 1	25
Tetracaine	9 ± 1	40	4 ± 0.25	50	4.5 ± 1	25
Dibucaine	6.5 ± 0.7	40	2.8 ± 0.2	40	2.8 ± 0.5	25

(From Beyer, K. H., Latven, A. R., Freyburger, W. A., and Parker, M. P.: A Comparative Study of the Activity and Toxicity of Hexylcaine (1-Cyclohexylamino-2-Propylbenzoate); A New Local Anesthetic Agent. J. Pharm. & Exper. Therap., *388*, 93, 1948.)

Table 13–4.—The Subcutaneous Toxicity of Local Anesthetic Agents Dissolved in Aqueous Solution and (for Guinea Pigs) in 1 : 50,000 Solution of Epinephrine Hydrochloride (Results Are Expressed as LD_{50} in Terms of Mg. of Base/Kg. of Body Weight)

	Mice		Guinea pigs				Rabbits	
Agent	Aqueous soln.	No. of animals	Aqueous soln.	No. of animals	Epinephrine soln.	No. of animals	Aqueous soln.	No. of animals
Procaine	720 ± 64	70	353 ± 18	25	500 ± 146	25	595 ± 56	20
Neothesin	1140 ± 96	50	255 ± 33	20	305 ± 98	20	385 ± 45	25
Hexylcaine	1080 ± 213	60	146 ± 15	25	385 ± 40	25	164 ± 31	25
Cocaine	140 ± 21	40	27 ± 3	25	87 ± 7	25	70 ± 2	25
Butacaine	110 ± 12	70	39 ± 8	25	71 ± 7	20	30 ± 8	30
Tetracaine	64 ± 8	70	19 ± 6	20	78 ± 11	20	13 ± 2	20
Dibucaine	32 ± 3	90	18 ± 2	20	35 ± 4	30	7 ± 1	25

(From Beyer, K. H., Latven, A. R., Freyburger, W. A., and Parker, M. P.: A Comparative Study of the Activity and Toxicity of Hexylcaine (1-Cyclohexylamino-2-Propylbenzoate); A New Local Anesthetic Agent. J. Pharm. & Exper. Therap., *388*, 93, 1948.)

Table 13–5.—*Historical and Clinical Data of the Regional Anesthetic Agents*

Agent (Generic Name)	Cocaine	Chloroprocaine	Dibucaine	Hexylcaine	Lidocaine	Piperocaine	Procaine	Tetracaine
Chemical Formula	$C_{17}H_{21}NO_4 \cdot HCl$	$C_{12}H_{23}N_2O_2C_1 \cdot HCl$	$C_{20}H_{29}N_3O_2 \cdot HCl$	$C_{16}H_{23}NO_2 \cdot HCl$	$C_{14}H_{22}N_2O \cdot HCl$	$C_{16}H_{23}NO_2 \cdot HCl$	$C_{1}H_{30}N_2O_2 \cdot HCl$	$C_{15}H_{24}N_2O_2 \cdot HCl$
Trade Name		NESACAINE ® Wallace & Tiernan, Inc.	NUPERCAINE ® Ciba Pharmaceutical Products	CYCLAINE ® Sharp & Dohme	XYLOCAINE ® Astra Pharmaceutical Products	METYCAINE ® Eli Lilly & Company	NOVOCAINE® Winthrop Laboratories	PONTOCAINE ® Winthrop Laboratories
Discovery of Compound	1860 by Niemann	1943 by Marks and Rubin	1929 by Uhlmann	1944 by Cope and Hancock	1943 by Löfgren	1927 by McElvain	1905 by Einhorn	1928–29 by Eisleb
Discovery of Anesthetic Properties	1879 by Van Anrep	1944 by Marks	1929 by Uhlmann	1948 by Beyer	1943 by Löfgren and Lundquist	1927 by Rose	1905 by Biberfeld	1930 by Fussganger & Schaumann
First Used Clinically	1884 by Koller	1950 by Foldes	1929 by Killian	1948 by Wylde	1944 by Gordh	1930 by Meeker	1905 by Braun	1930 by Kiess
Type of Compound	Ester of benzoic acid and nitrogen containing base	Amino-ethyl ester of chloro-amino benzoic acid	Amine derivative of quinoline	Cyclohexylamine derivative of propyl benzoate	Diethylamine derivative of acetanilide	Substituted piperidino-alkyl benzoate	Amino-ethyl ester of benzoic acid	Dimethyl amino-ethyl ester of benzoic acid
Molecular Weight	339.81	307.2	343.45	297.85	234.33	292.82	272.77	300.46
Soluble in	Water	Water	Water	Water	Water	Water and alcohol	Water and alcohol	Water
pH of Solution in 0.9% NaCl	4% pH 5–5.5	3–4	0.06% pH 4.5–5	1% pH 3.9–4.4	1% pH 6.5–7	1% pH 4–5	1% pH 3.5–4	0.1% pH 3.5–4

Thermostability	Crystals and solution stable	Crystals stable Solution may lose potency during autoclaving	Solution stable Crystals melt at 97°C.	Crystals and solution stable	Crystals and solution stable	Crystals and solution stable	Crystals and solution stable	Crystals stable Solution may lose potency during autoclaving
Potency (Procaine = 1)	4:1	2.4:1	20:1	1.2:1	1.5–2:1	1.4:1	1:1	10:1
Toxicity (Procaine = 1)	4:1	0.5:1	20–30:1	1.2:1	Varies in direct proportion to concentration (0.5% 1:1) (1.0% 1.4:1) (2.0% 1.5:1)	1.4:1	1:1	10:1
Recommended Concentration For:								
Spinal	Not Recommended For Use Other Than Topical	Not recommended	0.5%	1.5–2%	2%	Not recommended	2–5%	0.2–0.5%
Epidural		2–3%	2%	1–1.5%	1–2%	1–2%	2–4%	0.2%
Block of Large Nerve		2%	0.1%	1%	2%	2%	2%	0.2%
Block of Small Nerve		1%	0.05%	0.5–1%	1%	1–1.5%	1%	0.1%
Infiltration		0.5–1%	0.05%	0.5%	0.5%	0.5–1%	0.5%	0.1%
Topical	4–10%	Does not produce topical anesthesia	2%	2.5–5%	2–4%	2–4%	Does not produce topical anesthesia	2%

(Courtesy of Dr. W. H. L. Dornette and the Ohio Chemical and Surgical Equipment Company.)

(245)

In general, reactions are avoided by: (1) limiting the total quantity of drug used, (2) use of dilute solutions, (3) retarding absorption by addition of a vasoconstrictor, and (4) the administration of a central nervous system depressant prior to anesthesia.

When the concentration of local anesthetic in the general circulation reaches the toxic level, two types of symptoms may be seen either singly or together. These are: (1) vascular and (2) central nervous types.

The vascular type of reaction is caused by decreased cardiac output due to depression of the myocardium along with local vasodilatation. It is characterized by sudden collapse, pale mucous membranes, tachycardia, and disappearance of the pulse. Vasopressors administered intravenously will overcome the hypotension.

The central nervous type is caused by stimulation of the central nervous system, the cortex being affected first, then the subcortical centers, the midbrain, and finally the medulla. Apprehension, excitement, and nausea or vomiting usually are seen before convulsions occur. Barbiturates are used to counteract the convulsive action of local anesthetics. Care should be exercised in their use, since depression, coma, respiratory and circulatory failure follow the convulsive seizures. Barbiturates antagonize the central nervous system stimulation but do not neutralize local anesthetics or hasten their detoxification and elimination.

Respiratory stimulants (analeptics) are contraindicated in attempting to overcome apnea. Local anesthetics depress the central nervous system and it does not respond to these stimulants. Artificial respiration and oxygen should be administered.

Desirable Characteristics of Local Anesthetic Agents

From the foregoing it can be seen that a number of characteristics are desirable in a local anesthetic agent. They include:

1. Good penetrating qualities in body tissues.
2. High potency so that low concentrations can be used.
3. Rapid onset.
4. Long duration of action.
5. Low systemic toxicity.
6. No irritation to nerve and other body tissues.
7. Reversible action.
8. Availability in sterile solution or ability to be easily sterilized.

Unfortunately, no agent possesses all of these. Table 13–5 summarizes the characteristics of some local anesthetics employed today.

Cocaine Hydrochloride, U.S.P.

From a practical standpoint the significance of cocaine to veterinary anesthesiology is principally historical. Cocaine has the disadvantage of being toxic to the tissues when injected; therefore, newer less toxic, non-addictive, synthetic "caines" have supplanted it in the United States.

Cocaine in 2 to 4% aqueous solution produces good surface anesthesia of the cornea and conjunctiva. In addition it causes a vasoconstriction of superficial vessels and a mydriasis. Occasionally it may produce corneal irritation with cloudiness and even ulceration. For this reason butacaine or tetracaine are more generally used. Since cocaine and its derivatives are habit-forming, they are subject to the federal narcotic laws and may be purchased only by individuals possessing a narcotic license.

Procaine Hydrochloride, U.S.P. (Novocaine)

Procaine hydrochloride was first synthesized by Einhorn in 1905. Because procaine was the first of the synthetic local anesthetics to be used clinically, it has served as a criterion for newer local anesthetic drugs. Procaine is not as active as cocaine but is only about one-fourth as toxic.

Procaine hydrochloride is a white crystalline water-soluble powder. Solutions are relatively stable and can be sterilized repeatedly by boiling without loss of potency. Those which have begun to deteriorate have a yellowish tint and should be discarded. Procaine hydrochloride solutions have a pH of approximately 6.0 when fresh; on standing they become more acid.

Lethal doses of procaine for four species are listed in Table 13–6.

Intravenous procaine hydrochloride has been used in man for treatment of spastic muscles, inflammatory conditions, and cardiac arrhythmia. In dogs, Jones (1951) found that up to 6 mg./kg. could

Table 13–6.—Average Minimal Lethal Dose of Procaine Hydrochloride (in gm./kg.)

Species	Route of Administration	
	Subcutaneous	*Intravenous*
Guinea Pig	0.43	0.05
Rabbit	0.46	0.055
Cat	0.45	0.045
Dog	0.25	—

(Graubard, D. J. and Peterson, M. C.: *Clinical Uses of Intravenous Procaine.* Charles C Thomas, 1950.)

be safely injected intravenously in a 20-minute period without disturbing the animals. However, this dose did not produce analgesia and convulsive muscular contractions were seen at levels producing analgesic effect. The heart rate was increased and became very regular. For dogs the minimum lethal dose of intravenous procaine hydrochloride injected within 5 seconds was approximately 100 mg./kg. of body weight. At necropsy an enlarged liver and engorged spleen were found along with a variable hyperemia of the lungs and kidneys. Jones concluded that intravenous procaine hydrochloride is not suitable for analgesia in the dog.

Procaine is hydrolized in the body to para-aminobenzoic acid (PABA) and diethylaminoethanol. In the dog procaine is converted rapidly into these end-products which are then eliminated by the kidneys; the procaine blood level itself is not significantly lowered by the kidneys.

Procaine   PABA   Diethylaminoethanol

According to Dunlop (1935), in nephrectomized dogs the end-products may be found in the blood as long as the animal survives. The liver is not essential for the detoxification of procaine, other tissues being able to convert it into these end-products. However, the liver detoxifies procaine much more rapidly and efficiently than other tissues. The enzyme responsible for hydrolysis of procaine has been called procaine esterase but may well be cholinesterase (Kalow, 1952).

Procaine is used for infiltration, conduction, and spinal anesthesia in small animals. It is non-irritant and rapidly effective. Without added vasoconstrictor, the duration is relatively brief because of rapid absorption and destruction by the tissues. One or two per cent solutions are generally employed. One ml. of epinephrine hydrochloride solution, U.S.P. (1:1,000), added to each 99 ml. of anesthetic solution will give a concentration of 1:100,000. Procaine is not an effective surface anesthetic and therefore is seldom used for this purpose.

Excessive intravenous injection of procaine in dogs produces respiratory failure. According to Hulpieu and Cole (1951), central nervous system stimulants (nikethamide, pentylenetetrazol, picrotoxin, and lobeline) are of no value in respiratory failure due to procaine. Oxygen and artificial respiration are often life-saving.

To prolong the effect of procaine, oily solutions were introduced, the aim being to achieve slow release of the active procaine base. Claims for prolonged anesthesia with such solutions have not been substantiated and the oil increases the incidence of inflammatory reactions, suppuration, and necrosis.

Lidocaine Hydrochloride (Xylocaine)

Lidocaine is chemically unrelated to cocaine, procaine, or derivatives of these substances. It is quite stable, even when boiled with strong acids or alkalies, and solutions may be autoclaved repeatedly if necessary. Goldberg (1947) found the absolute toxicity was greater than that of procaine but the security coefficient, which takes into account the therapeutic efficacy of both drugs, was 2 to 4 times greater than that of procaine. Bremer *et al.* (1948) have indicated that the onset of anesthesia is twice as quick as that attained with procaine and the duration exceeds that of procaine by 50% or more. In dogs the dose for epidural anesthesia is from 2 to 10 ml. of 2% solution with epinephrine 1:100,000. For infiltration 0.5% without epinephrine is suggested. In cats for epidural anesthesia 2 ml. of 2% solution with 1:100,000 epinephrine is the average dose.

The LD_{50} of xylocaine for mice is 48, 170, and 360 mg./kg. of body weight when administered subcutaneously, intraperitoneally, and intravenously (Truant and Wiedling, 1958).

Hexylcaine Hydrochloride (Cyclaine)

Hexylcaine hydrochloride is soluble to a concentration of 12% in water; 1% solution is stable on boiling, autoclaving, and storage at room temperature. One per cent solution has a pH of 3.9.

Hexylcaine hydrochloride is four to eight times more active than procaine and produces anesthesia of longer duration probably because it is more slowly hydrolyzed. Experimental and clinical investigations have shown it to have a comparatively low order of toxicity (Beyer *et al.*, 1948).

One per cent solution is suggested for infiltration and nerve blocks. For topical anesthesia of the eye 1 or 2% solutions are recommended. Five per cent cyclaine is used in the ear for removal of grass awns and in the vagina for catheterization.

Dyclonine Hydrochloride (Dyclone)

Dyclonine hydrochloride is a white crystalline powder which is stable in acidic aqueous solutions. Chemically it is an organic ketone and has no relation to the "caine" type of local anesthetics. For this reason no cross-sensitivity has been observed.

In vitro studies have shown dyclonine hydrochloride has bactericidal and fungicidal properties with a phenol coefficient of 3.6. Solutions of dyclonine hydrochloride are considered self-sterilizing unless massively contaminated.

Dyclonine hydrochloride has excellent topical anesthetic properties and a wide margin of safety. In rabbits a 0.5% solution will give corneal anesthesia for 50 to 60 minutes. It has a wide variety of indications including urethral catheterization, itching dermatoses, bronchoscopy, esophagoscopy, and tonometry.

Concentrated solutions of dyclonine hydrochloride are irritating on injection; therefore, concentrations of over 0.5% are not recommended. When given parenterally it has no parasympatholytic action in animals. For epidural use in dogs and cats 1 ml./5 lb. of 0.5% solution is suggested; for infiltration the dose varies depending on the area involved.

Dyclonine hydrochloride is available as 0.5% solution, and as a 1.0% cream for topical application.

Butacaine Sulfate, U.S.P. (Butyn)

Butacaine sulfate is a white crystalline water-soluble powder which is closely related chemically to procaine. Solutions are com-

Table 13–7.—The Relative Corneal Anesthetic Activity of Local Anesthetic Agents

Compound	Corneal Anesthesia in Guinea Pigs			Corneal Anesthesia in Rabbits (Using Saline Washout)			Corneal Anesthesia in Rabbits (Without Saline Washout)		
	A.C. 100* per cent	Dur. at 1%† min.	Conc. prod. dur. = 2% coc.‡	A.C. 100 per cent	Dur. at 1% min.	Conc. prod. dur. = 2% coc.	A.C. 100 per cent	Dur. at 1% min.	Conc. prod. dur. = 2% coc.
Tetracaine§	$\frac{1}{64}$	52	$\frac{1}{8}$	$\frac{1}{64}$	98	$\frac{1}{64}$			
Butacaine	$\frac{1}{2}$	40	$\frac{1}{2}$	$\frac{1}{8}$	16	$\frac{1}{2}$	$\frac{1}{8}$	35	1
Hexylcaine	$\frac{1}{2}$	19	2	$\frac{1}{4}$	12	$\frac{1}{2}$	$\frac{1}{8}$	19	2
Cocaine	1	18	2	$\frac{1}{2}$	7	2	$\frac{1}{4}$	30	2
Neothesin	1	16	2	1	5	4	$\frac{1}{2}$	5	2
Procaine	4	0	7	8	0	16	4	0	8

* A.C. 100 = minimal concentration necessary to produce anesthesia in all animals.
† Duration of anesthesia when a 1% solution was instilled.
‡ Percentage concentration that produced a duration of anesthesia equivalent to 2% cocaine.
§ Corneal anesthesia in rabbits (without saline washout) was not determined.

(From Beyer, K. H., Latven, A. R., Freyburger, W. A., and Parker, M. P.: A Comparative Study of the Activity and Toxicity of Hexylcaine (1-Cyclohexylamino-2-Propylbenzoate); A New Local Anesthetic Agent. J. Pharm. & Exper. Therap., *388*, 93, 1948.)

monly used for surface anesthesia of mucous membranes and the cornea (Table 13–7). It is a good substitute for cocaine in that it possesses most of the advantages of the latter without the disadvantages. It has a rapid onset of action, penetrates well, and has a fairly long duration of anesthesia. It does not cause mydriasis or damage to the cornea, as is sometimes produced by cocaine, but does slow corneal healing. It has the advantage over cocaine that it does not require a narcotic license for its use. Because it is approximately nine times more toxic than procaine it is never used for infiltration anesthesia.

Butacaine sulfate is usually used as a 2% solution which is instilled in the eye or applied on any mucous membrane. When applied in the eye once, minor anesthesia is produced. If instilled four times at 1-minute intervals, surgical anesthesia is produced.

Solutions must be stored in brown bottles to prevent deterioration.

Butacaine sulfate ointment, N.N.R. for local use, contains 1% of the anesthetic.

Tetracaine Hydrochloride, U.S.P. (Pontocaine)

Tetracaine hydrochloride is a white crystalline substance easily precipitated from solution by bases. Crystals or solutions should not be autoclaved.

While it has been employed as an all-purpose anesthetic, its systemic toxicity is 12 to 20 times that of procaine and its anesthetic potency is no more than 10 times the latter. For this reason its use is confined chiefly to topical application. As a surface anesthetic its potency is 10 times greater than cocaine. It interferes less with corneal healing than other commonly used agents, and therefore is a drug of choice for corneal anesthesia. For this purpose a 0.5% solution is quite adequate.

Ethyl Alcohol

When injected into soft tissue, 5 ml. of absolute alcohol will cause an area of necrosis 1 cm. in diameter. When injected around a nerve, neuritis and degeneration will occur, followed by sclerosis. Thirty per cent alcohol temporarily destroys sensory nerves which regenerate in time. The duration of block will depend on the size of the nerve and degree of destruction.

According to Adriani (1947) destruction of nerve tissue with alcohol is similar to that obtained by sectioning a nerve and is typical of Wallerian degeneration. Small unsheathed nerves may be permanently destroyed; whereas, large heavily sheathed nerves are only temporarily affected. Since nerves regenerate, after a variable period of time function may return. Fibrosis which accompanies the injection may predispose to neuritis.

Ethyl Chloride, U.S.P.

Ethyl chloride is occasionally used as a local anesthetic. For this purpose it is marketed under pressure in containers equipped with a fine capillary nozzle and a control valve which allows the liquid to be sprayed from the container (Fig. 13–2). As it is sprayed on the skin it evaporates instantly, removing heat in the process and causing an area of skin to freeze. Surface anesthesia lasting from 30 to 60

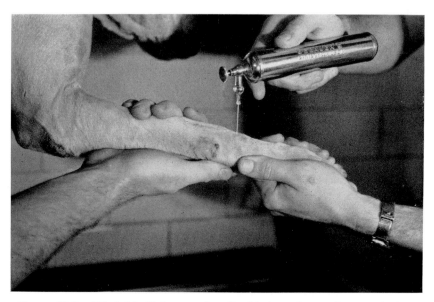

FIGURE 13–2.   Ethyl chloride is sprayed on the skin to produce surface anesthesia.

seconds is produced. Overzealous administration will produce frostbite. Because the anesthesia is quite superficial and of very short duration, and because frozen tissue is not easily dissected, its use is confined to simple incisions or punctures such as the drainage of abscesses.

For further information concerning ethyl chloride and its use as a general anesthetic see Chapter 8, page 129.

Topical Anesthesia

Local anesthetic agents applied to the unabraded skin surface have no effect, and even when applied to raw skin surfaces of small animals these agents are often of dubious value. This is due, in part, to the natural tendency of animals to lick wounds and keep them clean. On mucous surfaces the anesthetic effect is good. For example, anesthetic ointments are generally quite effective in treatment of pruritis ani. Jellies are useful in lubricating endotracheal catheters and help prevent postintubation cough. When instilled in the eye, local anesthetics produce good surface anesthesia. Solutions may be injected into the urethra of animals suffering from obstruction due to calculi with good results. By anesthetizing the mucous membrane, spasm is relieved and passage of stones facilitated.

Uses for Topical Anesthesia

Topical anesthesia is employed for many purposes:

1. To produce surface anesthesia of the conjunctiva and cornea for minor surgical procedures, tonometry, and beta ray therapy.
2. To produce surface anesthesia and thus prevent scratching and/ or licking in inflammatory conditions such as dermatitis, otitis externa, conjunctivitis, and pruritis ani. Here the anesthetic is usually combined with other therapeutic agents in a creme or jelly.
3. To produce anesthesia of tissues for superficial surgical procedures (ethyl chloride).
4. To lubricate and anesthetize mucous surfaces for procedures such as nasal, endotracheal, and urethral catheterization, and for otic examination.

Infiltration and Field Block

Infiltration and field block anesthesia are used chiefly for removal of small superficial tumors, debridement and suturing of wounds, cesarean section, and tail amputation in young puppies.

Tumors and Wounds

The surgical site should be clipped, washed, and a suitable antiseptic applied to the skin. Injection of local anesthetic is made with a glass syringe to which a fine caliber needle is attached. In most small animal patients a 1- or 1½-inch 22 gauge needle is suitable. The needle is held with the bevel against the skin and the shank at an acute angle as it is inserted. An intradermal wheal can be raised prior to insertion of the needle into the subcutaneous tissue. If injections are made with the needle in a fixed position, aspiration should be performed to determine that the point is not within a blood vessel. If on aspiration blood returns to the syringe, the point of the needle must be repositioned. Infiltration of subcutaneous tissue may be continuous if the needle is kept constantly in motion.

When removing a small tumor or similar lesion a diamond-shaped block is made by linear infiltration of anesthetic agent as shown in Figure 13–3. This is accomplished by holding the needle practically parallel to the skin surface and injecting anesthetic as the needle is

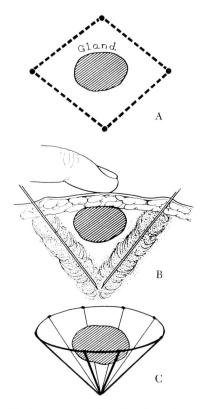

FIGURE 13–3.   Field block for biopsy of lymph node (or for equivalent operation). (*A*) Outline on cutaneous surface of diamond-shaped field block; (*B*) node is continuously palpated throughout the injection to avoid losing it; (C) a cone of anesthetic is deposited around the node. (From Lundy, J. S.:   *Clinical Anesthesia*. W. B. Saunders Co., 1942.)

advanced its full length. The deep tissues are then infiltrated by injections around the periphery so that they form a cone, the apex of which is directly beneath the lesion. Ten minutes should be allowed to elapse, following which the block should be tested prior to surgery.

Riser (1947) has advocated the use of field block anesthesia in removal of extensive mammary tumors in the dog. Most veterinarians, however, are of the opinion that a more deliberate and thorough resection can be accomplished with general anesthesia.

Infiltration anesthesia is contraindicated in malignant tumors since the infiltration procedure may transplant tumor cells to otherwise normal tissues.

Cesarean Section

For anesthesia in cesarean section in the dog, Schirmer (1960) has recommended administration of promazine intravenously "to effect" over a 10-minute period. This usually requires a dose of 1 to 3 mg./lb. When the dog appears tranquilized, lidocaine is injected at three levels along the incision line using a 1-inch 22 gauge needle. The first level is in the deep layer of the skin and produces a skin bleb. The second is in the deep subcutaneous tissue and the third in the muscle. The injection is fanned out at the ends of the incision. Approximately 3 ml. of 2% lidocaine are used for a 20 pound dog.

The bitch should be removed from the puppies for 3 or 4 hours postoperatively, since she may chew and kill them until tranquilization subsides.

Tail Amputation

A use for field block anesthesia is in amputation of puppies' tails. This is performed by depositing a ring of anesthetic around the tail proximal to the amputation site. Two precautions should be observed if this procedure is used. First, the small size of most puppies precludes the use of large quantities of local anesthetic agent. Toxic

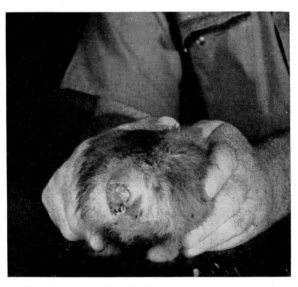

FIGURE 13–4.   Slough of a puppy's tail following injection of procaine-epinephrine for anesthesia during tail amputation.

symptoms and even death will occur with large doses. Second, vasoconstrictors should not be used in the anesthetic solution, since it is possible to compromise the blood supply of the tail close to the site of infiltration with resulting necrosis of tissue proximal to the amputation site (Fig. 13–4).

Conduction Anesthesia

Nerve blocks in small animals have never been popular among veterinarians because, even though good anesthesia of an area is achieved, restraint is often a problem. Since more satisfactory techniques are available, dental nerve blocks have largely been abandoned.

Dental Blocks in the Dog

The sensory nerves of the teeth are the maxillary and mandibular branches of the trigeminal nerve (fifth cranial nerve). The maxillary nerve leaves the cranium through the foramen rotundum, traverses the pterygopalatine fossa, and continues in the infraorbital canal as the infraorbital nerve. The first and second molars are supplied by branches which leave the main trunk before it enters the infraorbital canal. Other branches are given off in the canal to the four premolars and surrounding alveoli and gum. The canine and incisor teeth are supplied by branches originating in the infraorbital canal which pass forward in the maxillary and premaxillary bones (incisivomaxillary canal).

The mandibular alveolar nerve, a branch of the mandibular nerve, enters the mandibular canal on the medial aspect of the ramus through the mandibular foramen. In the canal it supplies branches to the molars and premolars and a branch passes forward, in the incisivo-mandibular canal, to supply the canine and incisor teeth of that side.

The Infraorbital Nerve

The infraorbital nerve supplies all upper teeth on its respective side. It can be blocked at two sites:

1. In the pterygopalatine fossa at its point of entry into the infraorbital canal (maxillary foramen). In the average dog a 2-inch 20 gauge needle is inserted about 1 inch below the lateral canthus of the eye with the point directed medially, between the malar bone anteriorly and the coronoid process of the mandible posteriorly, until the border of the malar bone has been passed. Then the needle is pointed anteriorly toward the gingival border of the upper incisor

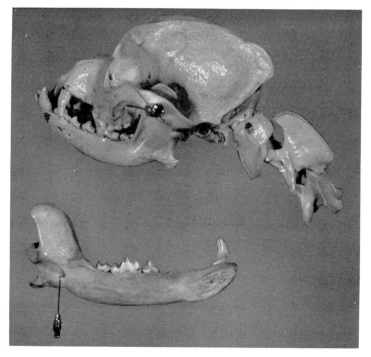

FIGURE 13–5.   Locations for blocking the maxillary and mandibular nerves.

teeth (Fig. 13–5). The maxillary foramen will be encountered at a depth of 1 to 1½ inches (Frank, 1928). Two ml. of 2% procaine are injected. All of the upper teeth on that side of the head will be desensitized.

Lacroix (1957) has described an alternative method in which the needle is inserted from within the mouth.

> "The syringe is introduced just posterior to and parallel with the long axis of the last molar tooth. The solution is injected slowly as the needle is pushed into the tissues. The depth of penetration varies with the size of the subject. A needle one inch in length is sufficient for the largest dog. . . ."

2. In the lower part of the infraorbital canal. The upper lip is retracted and the infraorbital foramen located by palpation of its border, dorsal to the third premolar, where the mucous membrane of the lip reflects on the gum. After preparation of the gum, the needle is inserted into the canal about ½ inch and 1 ml. of 2% procaine injected. The incisors, canine, and first two premolars of that side are desensitized.

17

The Mandibular Nerve

This nerve supplies the teeth of the lower jaw and can be blocked at two sites:

1. At the mandibular foramen. The depression just in front of the angular process of the mandible is palpated. A 1-inch 22 gauge needle is inserted at right angles to the ventral border of the jaw just medial to the bone, for a distance of $\frac{1}{2}$ to $\frac{3}{4}$ of an inch (Frank, 1928). Two ml. of procaine are deposited at this site. All of the teeth on that side of the lower jaw are desensitized.

Lacroix has described an alternative approach from within the mouth. The needle is inserted medial and parallel to the long axis of the sixth molar with the point inclined toward the mandible. The anesthetic is deposited in the tissues around the nerve by gauging the relative positions of the needle and nerve.

2. Through the mental foramen. There are three mental foramina, anterior, middle, and caudal. The middle one is used for this procedure. The foramen is situated immediately beneath the anterior root of the second lower premolar, about one-half the distance between the dorsal and ventral borders of the mandible. The opening cannot be felt with the finger and a search must be made with the needle point. The needle is inserted about $\frac{3}{8}$ inch into the foramen and 1 ml. of 2% solution is injected into the mandibular canal. The incisors, canine, and first two premolars on that side are desensitized.

There is considerable variation in the position of the various foramina in the three head shapes observed in dogs. In addition, there are anastomoses between sides so that complete block of the incisors on a given side may not occur.

Block of the Brachial Plexus

Anesthesia of the brachial plexus in the dog has been described by Tufvesson (1951) who states that it is indicated for operative interference of the foreleg at, or below, the elbow joint. He indicates that luxations and fractures are easily reduced due to complete muscular relaxation.

With the skin prepared, a 3-inch 18 gauge needle is inserted in the triangular depression bounded by the anterior border of the supraspinatus muscle, the thoracic wall, and the dorsal border of the brachiocephalicus muscle. The needle is directed caudally, lateral to the thoracic wall and medial to the subcapsularis muscle, until the point is even with the spine of the scapula. After aspirating to prevent intravascular injection, 10 ml. of 2% lidocaine is deposited around the brachial plexus. In puppies and toy breeds the dose is reduced accordingly. Paralysis is the first sign of anesthesia; full anesthesia requires 18 minutes and lasts 1 to 2 hours.

The Palpebral Nerve

The palpebral nerve is a branch of the auriculopalpebral which, in turn, is a branch of the facial nerve. It can be anesthetized by subcutaneous injection of 1 ml. of a local anesthetic approximately 1 cm. dorsal to the zygomatic arch at its most lateral projection (Fig. 13–6). Anesthesia of all the muscles of the eyelids except

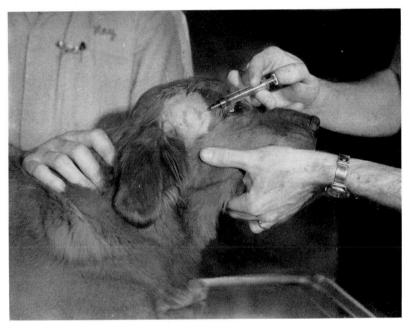

FIGURE 13–6. Block of the palpebral branch of the auriculopalpebral nerve will prevent closure of the eyelids.

the levator palpebrae will be produced. This is helpful in application of beta ray therapy to the cornea or in ocular surgery. Unless general anesthesia is also used, the animal is unable to close the eyelids but can still rotate and retract the eyeball.

The Radial Nerve

The radial nerve can be blocked where it spirals around the humerus from the medial to the lateral surface (Fig. 13–7A). In some dogs the nerve can be palpated at this site which is one-half the distance from the olecranon to the acromion. This is distal to the

branches to the triceps brachii and will produce paralysis of the ex
tensors of the carpus and digits with anesthesia of the dorsal and
lateral aspect of the forearm and the dorsal aspect of the paw.

The Median, Ulnar, and Musculocutaneous Nerves

Together, the median and ulnar nerves supply all flexors of the
carpus and digits and are sensory to the carpal, metacarpal, and
digital pads. The ulnar nerve supplies sensation to the caudal surface of the forearm and lateral side of the fifth digit. The musculocutaneous nerve supplies the biceps brachii and brachialis muscles

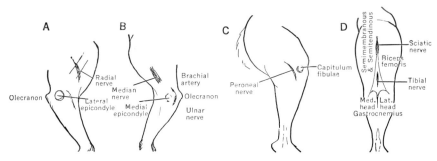

FIGURE 13–7.   Location of the radial, median, and ulnar nerves in the foreleg of the
dog (*A* and *B*). Location of the peroneal, sciatic and tibial nerves in the hind leg of the
dog (*C* and *D*). (From Allam, M. W., Nulsen, F. E., Lewey, F. H.: Electrical Intra-
neural Bipolar Stimulation of Peripheral Nerves in the Dog. J.A.V.M.A., *114*, 87, 1949.)

and is sensory to the medial aspect of the forearm. In the middle of
the true arm all three nerves lie around the brachial vessels, the
median and ulnar posterior to the brachial artery and the musculocutaneous anterior.

For complete loss of sensation in areas supplied by the median and
ulnar nerves, it is necessary to block both plus the musculocutaneous
nerve which supplies a branch to the median at the elbow. This is
best accomplished by injecting the three nerves on the medial aspect
of the arm, as they course distally accompanied by the brachial
artery (Fig. 13–7*B*). Pulsation of the artery may serve as a guide.
At least 2 ml. of 2% solution should be infiltrated around the vessel,
care being taken to prevent intravascular injection.

The Saphenous Nerve

This is a branch of the femoral nerve and is motor to the sartorius
muscle and sensory to the medial surface of the thigh, stifle, and leg.
It can be reached in the femoral triangle as it runs distally just

cranial to the femoral artery. Using the arterial pulse as a land-mark, injection is made anterior to the artery being careful to prevent intravascular injection.

The Fibular (Peroneal) Nerve

The fibular nerve, a terminal branch of the sciatic nerve, supplies the flexors of the hock and extensors of the digits. It is sensory to the dorsal aspect of the tibial region, hock, and paw. It passes laterally, under cover of the biceps femoris, around the fibula just below its head (Fig. 13–7C). It can be infiltrated by injecting just posterior and dorsal to the head of the fibula.

The Tibial Nerve

The tibial nerve is the other terminal branch of the sciatic. It is motor to the extensors of the hock and flexors of the digits and sup-plies sensation to the plantar surface of the paw. It can be blocked just above the stifle joint by inserting the needle from behind into the popliteal space between the two heads of the gastrocnemius muscle (Fig. 13–7D).

The Sciatic Nerve

The terminal branches of the sciatic nerve have been described above. In addition, it supplies the caudal thigh muscles which extend the hip and flex the stifle. Sensory branches innervate the skin on the caudal and lateral aspect of the true leg. The nerve can be blocked most easily where it passes over the lesser sciatic notch. The needle is inserted at a right angle posterior to the femur for a variable depth depending upon the size of the animal.

Epidural Anesthesia (Extradural, Peridural, Caudal Anesthesia)

According to Brook (1935), Cuillé and Sendrail were first to use epidural anesthesia in veterinary medicine. They published an article on its use in 1901. In the United States Frank (1927) popu-larized this technique.

Epidural anesthesia is accomplished by injection of anesthetic sol-tion into the spinal canal so that it lies outside or upon (epi) the dura mater. This temporarily paralyzes the spinal nerves which are con-tacted by the solution and produces anesthesia of the tissues supplied by them. In humans this type of anesthesia is termed caudal an-esthesia, and is widely used, particularly in obstetrics.

The injection in the dog and cat is commonly made at the lum-bosacral space (Fig. 13–8). Early workers injected the dog at the sacrococcygeal space but abandoned this technique since it was difficult. Brook (1935) has pointed out that the dimensions of the sacral meningeal cul-de-sac are so small that a needle penetration at this point is highly improbable and thus the injection is extradural. In the dog the greater splanchnic nerve arises from the twelfth thoracic sympathetic ganglion. If anesthetic solution passes cranially past the first lumbar segment a serious fall in blood pressure may occur. Brook has suggested that the animal be restrained on its back immediately following injection so that the sensory dorsal spinal nerve roots are more profoundly affected than the ventral roots containing the vasomotor fibers.

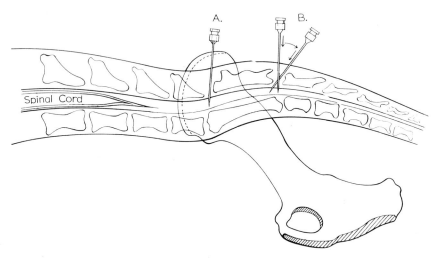

FIGURE 13–8. Sites for epidural injection in the dog: (A) at the lumbosacral space and (B) at the sacrococcygeal space. The latter is not used clinically.

In man continuous caudal or peridural anesthesia is sometimes administered by insertion of a ureteral catheter or plastic tube into the spinal canal. The anesthetic is then injected intermittently as needed (Adriani, 1947). Nothing in the veterinary literature indicates that continuous epidural anesthesia has been attempted in small animals; however, this possibility should, perhaps, be investigated.

Epidural Anesthesia in the Dog

Bone and Peck (1956) have listed indications for epidural anesthesia in dogs as follows:

1. Cesarean section.
2. Ovariohysterectomy.

3. Castration.
4. Reduction of rectal prolapse.
5. Caudectomy.
6. Mammectomy.
7. Excision of skin tumors of the hindquarters.
8. Fracture repair.
9. Relaxation of the abdomen to facilitate palpation.
10. Repair of wounds of the hindquarters.

Preanesthetic administration of a narcotic or tranquilizer will aid in restraint during injection but is not essential. The area over the lumbosacral space is clipped and scrubbed with a suitable antiseptic. Table 13–8 gives a dose schedule for three commonly used agents.

Table 13–8.—Dosage for Epidural Anesthesia

Agent	Per cent Solution	Epinephrine	Dog	Cat	Duration
Procaine	1 2 2.5	None None 1:10,000	1 ml./5 lbs. 1 ml./5 lbs. 1 ml./5 lbs. Reduce as weight increases over 20 lbs.	1 ml./5 lbs. 1 ml./5 lbs. 1 ml./5 lbs.	15–20 minutes 20–25 minutes 25–35 minutes
Hexylcaine (Cyclaine)	1 2 5*	None None None	1 ml. (puppies) 1 ml./12.5 lbs. 0.5 to 2.0 ml. (Approximately 1 ml./25 lbs.)		30–60 minutes 6–12 hours
Lidocaine (Xylocaine)	2	1:100,000	2 to 10 ml.	2 ml.	

* Not recommended because prolonged paralysis may occur.

Two techniques may be used for restraining dogs during the injection procedure. In the first, an assistant places the dog's head under one arm and grasps a hind leg in the stifle area with each hand (Fig. 13–9). With the second technique the dog is held by an assistant with the hind quarters bent over the edge of the table. The injection site is located with the left hand, by placing the thumb and second finger on the ilial crests while the index finger palpates and marks the lumbosacral space.

A $\frac{3}{4}$-inch 24 gauge needle is used for puppies, a $1\frac{1}{2}$-inch 20 gauge needle for medium sized dogs and a 3-inch 20 gauge needle for large or obese dogs. The needle is slanted forward at a slight angle. A subcutaneous wheal of anesthetic at the injection site is optional.

As the needle is inserted through the intervertebral ligament a distinct popping sensation is felt. The needle is introduced further until it touches the floor of the spinal canal and is then withdrawn approximately $\frac{1}{8}$ inch. Back pressure is first exerted on the syringe to insure against a bloody tap and the injection is then made. *There should be no resistance* to the injection; if it occurs the needle must be repositioned.

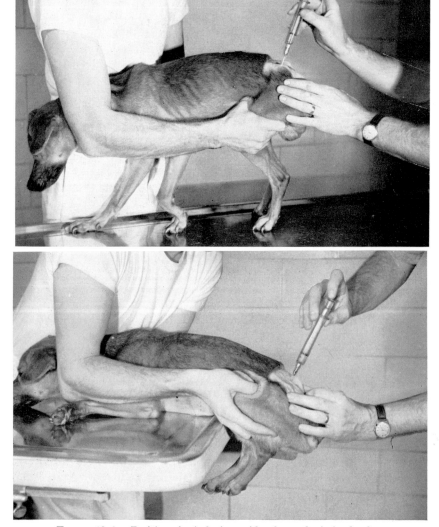

FIGURE 13-9.   Positions for inducing epidural anesthesia in the dog.

When injection is properly performed anesthesia begins almost immediately. The tail relaxes, followed by the anal sphincter, and soon the rear quarters collapse. Injection in an improper location results in:

1. Delay in onset of anesthesia.
2. Unilateral hind limb paresis due to anesthesia of one sciatic nerve, at or near the sciatic foramen.
3. Partial anesthesia of tail or perineal region due to injection of dorsal branches of sacral nerves.
4. Shock and/or death from injecting subarachnoid space.

Reinjection after 1, 2, and 3 above can be performed without adverse results.

Epidural Anesthesia in the Cat

Epidural anesthesia in the cat has been described by Garcia (1953). The patient is restrained on the operating table with tapes, the head facing toward the anesthetist's right (Fig. 13–10). The crest of the ilium on either side is used as a landmark. The thumb and second finger of the left hand are placed on the two crests, and the left index finger is used to palpate the depression of the lumbo-sacral fossa in the median line.

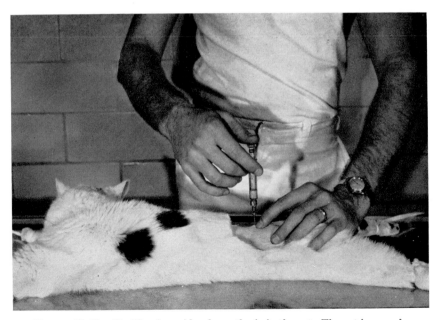

FIGURE 13–10.   Position for epidural anesthesia in the cat. The cat is spread-eagled on the table with gauze tapes.

Following preparation of the area a 1-inch 22 gauge needle held in the right hand is introduced into the fossa, leaving the left index finger in position to serve as a guide. The needle is inserted in a vertical position just behind the anterior boundary of the fossa. As the needle passes through the fibrotic intervertebral ligament a definite pop is usually felt and resistance to passage of the needle ceases. In an adult cat about one-third of the needle shank is visible above the skin surface. Back pressure is applied on the plunger of the syringe to insure against an intravenous tap. Garcia recommends use of a 2.5% procaine hydrochloride solution containing epinephrine 1:10,000. The dose is calculated on the basis of 1 ml./5 lb. of body weight. The injection should be made very slowly. When the needle is correctly placed and injection commenced, the cat's tail will usually fibrillate. This is indicative of proper positioning of the needle. Relaxation begins almost immediately, reaches its full effect in 5 to 10 minutes, and lasts from 20 to 30 minutes. Again, improper injection may result in unilateral hind limb paresis or partial anesthesia of the tail or perineal region. In the event poor anesthesia is obtained, the patient can be reinjected.

Garcia states that he has never experienced a fatality with epidural anesthesia in cats and recommends it for orchiectomy, hysterectomy, hysterotomy, and treatment of urolithiasis.

Others have found this type of anesthesia leaves much to be desired. Even when done well the restraint problem still exists. While observing the performance of this procedure by veterinary students, several fatalities have been witnessed. Unfortunately, no records exist to indicate the mortality associated with this technique.

Advantages of epidural anesthesia in both dogs and cats are:

1. The animal does not run the risks of general anesthesia.
2. Short recovery period.
3. Good muscle relaxation.
4. No depression of the fetuses in cesarean section.

Disadvantages are:

1. The animal is conscious and may struggle.
2. The effect is short-lasting and may need to be repeated depending upon the agent used. This is a distinct disadvantage in operations where the animal is fastened in dorsal recumbency.
3. It is not without fatality. If the filum terminale is elongated, it is possible to inject the subarachnoid space and the animal may collapse and die immediately. (This is a true spinal injection.)
4. Large quantities of anesthetic solution may cause paralysis of

the sympathetic vasoconstrictors with precipitant drop in blood pressure.

5. Fast injection may cause a convulsion.

6. In some dogs the lumbosacral space is absent or underdeveloped (Grafe and Schulze, 1949).

Spinal Anesthesia

Spinal anesthesia is induced by injection of local anesthetics in the subarachnoid space (intrathecal injection). The solution is deposited in the cerebrospinal fluid between the pia mater and the arachnoidea. While this method of anesthesia has met with excellent success in humans, it has certain inherent disadvantages for use in animals and for this reason has never been universally adopted.

The greatest deterrent is the problem of restraint, during both introduction of the needle and the subsequent period of anesthesia. The intervertebral space in pet animals is relatively small as compared to man. The human patient is asked to arch the back while the needle is being introduced. This, of course, is impossible in animals. Struggling during introduction of the needle is dangerous because injury to the spinal cord can easily occur.

According to O'Connor (1931), Mennerat used spinal anesthesia in the dog with complete success. The site for injection in the dog was through (sic) the sixth lumbar intervetebral space. O'Connor went on to say, "The method is not much in vogue so far in veterinary practice." He stated the dose of procaine for dogs is $\frac{1}{3}$ to 3 grains administered in a 2 to 5% solution (1 to 5 cc. of 2% procaine). A quantity of fluid equal to that which is to be introduced should first be withdrawn.

It is interesting to note that barbiturates can be used as spinal anesthetics, although they are not advocated for this purpose. Purdy and Westfall (1956) injected four barbiturates, pentobarbital, secobarbital, barbital, and thiopental, at a rate of 0.05 ml. of 5% solution in 6% dextrose/kg. as spinal anesthetics in the dog. Injection was made by first administering nitrous oxide-oxygen following which the spinal puncture was made between the third and fourth lumbar vertebrae. Cerebrospinal fluid was aspirated prior to injection. It was found that the four barbiturates produced complete spinal block, which persisted approximately the same length of time as resulted from an equal volume of 2% procaine. No undesirable side effects were observed. Complications have been reported from the intrathecal use of these drugs in man, however.

References

ADRIANI, J.: *Techniques and Procedures of Anesthesia*. Charles C Thomas, Springfield, Illinois, 1947.

ADRIANI, J.: *Local Anesthetics*. Merck, Sharpe and Dohme Seminar Report, Fall, 1956

BEYER, K. H., LATVEN, A. R., FREYBURGER, W. A., and PARKER, M. P.: A Comparative Study of the Activity and Toxicity of Hexylcaine (1-Cyclohexylamino-2-Propylbenzoate): A New Local Anesthetic Agent. J. Pharm. & Exper. Therap., *93*, 388, 1948.

BONE, J. K. and PECK, J. G.: Epidural Anesthesia in Dogs. J.A.V.M.A., *128*, 236, 1956.

BREMER, G., EKMANNER, S., PERSSON, H., and STANDBERG, N.: Xylocaine, a New Local Anesthetic. Brit. Dent. J., *85*, 278, 1948.

BROOK, G. B.: Spinal (Epidural) Anaesthesia in the Domestic Animals. Vet. Rec., *15*, 664, 1935.

DUNLOP, J. G.: The Fate of Procaine in the Dog. J. Pharm. & Exper. Therap., *55*, 464, 1935.

ECKENHOFF, J. E. and KIRBY, C. K.: The Use of Hyaluronidase in Regional Nerve Blocks. Anesthesiology, *12*, 27, 1951.

FRANK, E. R.: Dental Anesthesia in the Dog. J.A.V.M.A., *73*, 232, 1928.

FRANK, E. R.: Regional Anesthesia in the Dog and Cat. J.A.V.M.A., *72*, 336, 1927.

GARCIA, J. G.: Epidural Anesthesia in the Cat. The Allied Vet., July-August, 20, 1953.

GRAFE, W. and SCHULZE, W.: Zur Technik der Lumbo-sacren Extraduralanaesthesie beim Hund. Berl. Münch. Tierarzt. Wchnschr., *10*, 140, 1949.

GOLDBERG, L.: Pharmacological Properties of Xylocaine. Svensk Tandl.-Tidskr., *40*, 819, 1947.

HEINBECKER, P., BISHOP, G. H., and O'LEARY, J.: Allocation of Function to Specific Fiber Types in Peripheral Nerves. Proc. Soc. Exper. Biol. & Med., *30*, 304, 1932.

HEINBECKER, P., BISHOP, G. H., and O'LEARY, J.: Analysis of Sensation in Terms of the Nerve Impulse. Arch. Neurol. & Psychiat., *31*, 34, 1934.

HULPIEU, H. R. and COLE, V. V.: Effects of Oxygen, Analeptics and Artificial Respiration on the Toxicity of Procaine. Proc. Soc. Exper. Biol. & Med., *76*, 62, 1951.

JONES, L. M.: The Toxic and Analgesic Effects of Procaine Hydrochloride Administered Intravenously in the Dog. Vet. Med., *46*, 93, 1951.

KALOW, W.: Hydrolysis of Local Anesthetics by Human Serum Cholinesterase. J. Pharm. & Exper. Therap., *104*, 122, 1952.

LACROIX, J. V.: In *Canine Surgery*. 4th ed. Edited by Mayer, K., Lacroix, J. V., and Hoskins, H. P. American Veterinary Publications, Inc., Evanston, Ill., 1957.

MOORE, D. C.: An Evaluation of Hyaluronidase in Local and Nerve Block Analgesia: A Review of 519 Cases. Anesthesiology, *11*, 470, 1950.

O'CONNOR, J. J.: *Dollar's Veterinary Surgery*. 2d ed. Alexander Eger, Chicago, 1931.

PURDY, F. A. and WESTFALL, B. A.: Barbiturates as Spinal Anesthetics. J. Pharm. & Exper. Therap., *118*, 318, 1956.

RISER, W. H.: Surgical Removal of the Mammary Gland of the Bitch. J.A.V.M.A., *110*, 86, 1947.

SCHIRMER, R. G.: Personal Communication. Michigan State University, East Lansing, Michigan, 1960.

SEIFTER, J.: Studies on the Pharmacology and Toxicology of Testicular Hyaluronidase. Ann. N. Y. Acad. Sci., *52*, 1141, 1950.

TAINTER, M. L., THRONDSON, A. H., and MOORE, S. M.: Vasoconstrictors on the Clinical Effectiveness and Toxicity of Procaine Anesthetic Solutions. J.A.D.A., *25*, 1321, 1938.

TRUANT, A. P. and WIEDLING, S.: A Contribution to the Pharmacological and Toxicological Evaluation of a New Local Anesthetic, dl-N-Methylpipecoly!-2-6-Xylidide. Acta. chir. scandinav., *116*, 351, 1958.

TUFVESSON, G.: Anestesi av Plexus Brachialis. Nord. Vet.-Med., *3*, 183, 1951.

ANESTHESIA
OF
LABORATORY
AND
ZOO ANIMALS

Chapter 14

VETERINARIANS are occasionally called upon to anesthetize a wide variety of mammals, birds, reptiles, and fish. Some of the lower species of mammals, such as rabbits, rats, and mice, have been used through the years to assess anesthetic agents and a great mass of data is available concerning these species. Others have been anesthetized rarely if at all, and little specific information is available; that which follows may serve as a basis for further investigations.

Fish

A number of agents have been used to anesthetize fish, including ether, sodium amytal, tricaine methanesulfonate, carbon dioxide, urethane, and cresol.

In handling fingerling trout for fin-clipping, ether anesthesia was found to increase efficiency markedly. A 1% aqueous solution was placed in a basin and additional ether added as required; thus, the concentration varied considerably after the initial fish were anesthetized (Eschmeyer, 1953).

Sodium amytal (0.5 gr./gal.) can be used to anesthetize fish for transportation. With this method only one-third to one-fourth the water normally required is needed, since the fish become calm and

(269)

use less oxygen. The small water volume facilitates transplanting operations by airplane. Because of its slow action sodium amytal has no practical value in spawning or fin-clipping operations.

Tricaine methanesulfonate, a crystalline water-soluble powder, was synthesized by M. Sandoz and is marketed under the commercial name M.S. 222. It is used as an anesthetic to immobilize fish and other cold-blooded animals by complete bathing of small subjects, by gill spraying in large fish, or by injection in large animals. It exerts a prompt and intense action and has a low degree of toxicity, being approximately three times less toxic than procaine and about ten times less toxic than cocaine. A 1:1000 solution may be autoclaved without loss of narcotic properties or increase in toxicity.

In anesthetizing most common fishes (teleosts), concentrations of 0.5 to 1.0 gm./gal. of fresh water are used and the temperature is maintained at 40 to 60°F. Induction time varies depending on concentration and the period of exposure to the solution.

The fish is immersed until it becomes immobilized at which time it can be removed for examination, treatment, or surgery. While the fish is exposed to the air provision should be made to keep it wet. For longer anesthesia the fish can be re-immersed or the gills sprayed with solution. Repeated use tends to reduce the concentration; for best results, therefore, fresh solutions should be used. Bluegills, bass, trout, and salmon have been anesthetized in concentrations of 1:3000 to 1:25,000 for weighing, tagging, and spawn collection, with anesthesia varying in duration from 3 minutes to several hours depending again on concentration and immersion time. For large numbers of fish a closed recirculating system may be advantageous (Hublou, 1957).

Tricaine methanesulfonate can be used for transporting fish without water (Martin and Scott, 1959). A dilution of 0.25 gm./gal. with water temperature of 5°C. is used. When the fish turn over in the water they are allowed to remain 8 minutes, following which they are transferred to tanks containing layers of moss and chipped ice. Fish so anesthetized can be held for 4 to $4\frac{1}{2}$ hours with a mortality of approximately 10%.

Treatment of fungus infections and other localized diseases in pet or ornamental fish can be performed with tricaine methanesulfonate. For "tranquilization" of pet or ornamental fish for transportation low concentrations are used. Gossington (1957) employs 0.14 to 0.32 gm./gal. depending upon the species of fish, size of container, and presence or absence of oxygen (Table 14–1).

Large fish, such as sharks and rays, cannot be conveniently immersed in a solution. Therefore, Gilbert and Wood (1957) developed a method by which these fish can be anesthetized while struggling behind a boat either on a hook or harpoon. M.S. 222 in a concentration of 1:1000 (1 gm./liter of sea water) is used. The head of the fish is held above the water level by means of a gaff or leader; small fish may be temporarily removed from the water. By means of a water pistol, rubber bulb syringe, or small hand pump, the solution is introduced into the mouths of fish or the spiracles of rays and sprayed over the gill exits of the pharynx. Small species require approximately 100 ml. and larger fish up to 1 liter of solution.

Table 14–1.—Dose of Tricaine Methanesulfonate for Ornamental Fish

Variety of Fish	Concentration	Anesthesia Time
Tropicals at 75° to 80° F.:		
Live Bearers	0.32 gm. per gal.	to 12 hrs., uncrowded
Egglayers	0.24 gm. per gal.	to 12 hrs., uncrowded
For uncrowded shipment of pugnacious species, without oxygen:		
Bettas, Pirhanas	0.25 gm. per gal.	to 48 hours
For Goldfish, with oxygen:		
Goldfish variety	0.14 gm. per gal.	to 48 hours.

(From Gossington, R. E.: An Aid to Fish Handling—Tricaine. Aquarium J., *28*, 318 1957.)

The action of the drug is quite rapid, 15 seconds being required for a visible effect to take place. A 400-pound shark may be anesthetized in 1 minute or less. The fish may then be manipulated either in or out of the water until recovery begins to take place. If additional anesthesia is required it may be given, or recovery may be hastened by washing the gills with fresh sea water. This can be accomplished with large fish by "walking" the fish in a pool with its mouth open or by spraying a stream of fresh sea water into the mouth. Recovery usually begins to take place within 5 to 30 minutes after the fish is returned to the water.

The time elapsing before loss of muscular activity appears to be directly proportional to the concentration of drug which is used. Figure 14–1 shows the suggested dose for sharks. The effect of a given concentration varies inversely with the size of the fish. An increase in toxicity has been observed and correlated with a marked rise in temperature of the immersing solution.

The use of M.S. 222 on fish does not affect their palatability and has no adverse effect on persons consuming them.

A very inexpensive method for anesthetizing large fish in tank trucks or other large volumes of water is by the use of carbon dioxide (Fish, 1942). This is produced by addition of calculated amounts of technical grade sodium bicarbonate and sulfuric acid to water with a temperature between 45° and 60°F. The carbon dioxide content of the water is determined by titration with N/44 sodium hydroxide. Some type of recirculating equipment must be available to disperse the reagents when added. Care must be taken in the storage and handling of sulfuric acid.

Carbon dioxide concentrations of 400 ppm for as long as 20 minutes of anesthesia appear to cause no permanent ill effect. The optimum carbon dioxide concentration for anesthetizing salmon and steelhead trout is 200 ppm. At this concentration the fish gradually lose consciousness, turn over, and sink to the bottom of the tank within 90 seconds after the solution reaches full strength. The depth of respiration is used as a measure of the approaching lethal end point. Respiratory movement gradually lessens and finally

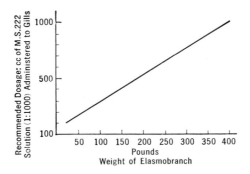

FIGURE 14–1.   Dose of M. S. 222 solution (1:1000 concentration) recommended to anesthetize a shark or ray in 60 seconds or less. The solution should be sprayed over the gill exits of the pharynx while the head of the elasmobranch is held above the water level. If the head remains under water, proportionally stronger concentrations must be utilized. (From Gilbert, P. W. and Wood, F. G., Jr.:   Method of Anesthetizing Large Sharks and Rays Safely and Rapidly. Science, 126, 212, 1957.)

ceases at which time the fish will not revive when placed in fresh water.

After the period of exposure during which the fish are sorted or otherwise handled (which should not exceed 5 minutes), the carbon dioxide is neutralized by addition of the proper quantity of sodium carbonate. This quickly restores the original carbon dioxide concentration. Following neutralization with sodium carbonate the fish remain anesthetized for an additional 5 to 10 minutes.

Urethane in concentrations of 1 to 5% can be used to anesthetize trout (Savage, 1935; Cuerriere, 1953). Because of its carcinogenic potential, however, its use has largely ceased.

Cresol is cheap but has wide variation in effect and subsequent toxicity (Fish, 1942).

A tumor operation on a 500 pound Jewfish, performed while submerged 16 feet under water in a 500,000 gallon tank, has been reported (————, 1958). By feeding small fish containing tranquilizers and then injecting a local anesthetic, the fish was prepared for operation.

Amphibians and Reptiles

Tricaine methanesulfonate (M.S. 222) has been used in laboratories to immobilize cold-blooded animals such as frogs, toads, newts and salamanders during demonstrations and experiments. For this purpose it is used in dilutions varying from 1:1000 to 1:10,000 depending on immersion time, temperature, and the needs of the situation. Species which respire with gills are more susceptible than those which have no gills and must absorb the drug through the intact skin.

Ten per cent ethyl alcohol can be used to anesthetize frogs, since it is absorbed through their intact skin (Kaplan and Kaplan, 1961). Three-inch frogs (*Rana pipiens*) are placed in a container filled with alcohol to a depth of 8 to 10 mm. When deep anesthesia is reached, the frog is washed with tap water and placed in water 8 to 10 mm. deep to recover. About 10 minutes is required to induce surgical anesthesia which lasts about 20 minutes. Variations in induction and duration of anesthesia occur, depending upon the frog's size and the ambient temperature. Higher concentrations of alcohol or a longer immersion time may prove fatal.

Mosby and Cantner (1955) have administered tribromoethanol orally with a syringe to snakes and turtles (Table 14–2). These responded quickly and remained narcotized longer than warm-

Table 14–2.—Reactions of Various Forms of Wildlife to Orally Administered Tribromoethanol

Type of Specimen	Dosage in gm./lb.	Time required to anesthetize in minutes	Time required to recover in hours	Remarks
Turtle, snapper	0.08	5	48	Still drowsy 3.5 days later.
Snake, copperhead	0.05	3	6+	
Snake, coachwhip	0.08	3–5	6+	
Blackbird, rusty	0.15	7	1.5	
Starling	0.12	1	3+	
Chipmunk	0.02	1	3.5	Resp. rate changes 132-34-60.
Opossum	0.11	6	10+	Still drowsy after 24 hrs.
Woodchuck	0.09	2	0.5	Easily handled for 1 hour.
Cat, domestic	0.09	4	24	Resp. rate changes 35-14-20.
Skunk, striped	0.06	3	2.5	

(From Mosby, H. S. and Cantner, D. E.: The Use of Avertin in Capturing Wild Turkeys and as an Oral-Basal Anaesthetic for Other Wild Animals. Southwest Vet., *9*, 132, 1955.)

blooded animals. A snapping turtle remained anesthetized more than 2 days after 0.08 ml./lb., and did not fully respond to stimuli for 5 days.

For anesthetizing small snakes with ether, a wide-mouth jar, such as a pickle jar, is suitable. Ether-soaked cotton is placed in the jar, the snake inserted, and the lid fastened securely. Anesthesia usually develops in about 3 minutes. There is a wide margin of safety, approximately 1 hour being required to kill a snake in a closed jar containing ether vapor. Three minutes within the jar will produce roughly 15 minutes of anesthesia. The ambient temperature is important since snakes are poikilothermic and anesthesia should be induced at room temperature. In no instance should this procedure be done at very high temperatures. Anesthesia is not accompanied by muscle relaxation, hypertonicity usually resulting (Van Stee, 1960).

Snakes become very sluggish at low temperatures and Vierheller (1959) has reported an instance in which advantage was taken of this fact to facilitate radiography of a Pacific Rattler. The snake was placed in a refrigerator at about 45° F. for 1 hour following which it was transported in a sack containing ice cubes from the owner's home to a veterinary hospital. Though tractable, the snake was still able to coil and raise its head! Three weeks following hypothermia the snake gave birth to eight living young.

Caged Birds

With the recent increase in popularity of pet birds, veterinarians are frequently confronted with the necessity for administration of anesthesia to various avian species. Agents commonly employed in dogs and cats have also been used in birds; among these are ether, ethyl chloride, pentobarbital, chloral hydrate and tribromoethanol.

Volatile anesthetics have not proved very satisfactory due to the bird's air sac system which may allow a dangerous over-concentration of the anesthetic before the anesthetist realizes this has occurred. Gandal (1956) recommends that volatile anesthetic agents such as ether be given by intermittent administration, brief periods of access to air being allowed both during induction and after anesthesia is attained. Thus the danger of over-concentration within the air sacs is lessened.

Ether can be used for brief anesthesia, the bird being held in a recumbent position and ether sprayed from a 2 ml. syringe, equipped with a 26 gauge ¼-inch needle, into a nostril from a distance of about 1 inch. Administration must be discontinued as soon as struggling ceases and resumed at intervals as the bird begins to regain consciousness (Friedberg, 1961). Ethyl chloride also can be administered in much the same fashion from a dispenser. Its safety margin is greater than that of ether when used on birds. Ferguson (1961) has recommended the use of preanesthetics plus ethyl chloride for parakeets. A tablet containing $\frac{1}{4}$ gr. of morphine sulfate and $\frac{1}{150}$ gr. of atropine sulfate is diluted in 3 ml. of sterile water and 0.1 ml. is given subcutaneously. After 30 minutes the bird is anesthetized with ethyl chloride sprayed on cotton and held over the nostrils.

It is quite difficult to administer anesthetics intravenously to birds (Gandal, 1956). In addition to the very small caliber of the accessible veins in small birds, restraint of a bird in an unnatural position is likely to induce shock which is frequently fatal. Because the wing must be held extended, sudden movements by the bird may result in fracture or luxation of the wing bones. Even when venipuncture is accomplished, bird veins are so thin-walled that any struggling during injection is likely to cause their rupture.

Following considerable experimentation Gandal (1956) has suggested that Equithesin* be used. This solution is given intramuscularly in the breast on either side of the keel bone at the rate of 2.5 ml./kg. of body weight. Gandal reported no sloughing occurred with Equithesin in 22 trials conducted in various species of birds. No fatalities occurred in this group which varied in weight from 0.018 to 5.1 kg. A dose of 3.0 ml./kg. of Equithesin resulted in a 19.5% mortality in a group of mixed species. Birds that are weak, debilitated, senile, or suffering from shock will not require as much anesthetic. In these patients the dose should be reduced to as little as 2.0 ml./kg.

To prolong the period of surgical anesthesia an additional 25% of the original dose may be given after 45 minutes to 1 hour has elapsed. Induction time varies from 10 to 35 minutes and the duration of satisfactory anesthesia from 25 to 90 minutes. An interval of 180 minutes was the longest time recorded between injection and return of ability to stand.

The average parakeet requires about 0.08 ml. of Equithesin since it weighs about 35 gm. Canaries weigh about 20 gm. The anesthetic stage is reached in 5 to 15 minutes and lasts 30 minutes to 1 hour.

Stone (1959) has advocated the use of Sedax† in birds. The bird is weighed and the dose calculated by multiplying the weight in grams by 0.002 ml. in the case of debilitated birds; 0.0025 ml. times

* Each 500 ml. contains 21.3 gm. chloral hydrate, 4.8 gm. pentobarbital sodium, and 10.6 gm. magnesium sulfate in aqueous solution of propylene glycol with 9.5% alcohol. See Appendix A, p. 402 for manufacturer.

† Sedax contains chloral hydrate, 164 grains; sodium pentobarbital, $37\frac{1}{2}$ grains; magnesium sulfate, 82 grains; alcohol $9\frac{1}{2}\%$, v/v in each 250 ml. and is in a propylene glycol vehicle. See Appendix A, p. 402 for manufacturer.

the weight of the bird is used in good anesthetic risks. Using a tuberculin syringe with a 25 gauge needle the anesthetic is injected approximately $\frac{3}{16}$ of an inch into the breast muscle.

If intramuscular pentobarbital sodium is used, it should be diluted so that 1 ml. is added to 8 ml. of sterile water. This gives a concentration of approximately 7 mg./ml. A 35 gm. bird will require 0.2 ml. of this diluted solution which is injected into the pectoral muscle or the abdominal cavity with a 25 gauge needle. This dose is approximately 1.5 mg. of the drug. The anesthetic stage is reached in 2 to 3 minutes and persists for about 30 minutes. Equithesin is the safer of the two drugs according to Friedberg (1961).

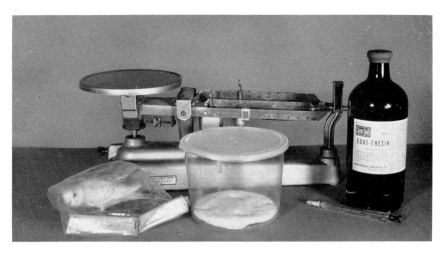

FIGURE 14–2.   Equipment for anesthetizing small birds. The bird is placed in a plastic bag or container for weighing.

For administration of anesthetic to small species, a 1 ml. glass tuberculin syringe and 25 gauge needle are recommended. Larger needles and syringes are used with correspondingly larger birds. Small birds, such as canaries and parakeets, may be weighed on a small two-pan scale by placing the bird head first in a cone made of paper toweling or in a small cardboard box or ice cream carton (Fig. 14–2). If a container is used frequently, time will be saved by marking its weight on the outside to avoid repeated weighing.

Following injection of anesthetic the bird should be released in a small well-ventilated confined area. Small caged birds can be returned to the cage. As anesthesia develops, these birds will become unable to maintain themselves in an upright position, and if sitting on perches will rotate and become suspended head down until deeper anesthesia causes them to fall to the floor of the cage.

Leonard (1960) believes oral pentobarbital is safer for parakeets and canaries than that given parenterally. He suggests that birds fasted for 24 hours be given 2.0 mg. of pentobarbital sodium diluted in 0.25 ml. of water orally. A second dose may be given in 15 minutes if necessary.

During the recovery period it is important that birds be kept warm; a temperature of 85° to 90° F. is optimum.

Occasionally small birds will evidence handling shock. If this develops, a heat lamp should be judiciously applied until arousal occurs. Oxygen administration may also be of value.

Procaine is toxic for parakeets and should *never* be used in this species. Procaine penicillin is also contraindicated.

Falcons

Reserpine has been found by Dodge (1963) to be quite useful in taming and training falcons. Newly caught haggard prairie falcons (*Falco mexicanus*) are given 1 to 2 mg./lb. orally in meat the first day, and a second dose of 0.5 mg./lb. is given the following day. Vomiting may reduce the effectiveness of the first dose. The birds become progressively relaxed and in about 8 hours a hypnotic state develops from which they can be aroused. The temperature drops from approximately 108° F. to below 100° F. During the period of tranquilization, which lasts 5 to 6 days, the birds will not eat and must be force-fed daily. After effects of the drug have ceased, most birds remain tame and tractable.

When meprobamate was used for the same purpose, some muscular relaxation was produced and the wings of the bird drooped. This has not been observed with reserpine. Chlorpromazine derivatives have produced excitement.

Because the breast muscles are so important in flying, falcons should never be injected in the breast, but rather in the leg muscles if intramuscular injection is to be performed. The femoral and jugular veins are readily accessible in falcons for intravenous injection.

Poultry

Sanger and Smith (1957) have used both Equithesin and Combuthal for general anesthesia in birds. Combuthal, composed of equal parts of sodium pentothal and sodium pentobarbital, was prepared for injection by adding 30 ml. of sterile water to 1 gr. of powder, providing a concentration of 0.5 gr./ml. Both drugs, Equithesin and Combuthal, were injected in the pectoral muscle. The dose of Combuthal needed to induce good surgical anesthesia in chickens was found to be 0.5 gr./lb. of body weight. Turkeys weighing from 7 to 13 pounds required 1.5 gr./lb. of body weight and with 0.5 gr./lb. only light anesthesia was produced. In day-old chicks surgical anesthesia was induced in 2 to 3 minutes and lasted 20 to 30 minutes. In broilers, induction required 20 to 25 minutes and surgical anesthesia lasted 25 to 30 minutes. Surgical anesthesia in turkeys was reached in 15 to 30 minutes and lasted 50 to 60 minutes.

Equithesin at a rate of 2.5 ml./kg. was found to be satisfactory in chickens, but in heavier birds, such as turkeys, the dose had to be increased to 2.85 ml./kg. With both Equithesin and Combuthal there was never any sign of swelling, pain, or necrosis at the injection site; however, in birds destroyed after 24 hours hemorrhage, fibrin, edema, and degenerative changes were present in the muscle tissue. Healing occurred rapidly and in 14 days no lesion could be found. There was no abscess formation in any of the birds. It was concluded that there was no difference between the action of these two anesthetics.

Geese are extremely sensitive to reserpine, 0.5 gm. per ton of growing ration causing excessive tranquilization, reduced feed intake, and loss of weight (Wilgus, 1960). Even as little as 0.0625 gm. per ton of feed for a period of 7 days causes inanition. This level for 3 or 4 days at 6 weeks of age results in a lasting degree of tranquilization.

For handling wild pheasants on game farms, reserpine can be added to the feed at a ratio of 8 gm./30 lbs. This amount will be sufficient for approximately 200 birds (40 mg./bird) and if fed in the afternoon will be consumed by the following morning. When fed on the day prior to handling, it will increase efficiency and reduce injuries to birds and handlers (Hewitt, 1959).

Young (1948) in describing wing amputation in birds suggests the use of local anesthesia. The feathers are removed over a 2-inch area around the outer joint of the wing. Using a 1-inch 20 gauge needle, 2% procaine is injected on the upper and lower surfaces of the wing medial to the joint. The needle is pointed toward the body and nearly parallel to the wing as it is inserted. One milliliter divided into equal parts on the upper and lower surfaces of the wing is usually sufficient for small birds such as ducks. Two milliliters are required for a bird the size of a pelican.

Tribromoethanol has been used by Mosby and Cantner (1955) in capturing wild turkeys. The dose of undiluted tribromoethanol was 0.75 ml. on approximately 60 kernels of whole corn. Since the amount taken by an individual bird could not be controlled, an estimate was first made of the number of feeding birds and the amount of bait required was then determined. The area was inspected 5 to 10 minutes after the turkeys had eaten, and following collection of anesthetized birds their crops were irrigated as quickly as possible.

The oral dose of tribromoethanol for turkeys, administered with a hypodermic syringe, is 60 to 90 mg./lb.

Mice

Ether is generally employed to anesthetize mice. The animal is placed in a bell jar or other container with a pledget of ether-soaked cotton and is removed when anesthetized.

It is possible to inject mice in the lateral vein of the tail, though extensive practice is necessary for proficiency (Croft, 1960).

Table 14–3.—Duration of Surgical Anesthesia and Survival Rates in Female Albino Mice (Harlan) After Intraperitoneal Injection of 0.5% Pentobarbital Sodium

Group*	Pentobarbital Na (mg./kg.)	Animals in surgical anesthesia (%)	Survivors (%) 1 day	Survivors (%) 1 week	Av. duration and range of surgical anesthesia in survivors (min.)
1	65	20	90	90	3.6 (0–8)
2	80	30	100	80	3.6 (0–19)
3	90	80	80	80	6.0 (0–20)
4	100	100	70	70	111.0 (109–115)
5	110	100	40	40	124.0 (84–168)
6	120	100	20	20	127.0 (123–132)

* Ten animals were used per group.

(From Dolowy, W. C., Mombelloni, P., and Hesse, A. L.: Chlorpromazine Premedication with Pentobarbital Anesthesia in a Mouse. Am. J. Vet. Res., *21*, 156, 1960.)

Table 14–4.—Duration of Surgical Anesthesia and Survival Rates in Female Albino Mice (Harlan) After Injection of 0.5% Chlorpromazine Hydrochloride Intramuscularly, Followed by 0.5% Pentobarbital Sodium Intraperitoneally 30 Minutes Later

Group	No. of animals	Chlorpromazine hydrochloride (mg./kg.)	Pentobarbital Na (mg./kg.)	Animals in surgical anesthesia (%)	Survivors (%) 1 day	Survivors (%) 1 week	Av. duration and range of surgical anesthesia in survivors (min.)
7	5	25	40	40	80	80	82 (0–95)
8	5	50	40	20	80	80	95 (0–95)
9	30	50	50	80	87	87	22 (0–51)
10	10	60	50	50	100	80	17 (0–56)
11	10	60	60	100	80	60	78 (67–99)

(From Dolowy, W. C., Mombelloni, P., and Hesse, A. L.: Chlorpromazine Premedication with Pentobarbital Anesthesia in a Mouse. Am. J. Vet. Res., *21*, 156, 1960.)

Intraperitoneal pentobarbital sodium can be used in mice. The dose is 90 mg./kg. and is administered using a tuberculin syringe and 24 gauge needle. A mortality of approximately 20% will occur since there is wide variation in the response of mice to pentobarbital sodium (Table 14–3). Dolowy *et al.* (1960) have advocated use of preanesthetic chlorpromazine to increase the duration of surgical anesthesia and lower the mortality rate (Table 14–4).

Anesthetized mice are particularly susceptible to cold and, therefore, should be kept in a warm draft-free location until fully conscious.

Rats

Rats which are not tame are difficult to manage without a little experience. While gloves can be worn, it is preferable to avoid their use since they impede the fingers and there is a tendency to crush the animals rather than grasp them securely. Using the thumb and forefingers of the left hand, the tail is grasped, the animal lifted out of the cage quickly, and placed head-down on the upper surface of the right thigh. With the thumb and forefinger of the right hand, the animal is then quickly grasped by the scruff of the neck and, without the left hand releasing its hold on the tail, is turned on its back. The rat when placed on the thigh will strain to pull away from the hand grasping the tail. If, however, the animal is not caught immediately in the right hand, it cannot be carried by the tail any length of time, as it will turn and climb its own tail far enough to bite the hand restraining it. A second method, which utilizes gloves, is to grasp the animal with the palm of the hand over the back and, with the thumb and forefinger, to fold the forelegs across each other under the animal's chin. With the legs held correctly, the animal cannot depress its chin to bite.

A turkish towel may be used for restraint while making intravenous injections into the tail veins or obtaining blood samples from them. The unanesthetized rat is rolled in a turkish towel as shown in Figure 14–3. The towel is folded over the rat, rolled, and pinned with safety pins, making sure the legs are secure. Rats may be left so restrained for hours without harm. A commercial rat restraining cage is shown in Figure 14–4.

The best agent for prolonged anesthesia in rats is pentobarbital sodium. The animal's weight in grams is determined. For convenience pentobarbital solution should be diluted so that each ml. contains 30 mg. (3% solution). A $\frac{1}{4}$ ml. syringe with a scale of $\frac{1}{100}$ ml. should be used. The dose on the scale is then the same as the animal's weight in grams divided by 10. Three mg./100 gm. is sufficient for light anesthesia; 4 to 5 mg./100 gm. will produce deep surgical anesthesia. The solution is given intraperitoneally just lateral to the umbilicus. Complete anesthesia will develop in 5 to 15 minutes and will be effective for approximately 45 minutes. Injection can be made subcutaneously but the effect develops more slowly and is of longer duration. If anesthesia lightens before the desired time has elapsed, a second dose approximately one-quarter of the first can be given after 45 minutes.

For short operations a solution containing 10 mg./ml. of evipal sodium has been used. When injected intraperitoneally the anes-

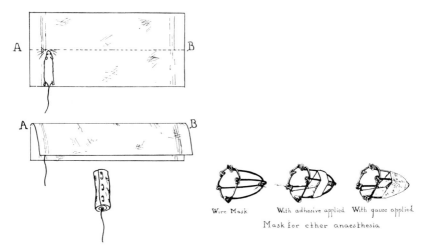

Wire Mask   With adhesive applied With gauze applied

Mask for ether anaesthesia

FIGURE 14–3. Wrapping the rat in a towel (left). Steps in making an ether mask (right). (From Griffith, J. Q., Jr. and Farris, E. J.: *The Rat in Laboratory Investigation.* J. B. Lippincott Co., 1942.)

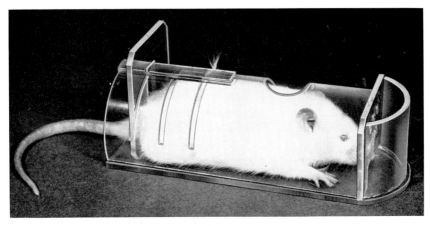

FIGURE 14–4. A plastic restrainer for rats. Ether-soaked cotton can be placed in the well at right to anesthetize the animal. (Courtesy of Fisher Scientific Company, Pittsburgh, Pennsylvania.)

thetic dose is 10 mg./100 gm. Young rats are intolerant to evipal
sodium according to Griffith and Farris (1942).

For procedures of short duration ether is probably preferable.
Rats may be placed in a bell jar containing a pledget of ether-soaked
cotton. If longer anesthesia is desired, a mask such as shown in
Figure 14–3 may be used after the animal is removed from the bell
jar. Ether anesthesia may be induced using only the mask if the
animal is held as shown in Figure 14–5. To prevent excessive
mucus formation in the respiratory tree, atropine may be given
preanesthetically but is not essential.

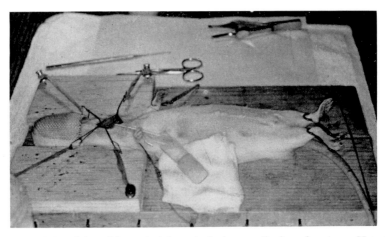

Figure 14–5.   A board for restraining rats during anesthesia and surgery. Note the
mask over the head. In addition a tracheotomy has been performed and a glass endotracheal catheter inserted. This in turn is placed in a small vial which contains ether-
soaked cotton. Maintenance of anesthesia may be performed by either of these two
methods.

An endotracheal insufflation technique can be used in rats.
Anesthesia is first induced by means of the bell jar or mask, following which a midline longitudinal cervical incision is made exposing
the trachea. A small hole is clipped between two cartilage rings and
a glass tube drawn to a diameter of 1 mm. at one end is then introduced into the lumen of the trachea. The other end is connected to
an apparatus shown in Figure 14–6. By raising tube A, pressure in
the tracheal tube is decreased; by lowering tube A it is increased.
The per cent of ether in the mixture can also be varied by raising or
lowering tube B. A water pressure of 1 cm. and a distance of 4 cm.
between the surface of the ether and tube B is optimal. With this
method anesthesia may be maintained for periods of 2 hours or
longer. If open chest surgery is to be performed, curare at a dose of
0.1 mg./100 gm. may be used to prevent respiratory movements.

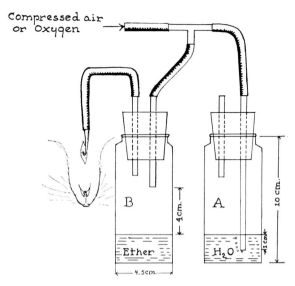

FIGURE 14–6. Sketch of apparatus for endotracheal ether anesthesia. (From Griffith, J. Q., Jr. and Farris, E. J.: *The Rat in Laboratory Investigation*. J. B. Lippincott Co., 1942.)

Weisner (1934) has used hypothermia for castration of 12-hour old rats. He states that it is practical only for operations on the newborn. The rat is wrapped in filter paper, placed in a test tube, and immersed in a thermos bottle filled with ice. The test tube must be dry or the rat will freeze to it. The rat is cooled until its body temperature falls to about 2° C. at which temperature it is immobile and shows no reaction to stimuli. Anesthesia will last for 3 to 10 minutes after the rat is removed from the thermos and the operation is performed during this period. Gradual rewarming is then allowed by placing the animal in a cool place for 10 to 30 minutes followed by warming in the palm of the hand for 20 minutes. When the animal has recovered, it is cleaned and returned to its mother. At least one young should be left in the nest with the mother during the procedure and the operated animal should be returned in front of the nest rather than placed in it. The mother then retrieves it.

Chloroform is not a satisfactory anesthesia for rats due to the high mortality rate.

Guinea Pigs

Ether and pentobarbital are commonly employed for anesthesia of guinea pigs.

When ether is used the animal should be fasted for 12 hours and given $\frac{1}{150}$ gr. of atropine sulfate subcutaneously approximately

30 minutes prior to anesthesia. Induction is usually performed in a bell jar or other closed container with ether-soaked cotton. Maintenance can be performed with a mask.

A peculiar sign exhibited by anesthetized guinea pigs occurs as the induction stage is complete. An extensive squirming movement, which develops in one hind leg and frequently spreads over the entire body, may occur once or twice. Croft (1960) has stated that this movement does not indicate returning consciousness; rather, if anesthesia is deepened at this point the animal may die. If this phenomenon occurs during laparotomy, the intestines are extruded; therefore, it may be preferable to wait until it has occurred before opening the peritoneal cavity. Generally speaking, ether is a safe and efficient anesthetic for guinea pigs.

When pentobarbital sodium is given by intraperitoneal injection, anesthesia requires approximately 15 minutes to develop and lasts 1 to 2 hours. Complete recovery may require as long as 12 hours and supplementary heat should be provided during this period. The recommended dose is 28 mg./kg.; the fatal dose is 56 mg./kg. (Croft, 1960).

Intravenous injection is difficult to accomplish and is seldom used. When necessary the marginal vein of the ear or the pudic vein in the male are possible sites.

For very short periods of anesthesia, such as needed for inoculation or cardiac puncture, carbon dioxide can be used effectively. Approximately 2 pounds of dry ice are broken into pieces 1 to 2 inches square and placed in the bottom of an open metal container, measuring $18 \times 12 \times 14$ inches deep. The guinea pig is placed on a removable wire platform 5 inches above the bottom of the container. Carbon dioxide liberated from the dry ice produces general anesthesia in 10 to 15 seconds following which the animal should be removed promptly. Anesthesia lasts approximately 45 seconds and recovery occurs in about 1 minute. In a group of 1460 guinea pigs anesthetized by this method, one death occurred from carbon dioxide (Hyde, 1962). There is no excitement on induction and no adverse side effects are seen. The respiration is increased temporarily. Chinchillas, rabbits, and mice also respond in a similar fashion to this method of anesthesia.

Rabbits

Wright (1957) has described ether anesthesia in the rabbit administered by a semi-closed technique. The respirations and degree of muscular relaxation are used to determine the depth of anesthesia. When it is becoming dangerously deep the eyeball becomes unusually prominent giving a "popeyed" appearance. Ether is not used for initial induction of anesthesia in rabbits because they evidence considerable laryngospasm. However, it may be used following induction.

The dose of pentobarbital usually recommended for rabbits is 30 mg./kg., but there is very wide variation in response. A dose of 15 mg./kg. may be sufficient for one, whereas another may require 50 mg./kg. The arousal time also varies widely ranging from 1 to 10 hours. Dolowy and Hesse (1959) have recommended that chlorpromazine be given as a preanesthetic agent when pentobarbital is used. This produces a more tractable animal for administration of the anesthetic and a much longer duration of surgical anesthesia (Table 14–5). The depth of respiration is the best sign of anesthesia; it should be regular, deep, and slower than in the unanesthetized animal.

Thiopental is also used in rabbits, the average dose being about 50 mg./kg.; using a 2.5% solution the dose will be 2 ml./kg. Recovery from thiopental anesthesia is quite rapid.

When barbiturates are administered to rabbits, they are usually given intravenously in the marginal vein of the ear. The animal

Table 14–5.—Duration of Surgical Anesthesia in Female New Zealand White Rabbits Preanesthetized with Chlorpromazine Hydrochloride Intramuscularly, Followed by Pentobarbital Sodium Intravenously (20 mg./kg. of Body wt.) 30 Minutes Later

Rabbit	Weight (kg.)	Chlorpromazine HCl (mg./kg.)	(total mg.)	Pentobarbital Na (mg.)	Induction time (min.)	Duration of surgical anesthesia (min.)
11	2.2	25	55	44	12	35
12	2.3	25	58	46	11	29
						Av. 32
13	2.2	50	110	44	25	33
14	2.0	50	100	40	18	28
						Av. 31.5
15	1.9	100	190	38	12	57
16	1.9	100	190	38	6	62
17	2.2	100	220	44	3	45
18	2.0	100	200	40	3	56
19	2.3	100	230	46	5	30
20	2.1	100	210	42	4	32
21	2.4	100	240	48	6	30
22	1.8	100	180	36	3	1 (died)
23	2.3	100	230	46	2	33
24	2.2	100	220	44	2	55
						Av. 44.4*

* Does not include rabbit 22 which died.
(From Dolowy, W. C. and Hesse, A. L.: Chlorpromazine Premedication with Pentobarbital Anesthesia in the Rabbit. J.A.V.M.A., *134*, 183, 1959.)

is weighed and prepared by plucking or clipping the hair over the vein. If rabbits are anesthetized only occasionally, it is recommended that the animal be wrapped in a towel with the four legs securely included.

With practice, use of a towel becomes unnecessary. An assistnat stands behind the animal and puts both hands over its eyes, directing the ear toward the anesthetist with his thumbs. The animal's rear is placed against the chest of the assistant, who leans forward with his forearms lightly restraining the animal on either side. The assistant can compress the marginal ear vein at the base of the

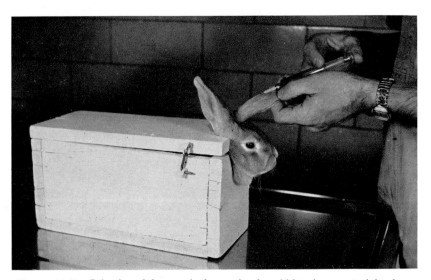

FIGURE 14–7.　Injection of the marginal ear vein of a rabbit using a restraining box.

ear. The anesthetist grasps the ear between thumb and second finger at its distal end, holding the index finger extended under the ear for support. The injection should be made toward the distal end of the ear so that if the first attempt is unsuccessful another may be made more proximal. A 24 or 25 gauge needle is inserted with the bevel upwards and is threaded up the vein for 4 or 5 mm. In laboratories where anesthetization of rabbits is carried out frequently, a restraining box will facilitate injection and will allow this procedure to be done by one person (Fig. 14–7).

The anesthetic is injected slowly. Often air bubbles may be seen traveling up the vein as injection is started. This assures that the needle is in the lumen and is not of any particular danger to the animal. During injection the respirations should be carefully observed. After the rabbit gives a deep sigh, about 0.75 ml. is injected very slowly. The anesthetist should then pause, leaving the syringe and needle in place gripped firmly between the thumb and forefinger of the left hand, and test the animal's reflexes. While the anesthetist holds the rabbit's head with his right hand, the assistant lightly pinches the Achilles tendon at the heel. If anesthesia is not deep, the animal may give a very forcible jerk and for this reason the head should be held firmly. Further injection of anesthetic is made until the Achilles tendon reflex produces only a moderate withdrawal response or tensing of the leg muscles. At this stage the animal is in surgical anesthesia, but the corneal reflex is still present and the pupil moderately dilated. In the rabbit, loss of the corneal reflex is a sign of dangerously deep anesthesia. With surgical anesthesia the respirations are regular. Using this technique anesthesia should be maintained for 1 to 2 hours. If the animal shows signs of awakening, more intravenous pentobarbital should be given since this is more effective than supplementary ether. When the needle is withdrawn, a cotton pledget can be held over the insertion site with slight compression between the thumb and forefinger for a minute or two. Should the need arise for supplementary anesthesia, the assistant should hold the head firmly when the ear is punctured since the rabbit may otherwise jerk violently at this time.

According to Field (1957), albino rabbits are very difficult to anesthetize to a satisfactory depth of anesthesia with intravenous pentobarbital. This is because there is a very small margin of safety between the surgical anesthetic dose and one causing respiratory arrest. He recommends that albino rabbits, and to a lesser extent "fancy breeds", should not be used for recovery experiments, and indicates that mixed breed animals give most satisfactory results.

When respiratory arrest does occur, it is usually due to too rapid administration of anesthetic. By holding the rabbit's chest in the hand so as to compress it *lightly*, the animal will resume respirations. This continues only as long as the chest is squeezed and stops when pressure is removed, thus it is only a temporary measure. To obtain more prolonged effect, a piece of rubber tubing can be placed in position around the chest to give moderate compression and held in position with forceps. Artificial respiration can be performed by rocking the animal alternately head-down and head-up. This can be continued gently and is usually effective. Oxygen administration and other resuscitative measures should also be undertaken if necessary.

When magnesium sulfate is used for anesthesia of rabbits, 20 gm. is dissolved in enough distilled water to make 100 ml. This solution is then given subcutaneously, intramuscularly, or intravenously at a rate of 5 ml./kg. The duration of anesthesia in rabbits is roughly $\frac{3}{4}$ to $1\frac{1}{2}$ hours with wide variation. Calcium gluconate or combined neostigmine (0.35–0.63 mg./kg.) and pentylenetetrazol (10 mg./kg.) intravenously will counteract the anesthetic effect almost immediately.

For acute non-recovery work in rabbits urethane may be used. The recommended dose is 1.75 gm./kg. subcutaneously or 1.6 gm./kg. intraperitoneally. This is 14 ml. of a 25% solution subcutaneously for a 2 kg. rabbit. Intravenous injection is made "to effect." There is a wide variation in dose, but less than with barbiturates. Because the recovery period lasts 36 hours or more, edema of the lungs usually develops before the animal recovers. The carcinogenic potential of urethane should be considered when it is used (Chapter 11, page 200).

Hamsters

Ether and pentobarbital sodium are the anesthetics commonly employed in hamsters. Induction and administration of ether anesthesia are performed similarly to the guinea pig, though fasting and atropine administration are not essential.

Pentobarbital is given intraperitoneally approximately $\frac{1}{4}$-inch lateral to the umbilicus. Intravenous injection is extremely difficult.

Chinchillas

Ether has been employed extensively as an inhalant anesthetic for chinchillas. Slow recovery with pulmonary complications has been the rule rather than exception. The chinchilla apparently does not tolerate ether as well as other domestic animals do.

For cesarean section in chinchillas, Hayes (1955) has advocated intramuscular administration of 15 mg. of meperidine approximately 30 minutes prior to operation, followed by 1% hexylcaine solution injected subcutaneously along the proposed line of incision. This produces sedation along with good local anesthesia. Recovery is almost immediate; the young will nurse within minutes and the mother will often eat within an hour.

Riddell (1952) has used epidural anesthesia for cesarean section and states the landmarks are easily located since the lumbosacral fossa is comparatively large. He reports one fatality in six cases.

Thiopental sodium in dilute solution has been given intravenously "to effect" for dental procedures (Boothe, 1953).

Squirrels

Heuschele (1960) has indicated that ether by inhalation is suitable for squirrels. Tribromoethanol has also been given orally in doses of 0.06 to 0.09 gm./lb. (Mosby and Cantner, 1955).

Mink

For restraint and anesthesia of mink, a metal tube such as described by Hummon (1945) is convenient. The dimensions vary according to the size of the mink being restrained. One end is covered with hardware cloth, the other remaining open (Fig. 14–8). The mink is inserted headfirst into the tube. Vaccinations or other injections can be given subcutaneously or intramuscularly on the inner surface of the hind leg while the animal is thus restrained. To anesthetize the animal, a pad of ether-soaked cotton is held over the screened end while the opposite open end is tightly covered.

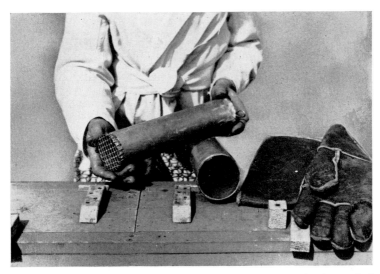

FIGURE 14–8. A holding tube for mink closed at one end with hardware cloth and reinforced at the open end with a heavy wire. Heavy leather gloves (right) are used in handling the animals. (From Hummon, O. J.: A Device for the Restraint of Mink During Certain Experimental Procedures. J.A.V.M.A., *106*, 104, 1945.)

Ferrets

Wright (1957) recommends intraperitoneal pentobarbital sodium for anesthetizing ferrets. The dose is 0.45 gr./500 gm. of body weight. Full anesthesia persists for 30 to 45 minutes followed by a recovery period of 3 to 4 hours. The safety margin is not wide and small ferrets are reported to have died after injection of 0.6 gr.

Skunks

Veterinarians are occasionally asked to de-scent skunks. Usually this operation is performed in young kittens. In general, either a volatile anesthetic, such as ether, or pentobarbital sodium is used.

For small skunks, a transparent plastic disposable obstetrical sleeve is an ideal container for induction of ether anesthesia. The skunk is placed in the sleeve with ether-soaked cotton and, after induction, the surgery is done through a small opening cut in the sleeve. On conclusion, the skunk is removed and the sleeve discarded, eliminating the problem of an odoriferous container.

Miller (1959) states an ether jar is the best insurance against "accidents" caused by the animal expressing the scent gland; however, because this anesthesia is fleeting he prefers pentobarbital. This is administered while holding the animal by the tail and "deftly" inserting a 4-inch needle into the abdomen.

According to Barry (1958), the best age for removal of the scent glands in skunks is between 5 and 6 weeks when the skunk's weight is about 2 pounds. The sacs may be emptied by turning the animal hindquarters away from the operator and pulling the tail up and forward forcing out their contents. Pentobarbital is given intraperitoneally using a 2 ml. syringe and 25 gauge needle; the usual dose is from 0.25 to 0.5 ml.

Intrathoracic injection of pentobarbital at the rate of 1 ml./5 lbs. has been advocated by Taylor (1961), who states induction requires 2 to 4 minutes and recovery occurs in approximately 4 hours.

Primates

In anesthetizing primates, the chief problem lies in restraint of the animals during induction because of their agility and often vicious nature. As an example, chimpanzees weighing over 30 pounds have tremendous strength coupled with a nasty disposition and are often extremely dangerous. For this reason they should never be handled by persons working alone. If large numbers are to be anesthetized, a squeeze cage will be found effective and time-saving. (Fig. 14–9).

Preanesthetic tranquilization or sedation is desirable. Promazine at the rate of 1 mg./lb. or meperidine at the rate of 5 mg./lb. will produce satisfactory results (Table 14–6). Caged monkeys that are hard to manage can sometimes be enticed to reach for fruit held close to the cage bars. By grasping the hand or forearm, intramuscular injection of these agents can be accomplished.

Perphenazine can be administered to chimpanzees by triturating the required number of tablets and suspending the powder in approximately 8 ounces of canned pineapple juice (Wallace et al., 1960). The effective dose for maximum restraint varies from 2.4 to 4.4 mg./kg. Optimum tranquilization occurs in approximately 3 hours and persists for 6 to 7 hours. Other tantalizing vehicles for drug administration include maple syrup and peanut butter.

After preanesthetics have taken effect, thiopental, thiamylal, or

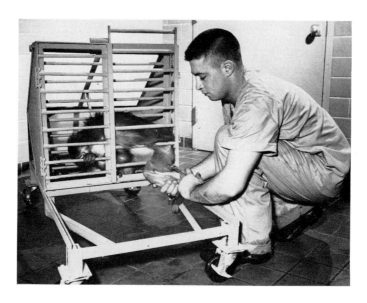

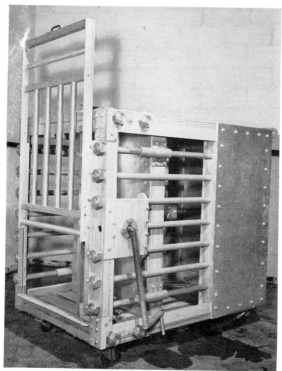

FIGURE 14–9.   Squeeze cage for monkeys (top) and chimpanzees (bottom) (Courtesy of Captain W. E. Britz, Jr., and the U.S.A.F. School of Aerospace Medicine, Brooks AFB, Texas).

Table 14-6.—*Promazine in Captive Wild Animals*

Species	Weight in lb.	Dose and Route of Administration	Reason for Administration	Effect
Artic Fox (*Vulpes lagopus*)	15	75 mg. I.M.	Apply cast to leg	Sleepy and gentle
Puma (*Felis concolor*)	50	100 mg. I.M.	Postsurgical sedation	Quieted but active if approached
Crested Ape (*Macaca nigra*)	30	75 mg. I.M.	Aggressive with mate	Drowsy
African Lion (*Felis leo*)	360	180 mg. I.M.	Venipuncture, caudal vein	Calm
Chimpanzee (*Pan troglodytes*)	30	75 mg. I.M.	E.C.G.	Calm
Greater Kudo Antelope (*Strepsiceros strepsiceros*)	700	1000 mg. I.M.	Hoof trimming	Calm
Guinea Baboon (*Papio papio*)	25	50 mg. I.M.	Venipuncture	Tranquil
Mule Deer (*Odocoileus hemionus*)	50	100 mg. I.V.	X-ray leg	Calm
Bennette's Wallaby (*Protemnodon ruficollis bennetti*)	25	50 mg. I.V.	Treat abscess	Quiet but required restraint

(From data of Heuschele, W. P.: Experiences with Promazine in Captive Wild Animals. Biochemic Review, *29*, 3, 1959.)

pentobarbital can be administered intravenously using either veins of the forearm or hind limb. Restraint for this procedure is necessary in most instances despite preanesthetic medication. The assistant can best hold small primates by grasping their arms and holding them behind the animal's back.

Newsome and Robinson (1957) have reported trial of a wide variety of agents for sedation and anesthesia of baboons. Among those used were morphine, amidone, chloral hydrate, chloralose, pentobarbital, hexobarbital, amobarbital, paraldehyde, chlorpromazine, ether, chloroform, and nitrous oxide.

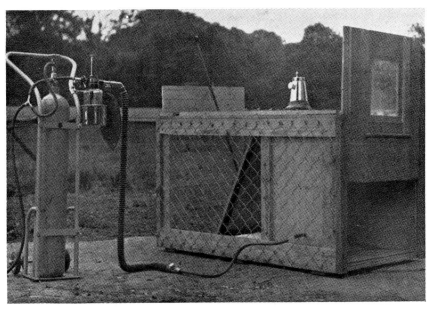

FIGURE 14–10. A box for administration of nitrous oxide. (From Newsome, J., and Robinson, D. L. H.: Sedatives and Anaesthetics for Baboons. Brit. Vet. J., *113*, 163, 1957.)

Morphine administered orally or by injection in doses up to 1 gr. produced very severe skin irritation of the palms and soles with loss of appetite. Sedation was not effected. Amidone was not particularly effective in doses of 80 mg. intramuscularly.

When chloral hydrate was offered orally, the animals refused it because of the bitter taste. Chloralose in doses of 1 to 1.5 grams was ineffective. Three grams/15 kg. or 4 gm./25 kg. produced heavy sedation in 30 minutes which lasted up to 3 hours. Rhythmic clonic spasms of the limbs and head, however, interfered with experimental procedures. Salivation and excessive sweating also occurred.

Pentobarbital sodium given by intramuscular injection was unpredictable, animals reacting differently to equal doses on different days. After several hundred injections it was deemed unsuitable. Hexobarbital and amobarbital given in tablet form were not effective because the animals rejected the tablets.

When paraldehyde was given intramuscularly in doses up to 5 ml., it produced a calming effect. It was most effective when combined with pentobarbital, reducing the dose of the latter. However, anesthetic emergencies and fatalities sometimes occurred.

Chlorpromazine proved the most valuable sedative, but there was a wide variation in the response of baboons. Doses of up to 3.5 mg./kg. made the animals apathetic and slow, but they could not be easily handled. When given intramuscularly the action was slow, maximum effect occurring at $2\frac{1}{2}$ to 6 hours after injection.

Induction by open ether, while used extensively, was difficult because of struggling. Nitrous oxide was found to be most satisfactory, the animal being enticed into a 6 cu. ft. box (Fig. 14–10). Nitrous oxide was allowed to flow into the box until anesthesia was induced, following which ether was also administered for a short period of time. The animal was then removed from the box and an ether-air mixture administered with a semi-closed system and face mask.

Swine

In recent years the pig has been used extensively as a laboratory animal. Under these circumstances, different anesthetic techniques are employed than are used "in the field."

According to Wright and Hall (1961) the pig is easily restrained for 45 to 60 minutes following an intramuscular injection of 0.5 mg./lb. of chlorpromazine. Intravenous doses of 75 to 100 mg. have been recommended in sows weighing 275 to 300 pounds (Hibbs, 1958).

The pig should be fasted 24 to 36 hours prior to general anesthesia. If not properly fasted, gaseous distention of the digestive tract may develop and cause death by interfering with ventilation and venous return to the heart. Magnesium sulfate or sodium sulfate (25 to 125 gm.) can be administered orally to assure complete evacuation of the gastrointestinal tract if abdominal surgery is to be done.

The animal is prepared for general anesthesia by administration of atropine sulfate (0.03 to 0.04 mg./lb.), meperidine hydrochloride (0.5 to 1.0 mg./lb.), and promazine hydrochloride (1.0 mg./lb.). These are injected intramuscularly in separate sites 45 to 60 minutes prior to anesthesia (Booth, 1963).

A 5% solution of thiopental is satisfactory for rapid induction of anesthesia. The intravenous dose varies considerably; swine weighing 10 to 50 and 50 to 100 pounds usually require 5.0 and 4.5 mg./lb. respectively.

When surgical procedures require only a few minutes of anesthesia, thiopental can be administered in the marginal ear vein using a 22 gauge 1-inch needle. Maintenance of anesthesia for prolonged periods is difficult because repeated punctures of the vein provoke head and ear shaking in animals lightly anesthetized.

Insertion of an indwelling polyethylene catheter (PE 190) provides a more satisfactory means for administering additional anesthetic when long periods are required. A 14 gauge thin-walled medium bevel 3-inch needle is used for making venipunctures in swine weighing 20 to 100 lbs. With the animal restrained in dorsal recumbency, the needle is inserted about 2 cm. to one side of the cariniform cartilage on a line from the point of the cartilage to the base of the ear. The needle is pushed inward, downward, and backward until its point enters the anterior vena cava (Carle and Dewhirst, 1942). The polyethylene catheter is then threaded through the needle into the vein. Following venipuncture, the catheter can be easily inserted into vena cava and right side of the heart for a distance of several centimeters. The needle is withdrawn by sliding it over the catheter. To prevent accidental withdrawal of the catheter from the vein, it can be taped or sutured to the animal's skin. An 18 gauge blunted needle is inserted into the catheter lumen and a 2- or 3-way valve is attached so injections can be readily made.

Because respiratory depression or paralysis can readily occur in swine following induction of anesthesia, an endotracheal catheter should be routinely inserted to establish an airway. With the animal properly anesthetized, the trachea is intubated by direct visualization using a lighted laryngoscope and porcine mouth speculum. Intubation is best performed with the animal secured in dorsal recumbency. A cuffed endotracheal catheter lubricated with 5% hexylcaine jelly is used.

In contrast to the dog, extremely deep pentobarbital anesthesia is required in the pig to abolish reflex activity. Moreover, recovery from a single anesthetic dose of pentobarbital is remarkably rapid. It is not uncommon to observe the return of violent motor activity within 10 or 15 minutes. According to Jones (1957), pentobarbital provides a considerable margin of safety in pigs weighing 25 to 30 pounds. An intravenous dose of 11 mg./lb. is sufficient to induce general anesthesia. Pentobarbital and atropine can be given intraperitoneally followed by an inhalant anesthetic, such as ether, to maintain surgical anesthesia. This method has been used by Wesolowski (1962) for experimental vascular surgery involving the thoracic vessels of the pig.

Trichloroethylene will provide satisfactory maintenance of anesthesia for short periods (30 to 45 minutes) following thiopental or pentobarbital anesthesia in swine. Booth (1963) has found that it can be conveniently administered using a glass beaker containing liquid trichloroethylene and cotton saturated with anesthetic. The beaker should be of sufficient size that it will fit over the snout of the pig but not too tightly. A polyethylene tube, connected to the flowmeter of an oxygen tank, is taped along the snout of the animal and extended into the liquid trichloroethylene in the beaker. Oxygen, flowing at a rate of 2 to 3 liters per minute, increases the volatilization of trichloroethylene and also displaces exhaled carbon dioxide accumulating inside the beaker. The beaker can be easily removed to discontinue anesthetic administration whenever respiratory depression is imminent. Recovery is rapid.

A disadvantage of trichloroethylene is that it fails to produce sufficient relaxation of skeletal muscle. Moreover, it causes cardiac arrhythmias and tachypnea. The severity of these conditions, however, can be greatly alleviated by using atropine, meperidine, and promazine.

Following premedication with a small dose of morphine (0.2–0.9 mg./kg.), the intravenous dose of chloralose necessary to produce hypnotic action in the pig is 55 to 86 mg./kg. of body weight (Booth et al., 1960). Paddling movements of the limbs are seen in the pig similar to those reported in sheep by Phillipson and Barnett (1939). Pentobarbital can be administered intravenously in small doses to prevent these without interfering greatly with baroreceptor activity.

Sheep and Goats

Sheep and goats are occasionally used as laboratory animals. The chief difficulties experienced during general anesthesia with these species are excessive salivation, tympanites, and regurgitation. The latter two can be eliminated to a great extent by fasting the animal for at least 24 hours and by administration of an antiferment one-half hour prior to induction.

Excessive salivation is controlled by intramuscular injection of atropine (15 mg./50 lbs.) 15 minutes before induction. To maintain control it should be given intravenously at 15 minute intervals. According to Booth (1963), a maintenance dose of 3 to 6 mg. will accomplish this in animals weighing 65 to 85 pounds.

Both thiamylal (4%) and thiopental (5%) have been used satisfactorily in sheep and goats. Since these anesthetics are detoxified at a rapid rate, the dose required for anesthesia varies greatly. An initial intravenous dose of 9 to 10 mg./lb. of body weight is usually effective.

Immediately following induction of anesthesia, a cuffed endotracheal catheter is inserted into the trachea to prevent aspiration of regurgitated ruminal contents.

Maintenance of anesthesia can be achieved by repeated injections of anesthetic through an indwelling catheter in the external jugular vein. An alternative is administration of ether, halothane, or methoxyflurane by means of a gas machine. Recovery from these volatile liquid anesthetics is rapid and uneventful.

Allam and Churchill (1946) used pentobarbital sodium intravenously in average-sized mature goats. They found that a total dose of 10 grains given in the jugular vein was sufficient to produce general anesthesia. The animals were able to stand in 2 or 3 hours. There is wide variation in the anesthetic dose and duration of anesthesia of pentobarbital in sheep (Phillipson and Barnett, 1939). Approximately 30 mg./kg. will produce a short period of surgical anesthesia (15 to 30 minutes) in adult sheep; in lambs it is of longer duration.

Triflupromazine (0.5 to 1 mg./lb. intravenously) is a satisfactory preanesthetic for goats when combined with either local or general anesthesia (Jha et al., 1961 a, b; Tyagi and Lumb, 1961).

Deer

Davis (1963) has had considerable experience in handling and anesthetizing Colorado mule deer. For tranquilization during transportation chlorpromazine at a rate of 2 mg./lb. is given intramuscularly. Good results have also been obtained in elk with this dose. The effect requires about an hour to reach its height and lasts 16 to 24 hours. If used as a preanesthetic prior to pentobarbital, it is injected intramuscularly at least 1 hour in advance. Deer given perphenazine as a tranquilizer have a tendency to chew on rocks during the recovery period.

For short periods of anesthesia (30 minutes), a 7% solution of chloral hydrate is given intravenously "to effect". The last part of the injection is made very slowly. No deaths occurred in a series of approximately 25 animals, though no attempt was made to starve the animals and no preanesthetic agents were used.

There is marked variation in the reaction of deer to intravenous pentobarbital and they must be watched very closely during the recovery period which is relatively long. Salivation and bloating are constant problems. If pentobarbital is to be used, it should be preceded by atropine and chlorpromazine, and the animal should be deprived of feed and water for 24 hours prior to induction. The dose of atropine is large, at least $\frac{1}{4}$ gr. is given initially, and additional increments up to 1 gr. may be necessary. In a series of approximately 50 deer, Davis reported one death and several cases of postoperative pneumonia due to regurgitation of rumen contents.

Undomesticated Cats

Treatment and handling of undomesticated cats are greatly facilitated by general anesthesia; however, anesthetics are difficult to administer and their results are variable. Chloroform can be used, the animal being confined in a small tarpaulin-covered cage and the anesthetic introduced by pouring it on the cage floor or on

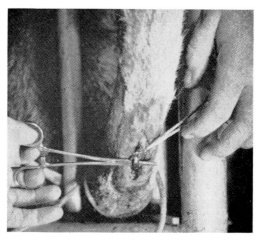

Figure 14–11. Following infiltration with a local anesthetic, the lateral caudal vein of a lion can be exposed for intravenous injection. (Clifford, D. H., Stowe, C. M., Jr., and Good, A. L.: Pentobarbital Anesthesia in Lions with Special Reference to Preanesthetic Medication. J.A.V.M.A., *139*, 111, 1961.)

cotton. As soon as the cat collapses the cage cover is removed and chloroform given by means of a mask on a long pole (Campbell, 1950).

Clifford (1958, 1961) has used combined meperidine and promazine as preanesthetic agents in an ocelot, a leopard, and in lions. In the latter, 11 mg./kg. of meperidine and 4.4 to 9 mg./kg. of promazine are recommended. Subcutaneous administration is facilitated by use of a squeeze-cage. After these take effect pentobarbital is given intraperitoneally, intrathoracically or intravenously. To accomplish the latter, a tourniquet is applied to the tail and the anesthetic injected into the caudal vein (Fig. 14–11).

According to Clifford, big cats require less anesthetic to produce surgical anesthesia, certain reflexes may persist longer, and the postanesthetic recovery period is longer. Pentobarbital is a dangerous anesthetic if used to abolish all reflexes in lions. The number and character of the respirations are important criteria with which to evaluate depth of anesthesia. Fewer than 10 respirations per minute should be the cause of grave concern. It is suggested that local anesthetics be employed, whenever possible, to avoid large doses of general anesthetic in undomesticated cats.

Bears

Small bears can be anesthetized with intravenous pentobarbital sodium given in the cephalic or saphenous vein. A squeeze cage will

Table 14–7.—Effect of Sucostrin-Toxital* Anesthesia on Bears

Sex	Est. Age	Wt.	Sucostrin Used	Effective Time (min.)	Re- covery Time (min.)	Toxital Used	Effective Time (min.)	Remarks
M	$2\frac{1}{2}$	200	$2\frac{1}{2}$ cc.	2	7	20 cc.	—	
F	$3\frac{1}{2}$	305	4 cc.	5	§	20 cc.	$9\frac{1}{2}$	Never went completely down with sucostrin.
F	$1\frac{1}{2}$	166	$1\frac{3}{4}$ cc.	$1\frac{1}{6}$	3	7 cc.	12	Sucostrin, 1 cc. had no effect.
F	$1\frac{1}{2}$	157	2 cc.	$1\frac{3}{4}$	§	10 cc.	6	8 cc. toxital not enough so gave 2 cc. more.
F	$3\frac{1}{2}$	292	3 cc.	2	3	12 cc.	$13\frac{1}{2}$	Recovered in $1\frac{1}{2}$ hours.
M	6+	680	7 cc.	4	§	8 cc.	—	Initial dose of 40 cc. had no effect. Kept adding at 15 min. intervals 10–15 cc. until anesthetized.
F	$1\frac{1}{2}$	146	2 cc.	$2\frac{1}{2}$	§	10 cc.	12	Did not completely relax under sucostrin.
M	$1\frac{1}{2}$	158	$2\frac{1}{4}$ cc.	$2\frac{1}{2}$	§	10 cc.	$7\frac{1}{2}$	Not out well with sucostrin but was under with toxital.
M	$2\frac{1}{2}$	245	3 cc.	3	8	12 cc.	13	
F	$3\frac{1}{2}$	350	$3\frac{1}{2}$ cc.	$2\frac{1}{2}$	9	31 cc.	—	Gave 16 cc. toxital; after 15 min. gave 15 cc. more.

§ Recovery time was not always known because toxital took effect before recovery from sucostrin. Effective time of toxital was not always known because bear had not recovered from sucostrin when toxital became effective.

* Sucostrin chloride (E. R. Squibb and Sons) contains 30 mg./ml. of succinylcholine chloride. Toxital (Jensen-Salsbery Laboratories, Kansas City, Missouri) contains 2.75 gr. of pentobarbital sodium/ml. and in conventional use is given for euthanasia of small animals.

(From Troyer, W.: Out for Bear. Jen-Sal J. April, 1960.)

facilitate the procedure. If not available, the caged animal is offered a favorite food and when it reaches for it the paw is grasped by an assistant wearing gloves. A rope is tied around the limb to act as a tourniquet and distend the vein. Fowler (1960) has described this procedure in a 75-pound Malayan sun bear. Eleven grains of pentobarbital produced surgical anesthesia for 2 hours. An average of 13.5 mg./kg. of pentobarbital intravenously permitted safe handling and minor surgery of American black bears and Himalayan black bears (Clarke *et al.*, 1963).

Oral administration of pentobarbital in food or drink has been described by Martyn (1955) but is not as reliable in producing anesthesia. In one instance, following oral pentobarbital as a preanesthetic, ether was administered by means of a large mask fastened on a long pole.

Troyer (1960) in trapping and tagging Kodiak bears has devised an efficient method for their management. Once the bear is caught by the foot in a special trap, succinylcholine is given intramuscularly in the hind leg by means of a syringe on a long aluminum pole. As soon as it takes effect, and the bear is tied in spread-eagle fashion, a special concentrated pentobarbital solution is injected intrapertoneally. Succinylcholine alone is less satisfactory. No deaths occurred in a series of 32 bears. Table 14–7 gives figures representative of effects obtained with this procedure.

Clifford *et al.* (1962) found that combined intramuscular injections of large doses of promazine and meperidine were not particularly effective in North American black bears (*Euartos americanus*). They suggested that 8.8 mg./kg. of morphine and 4.4 mg./kg. of promazine be given intramuscularly as preanesthetic agents prior to intravenous pentobarbital.

The Cap-Chur Gun

A useful development in capture and restraint of wild animals has been the Cap-Chur gun* which is essentially an air rifle, powered by carbon dioxide, that fires an automatic injecting syringe (Fig. 14–12). With this gun it is possible to inject from 1 to 10 ml. of any liquid into an animal for distances up to approximately 40 yards. It is also available in pistol form, the pistol being better at distances under 20 yards because lower muzzle velocity produces a softer impact on the animal with less contusion. In the open, and in large pens where the distance between the operator and animal is at least 20 yards, the rifle is most useful. The target area is usually the heavy muscles of the hip or neck.

* See Appendix A, p. 403 for manufacturer.

According to Thomas (1961), who uses the gun in a zoo practice, it seldom misfires or fails to inject the full quantity of drug. The range and accuracy vary somewhat and experience is necessary for best results. On cold days, with the ambient temperature between 20 and 40° F., it is difficult to get accurate shots over 30 yards unless the gun is pre-warmed. On hot days, with the ambient temperature between 80 and 100° F., accurate shots can be made up to 50 yards.

Wright (1962) reported that gunpowder was much more convenient and dependable for use in the automatic syringe than the chemical combustion method. He also emphasized that both the pistol and rifle required the same care and cleaning as other firearms.

The gun was originally designed for injection of nicotine as an immobilizing drug. As previously described in Chapter 12, the action of nicotine is dual depending upon the dose administered; large doses act as a stimulant producing convulsions in certain species, whereas, small doses have a pronounced tranquilizing action. Susceptibility to nicotine varies with each species, but, in most, a dose that will paralyze without producing convulsions can be determined (Table 14–8). Nicotine produces tachyphylaxis and a second injection given within 24 hours generally is ineffective.

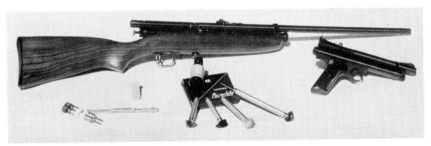

Figure 14–12. Palmer short and long range syringe projectors with projectile syringes and loading equipment. (Courtesy of Palmer Chemical and Equipment Company, Inc.)

Table 14–8.—Suggested Dosage for Cap-Chur Sol*

Species	Approximate Dosage Per Pound Body Weight	Species	Approximate Dosage Per Pound Body Weight
Dogs	2.0–4.0 mg.	Cattle	0.75–2.0 mg.
Cats	1.0–2.0 mg.	Swine	3.0 –5.0 mg.
Goats	2.0–5.0 mg.	Bears	3.0 –4.0 mg.
Sheep	2.0–4.0 mg.	Horses	1.5 –2.5 mg.
Deer (White Tailed)	1.5–2.5 mg.	Monkeys	2.5 –4.0 mg.

* Contains standardized alkaloidal nicotine; Palmer Chemical and Equipment Company, Inc., Atlanta, Georgia.

Table 14-9.—*Paralyzing Doses of Succinylcholine Chloride and Duration of Paralysis in Wild Animals*

Animal	Scientific name	Sex	No.	Age	Estimated weight (lb.)	Dose (mg.)	Av. latent period (min.)	Maximum latent period (min.)	Minimum latent period (min.)	Duration paralysis (min.)
Monkey, spider	*Ateles geoffroyi*	F	1	Adult	5	5	$4\frac{1}{2}$	—	—	20
Monkey, spider	*Ateles geoffroyi*	F	1	Adult	5	10	50 sec.	—	—	30
Monkey, spider	*Ateles geoffroyi*	F	1	Adult	5	20	$\frac{1}{2}$	—	—	45
Lion, African	*Panthera leo*	F	1	Adult	275	60	6	—	—	11
Lion, African	*Panthera leo*	F	1	Adult	275	120	$2\frac{1}{2}$	—	—	60
Goat, domestic	*Capra prisca*	M	1	Adult	110	70	$6\frac{1}{2}$	—	—	60
Goat, domestic	*Capra prisca*	M	1	Adult	110	40	9	—	—	30
Goat, domestic	*Capra prisca*	M	1	Adult	110	20	14	—	—	15
Goat, domestic	*Capra prisca*	F	3	Adult	50–80	20	11	14	9	15
Goat, domestic	*Capra prisca*	F	3	Adult	60	15	11	11	11	17
Goat (Tahr), Himalayan	*Hemitragus jemiahious*	M	2	Adult	165	$17\frac{1}{2}$	6	—	—	$21\frac{1}{2}$
Goat (Tahr), Himalayan	*Hemitragus jemiahious*	F	2	Adult	115	15	6	—	—	20
Sheep, Barbary	*Ammotragus lervia*	M	2	Adult	200	20	15	17	12	7
Antelope, pronghorn	*Antelope Capra Americana*	M	2	1 year	50	5	8	10	6	15

(302)

Deer, fallow	*Dama dama*	M	7	Adult	135	10	11½	17	17	7	13
Deer, axis	*Axis axis*	M	1	Adult	120	7	10	7	—	—	17
Deer, axis	*Axis axis*	F	1	Adult	120	7	8	7	—	—	19
Deer, sika	*Cervus nippon*	M	2	Adult	170	7	7	7	7	7	14
Deer, sika	*Cervus nippon*	F	4	Adult	130	7	7	7	7	7	14
Deer, barasingha	*Cervus dubauceli*	M	5	Adult	450	13	9½	11	7	7	15 7/10
Deer, barasingha	*Cervus dubauceli*	M	1	Adult	375	13	8½	—	—	—	20
Deer, barasingha	*Cervus dubauceli*	F	16	Adult	(170–360) Av. 227	6–10 / 7.2	8	12½	5	—	(10–30) 17½
Deer, barasingha	*Cervus dubauceli*	M	1	Adult	Emaciated 400	7	9½	—	—	—	20
Deer, barasingha	*Cervus dubauceli*	M	1	Adult	Emaciated 325	6	9	—	—	—	30
Wapiti (elk)	*Cervus canadinsis*	M	1	Adult	1,100	23	6	6	6	—	18
Wapiti (elk)	*Cervus canadinsis*	F	4	Adult	550	15	5–3/10	7½	3½	—	(18–25) 2½
Wapiti (elk)	*Cervus canadinsis*	M	1	Adult	450	15	5–3/10	7½	3½	—	21½
Deer, red	*Cervus elaphus*	M	5	Adult	260	15	7½	9½	(16–23) 6½	—	(14–18) 16
Bison	*Bison bison*	F	1	Adult	700	25	7	7	7	—	10
Antelope (eland)	*Taurotragus oryx*	F	1	Adult	250	6	9	—	—	—	14

(From Thomas, W. D.: Chemical Immobilization of Wild Animals. J.A.V.M.A., *138*, 264, 1961.)

Table 14-10.—Data on Immobilization of African Animals with a Projectile Syringe

Species	Drug	Dose	Mortality*	Remarks
Kob antelope (*Adenota kob thomasi*)	Succinylcholine chloride	Approx. 0.15 mg./lb. in adult males.	Approx. 10%	Add 5 mg. atropine per 100 lbs., if pregnant.
Hartebeest (*Alcelaphus lelwel jacksonii*)	Succinylcholine chloride		None	
	Gallamine triethiodide		None	Slower reaction than succinylcholine.
Waterbuck (*Kobus defassa ugandae*)	Succinylcholine chloride		None	
	Gallamine triethiodide		None	Slower reaction than succinylcholine.
Hippopotamus (*Hippopotamus amphibious*)	Succinylcholine chloride	0.08 mg./lb.	2/23	Avoid immobilizing in water, if possible, as animal may drown.
	Gallamine triethiodide	1.8 mg./lb.	0/2	May be safer than succinylcholine.

Buffalo (*Syncerus caffer*)	Gallamine triethiodide	1.2–1.3 mg./lb.	0/6	Average time to go down was 11 minutes.
	d-tubocurarine		1/4	Add atropine to solution.
Giraffe (*Giraffa camelopardalis*)	Gallamine triethiodide	1.7 mg./lb.	0/8	Wide variation in time required to go down.
Rhinoceros (*Diceros bicornis*)	Gallamine triethiodide	0.8–0.9 mg./lb.	2/10	Animals run long distances before going down.
Elephant (*Loxodonta africana*)	Gallamine triethiodide	1.2 mg./lb.	1/7	Appears quite effective.

* Fractions indicate number of deaths/number injected. Neostigmine methylsulphate was generally used as an antidote. (From Harthoorn, A. M. and Lock, J. A.: Advances in the Use of Muscle Relaxing Drugs for Immobilization and Handling of Larger Land Mammals. J. Small Anim. Pract., *2*, 163, 1961; Buechner, H. K., Harthoorn, A. M., and Lock, J. A.: Immobilizing Uganda Kob with Succinylcholine Chloride. Canad. J. Comp. Med., *24*, 317, 1960.)

When nicotine is used, immobilization usually occurs in 30 seconds to 12 minutes, though occasionally may require as long as 20 minutes depending on the position of the hit. Immediately following injection, the animal should be considered a patient and every effort made to afford maximum care until complete recovery has occurred. Paralyzed animals should be made as comfortable as possible and should never be forced to stand or exert themselves. Traumatic shock is easily induced under these circumstances. In ruminants, inhalation of regurgitated rumen contents commonly occurs; therefore, they should be placed in sternal recumbency with head and neck elevated. In dogs, intraperitoneal or intramuscular hits produce increased respirations and profuse salivation with retching and vomiting. In 1 to 3 minutes equilibrium is lost and catalepsy or flaccid paralysis develops. Occasionally artificial respiration is necessary. Most dogs return to normal in 6 to 12 hours (Jenkins et al. 1961).

No mortality rates are available for most animals immobilized with nicotine, but a relatively high death loss does occur. Hayes et al. (1957) reported the death rate in 162 deer given nicotine salicylate was 8.9%. They further stated, however, that this did not exceed that of some accepted trapping procedures. Davis (1963) concluded that alkaloidal nicotine, nicotine sulfate, and nicotine salicylate were all unsuitable for use in Colorado mule deer because of the excessively high mortality. Unsatisfactory results with alkaloidal nicotine, which include a fatality in a deer, have also been reported by Hatch et al. (1959) and by Hayes et al. (1959), who experienced some deaths in wild cattle.

Thomas (1961) has used succinylcholine chloride (20 mg./ml.) in the Cap-Chur gun for immobilization of a wide variety of zoo animals, and also for capturing wild animals in their native habitats (for the pharmacology of succinylcholine, see Chapter 12, page 224). The dose of succinylcholine is difficult to determine for various species because of differences in response; primates and goats have a great tolerance while deer and cattle have a low tolerance. Table 14–9 lists a wide variety of species which have been immoblized with this technique.

When succinylcholine is used in capturing wild animals the dose cannot be accurately determined; therefore, it is suggested that an oxygen tank connected to a rebreathing system be carried. If an overdose of succinylcholine produces respiratory paralysis, oxygen can then be given through an endotracheal catheter. Thomas recommends that all wild animals, while still paralyzed, be given prednisolone and antibiotics according to body weight. Amphetamine may be given if deemed necessary and a tranquilizer should be injected before the animal recovers.

Raccoons weighing 15 to 25 pounds are immobilized with the Cap-Chur gun approximately 7 minutes by 10 mg. of succinylcholine chloride (Farrell, 1963). Recovery is complete in 10 minutes.

Boyd (1962) injected succinylcholine chloride intrathoracically and intravenously into trapped Colorado mule deer with a conventional syringe. By the former route the effective dose was found to be 0.052 mg./lb. for adults and 0.078 mg./lb. for fawns. Intravenous administration caused severe respiratory paralysis and some deaths. The margin between a safe dose and a lethal one was found to be quite small with both methods.

When succinylcholine is used for restraint of wild elk, some deaths occur. Gallamine has been used in a limited number of elk to facilitate collecting blood samples (Wolff and Boyd, 1963). The average dose, 60 to 80 mg., was shot intramuscularly with a Cap-Chur gun. The shortest time for an elk to go down was approximately 80 seconds and the longest 150. Trembling and anxiety preceded collapse of the animals. After struggling ceased, they were securely tied and edrophonium given intravenously at a rate of 1.0 mg. for each 2.0 mg. of gallamine administered. The severe respiratory distress produced by gallamine was immediately relieved.

After blood collection, injected elk appeared dull and quiet and some remained in sternal recumbency for as long as $1\frac{1}{2}$ hours. No deaths occurred in a series of nine animals.

Harthoorn and Lock (1961) have used both succinylcholine and gallamine on wild African game with good results; (Table 14–10). It should be noted that often a considerable period of time elapsed before the animals went down.

In general, gallamine appears to be superior for use in the Cap-Chur gun to both nicotine and succinylcholine in that rapid-acting injectable antidotes, edrophonium and neostigmine, are available. These enable relief of the severe respiratory distress produced by this agent and lower the mortality rate.

References

ALLAM, M. W. and CHURCHILL, E. A.: Pentobarbital Sodium Anesthesia in Swine and Goats. J.A.V.M.A., *109*, 355, 1946.

BARRY, J. A.: Removal of Scent Glands in Skunk. M. S. U. Vet., *19*, 77, 1958.

BOOTH, N. H.: Personal Communication. Colorado State University, Fort Collins Colorado, 1963.

BOOTH, N. H., BREDECK, H. E., and HERIN, R. A.: Baroceptor Reflex Mechanisms in Swine. Am. J. Physiol., *199*, 1189, 1960.

BOOTHE, H. W.: Diseases of the Chinchilla. Proc. A.V.M.A., 19th Annual Meeting, p. 242, 1953.

BOYD, R. J.: Succinylcholine Chloride for Immobilization of Colorado Mule Deer. J. Wildlife Management, *26*, 332, 1962.

CAMPBELL, J. A.: Use of Anaesthesia in Treatment of Zoo Inmates. Canad. J. Comp. Med., *14*, 39, 1950.

CARLE, B. N. and DEWHIRST, W. H., JR.:   A Method for Bleeding Swine. J.A.V.M.A., *101*, 495, 1942.

CLARKE, N. P., HUHEEY, M. J., and MARTIN, W. M.:   Pentobarbital Anesthesia in Bears. J.A.V.M.A., *143*, 47, 1963.

CLIFFORD, D. H.:   Observations on Effect of Preanesthetic Medication with Meperidine and Promazine on Barbiturate Anesthesia in an Ocelot and a Leopard. J.A.V.M.A., *133*, 459, 1958.

CLIFFORD, D. H., GOOD, A. L., and STOWE, C. M., JR.:   Observations on the Use of Ataractic and Narcotic Preanesthesia and Pentobarbital Anesthesia in Bears. J.A.V.M.A., *140*, 464, 1962.

CLIFFORD, D. H., STOWE, C. M., JR., and GOOD, A. L.:   Pentobarbital Anesthesia in Lions with Special Reference to Preanesthetic Medication. J.A.V.M.A., *139*, 111, 1961.

CROFT, P. G.:   *An Introduction to the Anaesthesia of Laboratory Animals.*   The Universities Federation for Animal Welfare, London, 1960.

CUERRIERE, J. P.:   Transfer of Anesthetized Adult Lake Trout by Means of Aircraft. Progressive Fish Culturist, *15*, 42, 1953.

DAVIS, R. W.:   Personal Communication. Colorado State University, Fort Collins, Colorado, 1963.

DODGE, A. B.:   Personal Communication. Fort Collins, Colorado, 1963.

DOLOWY, W. C. and HESSE, A. L.:   Chlorpromazine Premedication with Pentobarbital Anesthesia in the Rabbit. J.A.V.M.A., *134*, 183, 1959.

DOLOWY, W. C., MOMBELLONI, P., and HESSE, A. L.:   Chlorpromazine Premedication with Pentobarbital Anesthesia in a Mouse. Am. J. Vet. Res., *21*, 156, 1960.

ESCHMEYER, P. H.:   The Effect of Ether Anesthesia on Fin-Clipping Rate. Progressive Fish Culturist, *15*, 80, 1953.

FARRELL, R. K.:   Personal Communication. Washington State University, Pullman, Washington, 1963.

FERGUSON, B. R.:   Personal Communication. Denver, Colorado, 1961.

FIELD, E. J.:   Anaesthesia in Rabbits. J. Animal Tech. Assoc., *8*, 47, 1957.

FISH, F. F.:   The Anaesthesia of Fish by High Carbon Dioxide Concentrations. Trans. Amer. Fisheries Soc., *72*, 25, 1942.

FOWLER, M. E.:   Extracting Canine Teeth of a Bear. J.A.V.M.A., *137*, 60, 1960.

FRIEDBERG, K. M.:   Problems Encountered in Pet Bird Practice. Vet. Med., *56*, 157, 1961.

GANDAL, C. P.:   Satisfactory General Anesthesia in Birds. J.A.V.M.A., *128*, 332, 1956.

GILBERT, P. W. and WOOD, F. G., JR.:   Method of Anesthetizing Large Sharks and Rays Safely and Rapidly. Science, *126*, 212, 1957.

GOSSINGTON, R. E.:   An Aid to Fish Handling—Tricaine. Aquarium J., *28*, 318, 1957.

GRIFFITH, J. Q., JR. and FARRIS, E. J.:   *The Rat in Laboratory Investigation.* J. B. Lippincott Co., Philadelphia, 1942.

HARTHOORN, A. M. and LOCK, J. A.:   Advances in the Use of Muscle Relaxing Drugs for Immobilization and Handling of Larger Land Mammals. J. Small Anim. Pract., *2*, 163, 1961.

HATCH, R. D., FERRIS, D. H., LINK, R. P., and CALHOUN, J.:   Unsatisfactory Results with Nicotine Immobilization of a Deer and Brahma Crossbred Cattle-2 Case Reports. J.A.V.M.A., *135*, 92, 1959.

HAYES, F. A.:   Modifications for Cesarian Section in Chinchillas. Vet. Med., *50*, 367, 1955.

HAYES, F. A., JENKINS, J. H., FEURT, S. D., and CROCKFORD, J. A.:   Observations on the Use of Nicotine for Immobilizing Semiwild Goats. J.A.V.M.A., *130*, 479, 1957.

HAYES, F. A., JENKINS, J. H., FEURT, S. D., and CROCKFORD, J. A.:   The Propulsive Administration of Nicotine as a New Approach for Capturing and Restraining Cattle. J.A.V.M.A., *134*, 283, 1959.

HEUSCHELE, W.:   Castration of a Squirrel. Modern Vet. Practice, *41*, 59, 1960.

HEWITT, O. H.:   *The Use of Serpasil in the Rearing and Handling of Pheasants.* Conference on the Use of the Tranquilizing and Antihypertensive Agent Serpasil in Animal and Poultry Production. Rutgers, The State University, New Brunswick, New Jersey, May 7, 1959.

HIBBS, C. M.:   Use of Chlorpromazine in Swine. Vet. Med., *53*, 571, 1958.

HUBLOU, W. F.:   A Method of Using an Anesthetic in Marking Fins. Progressive Fish Culturist, *19*, 40, 1957.

HUMMON, O. J.:   A Device for the Restraint of Mink During Certain Experimental Procedures. J.A.V.M.A., *106*, 104, 1945.

HYDE, J. L.:   The Use of Solid Carbon Dioxide for Producing Short Periods of Anesthesia in Guina Pigs. Am. J. Vet Res., *23*, 684, 1962.

JENKINS, J. H., HAYES, F. A., FEURT, S. D., and CROCKFORD, J. A.:   A New Method for the Live Capture of Canines with Applications to Rabies Control. Am. J. Pub. Hlth., *51*, 902, 1961.

JHA, S. K., LUMB, W. V., and JOHNSTON, R. F.:   Some Effects of Triflupromazine Hydrochloride on Goats. Amer. J. Vet. Res., *22*, 915, 1961.

JHA, S. K., LUMB, W. V., and JOHNSTON, R. F.:   Establishment of Permanent Carotid Loops in Goats. Amer. J. Vet. Res., *22*, 948, 1961.

JONES, L. M.:   *Veterinary Pharmacology and Therapeutics.* 2nd ed., Iowa State College Press, Ames, 1957.

KAPLAN, H. M. and KAPLAN, M.:   Anesthesia of Frogs with Ethyl Alcohol. Proc. Anim. Care Panel, *11*, 31, 1961.

LEONARD, R. H.:   Parakeet and Canary Practice. J.A.V.M.A., *136*, 378, 1960.

MARTIN, N. V. and SCOTT, D. C.:   Use of Tricaine methanesulfonate (M.S. 222) in the Transport of Live Fish without Water. Progressive Fish Culturist, *21*, 183, 1959.

MARTYN, N.:   Pentobarbital Sodium as an Anesthetic for Bears. J.A.V.M.A., *127*, 415, 1955.

MILLER, R. M.:   Personal communication. Thousand Oaks, California, 1959.

MOSBY, H. S. and CANTNER, D. E.:   The Use of Avertin in Capturing Wild Turkeys and as an Oral-Basal Anesthetic for Other Wild Animals. Southwest. Vet., *9*, 132, 1955.

NEWSOME, J. and ROBINSON, D. L. H.:   Sedatives and Anaesthetics for Baboons. Brit. Vet. J., *113*, 163, 1957.

PHILLIPSON, A. T. and BARNETT, S. F.:   Anaesthesia in Sheep. Vet. Rec., *51*, 869, 1939.

RIDDELL, W. K.:   Caudal Anesthesia in Canine Surgery. J. Small Animal Medicine, *1*, 159, 1952.

SANGER, V. L. and SMITH, H. R.:   General Anesthesia in Birds. J.A.V.M.A., *131*, 52, 1957.

SAVAGE, J.:   Copepod Infection of Speckled Trout. Trans. Amer. Fisheries Soc., *65*, 339, 1935.

STONE, R. M.:   Pet Bird Practice. Paper presented at the Michigan State University Veterinary Conference, January, 1959.

TAYLOR, M. E.:   Personal communication. Show Low, Arizona, 1961.

THOMAS, W. D.:   Chemical Immobilization of Wild Animals, J.A.V.M.A., *138*, 263, 1961.

TROYER, W.:   "Out for Bear", Jen-Sal J., *43*, 32, 1960.

TYAGI, R. P. S. and LUMB, W. V.:   Uterine Healing after Cesarotomy in Goats. Amer. J. Vet. Res., *22*, 1097, 1961.

VAN STEE, E. W.:   Personal communication. Michigan State University, East Lansing, Michigan, 1960.

VIERHELLER, R. C.:   What is Your Diagnosis? J.A.V.M.A., *134*, 9, 1959.

WALLACE, G. D., FODOR, A. R., and BARTON, L. H.:   Restraint of Chimpanzees with Perphenazine. J.A.V.M.A., *136*, 222, 1960.

WEISNER, B. P.:   The Post-Natal Development of the Genital Organs of the Albino Rat. J. Obstet. & Gynec., British Empire, *41*, 867, 1934.

WESOLOWSKI, S. A.:   *Evaluation of Tissue and Prosthetic Vascular Grafts.* Charles C Thomas, Springfield, Illinois, 1962.

WILGUS, H. S.:   *Reserpine for Tranquilizing Geese.* The Second Conference on the Use of Reserpine in Poultry Production. The Institute of Agriculture, University of Minnesota, St. Paul, Minn., May 6, 1960.

WOLFF, W. A. and BOYD, R. J.:   Personal Communication. Colorado State University, Fort Collins, Colorado, 1963.

WRIGHT, J. F.:   Immobilization of Wild Animals. Vet. Med., *57*, 331, 1962.

WRIGHT, J. G. and HALL, L. W.:   *Veterinary Anaesthesia and Analagesia.* 5th ed., Williams and Wilkins Co., Baltimore, 1961.

WRIGHT, J. G.: *Veterinary Anaesthesia.* 4th ed. The Williams & Wilkins Co., Baltimore, 1957.

YOUNG, W. A.: Wing Amputation of Birds in Lieu of Pinioning. J.A.V.M.A., *112*, 224, 1948.

—————: Dr. Bob Knowles Operates on Giant Fish and Makes News Headlines and T. V. Modern Vet. Practice, *39*, 17 (June 1), 1958.

MONITORING ANESTHESIA

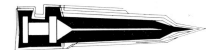

Chapter 15

In the past, response of the patient to an anesthetic has been assessed in large part by the senses of the anesthetist. As a result, anesthesia has been more an art than a science.

The veterinarian in practice often serves as both anesthetist and surgeon, and while operating may be the only person available to observe the anesthetized patient. Under these circumstances he develops a "6th sense" concerning the patient's status. By observing respiratory movements, the color of the tissues, pulsation of blood vessels, and the color of blood in the operative field, he continuously assesses cardiac and respiratory function.

In recent years, many types of monitoring equipment have become available to furnish objective data concerning the state of the patient. Some of these devices have practical use in small animal practice, while others, because of cost or the limited value of the information obtained, are restricted to the research laboratory.

Cullen (1961) has wisely pointed out that monitors are *not* a substitute for clinical observation and good judgement on the part of the anesthetist and surgeon.

> ". . . information provided by the instruments should be considered to be a portion, and most likely a small portion, of the data necessary for critical evaluation of the patient's condition. Unwarranted reliance on gadgetry can result only in restricted information, misleading information (at times), and deterioration of clinical acuity."

Body functions which can be monitored and which will give information to the anesthetist include:

1. Respiration.
2. Oxygen and carbon dioxide levels in the circulating blood.
3. Pulse and heart rate.
4. Blood pressure.
5. Temperature.
6. The electric potentials of the heart.
7. The electric potentials of the brain.

Simple Respiratory Monitors

Two simple respiratory monitors have been described in Chapter 9. The first is a piece of paper over the intake valve of an insufflation device (Fig. 9–6, p. 144). As the patient breathes, the paper flutters and gives a visual signal that respiration is occurring. The second is an accessory for the Ethaire apparatus (Fig. 9–9, p. 147) which whistles with each exhalation through the valve.

Tidal Volume

The ventimeter is a tidal volume indicating device for use in breathing circuits (Fig. 15–1). The volume, pressure, and pattern of each inspiration and expiration are directly visible in the movement of a volumetrically-calibrated bellows and an aneroid manometer. The breathing bag is not replaced by the bellows, the patient's respirations moving both reservoirs simultaneously. Little expiratory impedance is added by the ventimeter.

The patient's tidal volumes are monitored continuously during spontaneous respiration, or positive pressure breathing produced by compression of the rebreathing bag or a mechanical ventilator. Inadequate or excessive ventilation can be quickly recognized during inhalation anesthesia with closed, semi-closed, or non-rebreathing systems. The ventimeter incorporates a phased "pop-off" valve which, in all of these techniques, remains closed during inspiration; conventional "pop-off" valves are kept closed. Overflow of gas from the system occurs at low back pressure and is limited to a short interval immediately after expiration. Even when flows of 50 to 75 liters per minute are suddenly introduced (by an oxygen flush valve) into the circuit, total pressure never exceeds 3 cm. of water during expiration. Leaks in the system are indicated by a falling end-expiratory rest position of the ventimeter bellows. In addition, the need for adjustment of gas flow is obvious if the bellows either falls or remains fully extended.

Tidal volume can be read directly from the instrument. The ventimeter does not interfere with customary use of the rebreathing bag. By compressing the bag according to observed tidal volumes, it is possible to maintain the patient's ventilation within any desired limits, for example, within ± 5% of the measured tidal volume during a control or induction period.

To manually assist ventilation, the ventimeter is watched and the bag compressed synchronously with the inspiratory excursion of the bellows. With a closed system, the start of an active inspiration

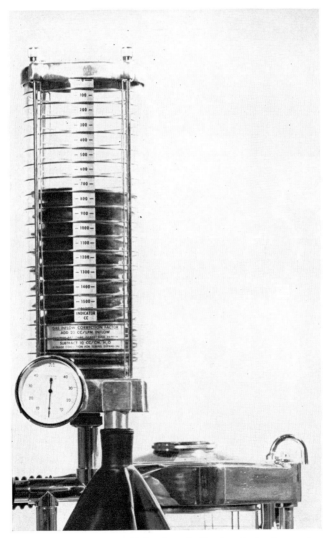

FIGURE 15–1.   The ventimeter, a tidal volume indicating device for use in anesthetic breathing circuits. (Courtesy of Ohio Chemical and Surgical Equipment Co.)

can be detected with the first 10 cc. inspired. Cardiac pulsations, which are sometimes transmitted to the bellows, are of lesser magnitude.

The ventimeter is made for routine use without removal from the gas machine. The anesthesiologist can thus detect hypoventilation, which is less obvious with the rebreathing bag alone. Hypoventilation is corrected in the conventional manner by squeezing the rebreathing bag and the ventimeter serves as continual objective evidence of performance.

Measurement of Respiratory and Anesthetic Gases

Gas analyzers have been devised to measure continuously such gases as carbon dioxide, halothane, cyclopropane, diethyl ether, and nitrous oxide during anesthesia. These operate on the principle of infrared absorption and measure any one gas in the anesthetic mixture.

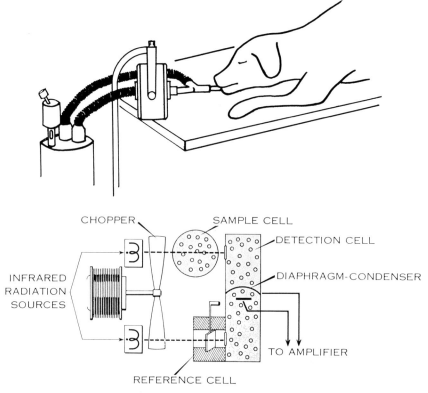

FIGURE 15–2. Breathe-through sampling cell, for measuring concentrations of respiratory and anesthetic gases, connected in a circle system. A schematic diagram of the apparatus is shown below. (Courtesy of Spinco Division, Beckman Instruments, Inc., Palo Alto, California.)

The detection unit contains two identical infrared sources which emit parallel beams of radiation, pulsed by a chopper (Fig. 15–2). One beam passes through the sample cell, the other through a reference cell. Both beams then pass into a detection cell, consisting of two rigid chambers divided by a diaphragm. Both chambers of the detection cell are charged to equal pressure with the gas being measured.

When the gas being measured enters the sample cell, it absorbs infrared radiation at the same wave lengths as gas in the detection cell. This reduces the amount of radiation reaching one side of the detection cell and produces a lower pressure in that side. The diaphragm moves toward the side of lower pressure, and this is translated into electrical impulses which actuate the indicating meter and recorder.

A breathe-through sampling cell is used in anesthetic circuits, the patient's exhaled breath passing through the cell.

Blood Oxygen

The efficiency of oxygen uptake in the lungs can be judged by determining the blood oxygen content. An oximeter composed of an

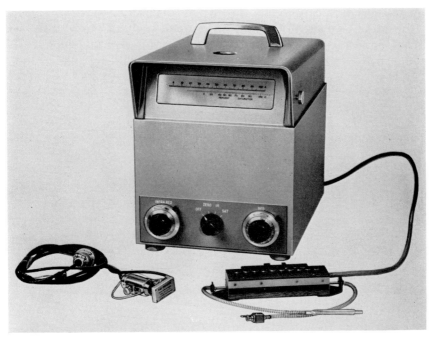

FIGURE 15–3. An oximeter for continuous determination of blood oxygen saturation. Readings may be taken either with the earpiece (lower left) or the cuvette (lower right). The latter enables immediate determination of saturation of whole blood samples, either flowing or stationary. (Courtesy of The Waters Corporation, Rochester, Minnesota.)

ear piece, amplifier with power supply, and recording device will measure the oxygen saturation of blood circulating through the ear (Fig. 15–3). This instrument operates on the principle that oxygenated hemoglobin transmits 70% of incident red light with a wave length of 6400 angstrom units, while transmission by reduced hemoglobin is negligible. In operation, the ear piece measures transmission of red light through a relatively translucent appendage such as the ear.

Pulse

The rate and force of the pulse have long been used as an indication of the state of the cardiovascular system. A fast weak pulse is present in shock and is a sign of impending vascular collapse.

The pulse in most small animals can be felt in the femoral artery midway between the hip and stifle on the inner surface of the thigh. Electronic pulse detection is discussed below in the section on blood pressure.

Heart Rate

The heart rate can be obtained by means of a stethoscope taped to the patient's chest in the area of the apex beat. A recent innovation is the esophageal stethoscope which is inserted in the esophageal lumen to the cardiac region (Fig. 15–4). It should be pointed out that heart and pulse rates are not always the same, since a pulse deficit may exist.

Electronic equipment to monitor the heart is discussed later in this chapter.

Blood Pressure

One of the most useful determinations made during anesthesia in man is of blood pressure. Unfortunately the method of indirect measurement used is not readily applicable to animals. Direct pressure readings can be made by cannulation of the femoral artery, but this is impractical except in the laboratory. For these reasons determination of blood pressure in anesthetized animals has been largely ignored. Treatment of shock has been done empirically based on symptoms observed in the patient. These include color of the mucous membranes and other tissues, rate and consistency of the pulse, respiratory rate and depth, and degree of reflex activity.

Recently two methods for indirect blood pressure measurement which have application in animals have been described. Both of these utilize a pressure cuff and an electronic pulse detection and

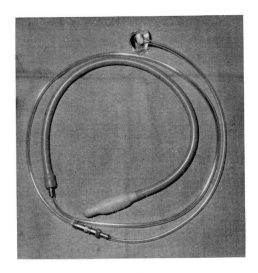

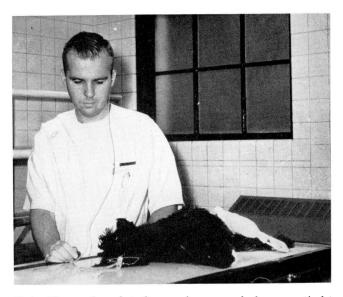

FIGURE 15-4. The esophageal stethoscope is composed of an acoustical transducer connected to an earpiece (top). In use the transducer is inserted in the esophagus to heart level (bottom). (Courtesy of Dr. N. R. Cholvin, Michigan State University, East Lansing, Michigan.)

indication system. One operates on the principle that the volume of blood in a vessel network fluctuates with each cardiac cycle. This can be detected by observing changes in the transmittance of a beam of light passing through the network (Robinson and Eastwood, 1959). With a sensitive crystal photocell, low intensity light source, and an amplifier, fluctuations can be detected in any tissue through which light can be transmitted (Fig. 15–5). In

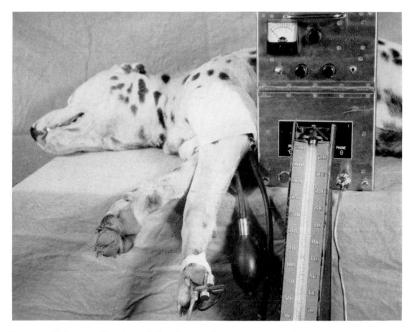

FIGURE 15–5. Application of the photo-sphygmometer to the measurement of blood pressure, showing blood pressure cuff and photocell in place. Controls on the monitor from left to right are power on-off, tone level, signal indicating meter, light intensity, and sensitivity. (From Robinson, R. E. and Eastwood, D. W.: Use of a Photo-Sphygmometer in Indirect Blood Pressure Measurements. Anesthesiology, *20*, 704, 1959.)

operation a photocell lamp assembly is clipped on a toe or other appendage and the light intensity and amplifier gain adjusted until fluctuations are recorded. A blood pressure cuff is then placed around the limb and inflated until fluctuations disappear. Pressure is slowly lowered until fluctuations reappear, at which point cuff pressure approximates systolic blood pressure. By proper connections the system can be attached to a recorder, oscilloscope, or speaker if so desired.

The second method operates on the same principle except it picks up the Korotkow sounds and pulse waves by means of a displace-

ment condenser microphone placed over an artery and held without
pressure by tape (Weinreb *et al.*, 1960) (Fig. 15–6).

Undoubtedly as these methods are refined their use will spread
from the physiology laboratory to clinical practice.

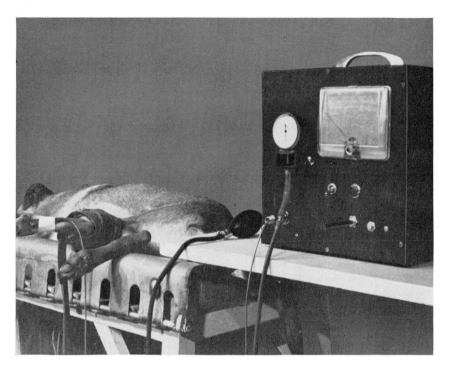

FIGURE 15–6.   Apparatus for indirect blood pressure measurement. A pressure cuff
is placed around the hock with a displacement condenser microphone taped below it on
the foot. As pressure drops in the cuff the needle on the gauge (right) fluctuates when
systolic pressure is reached. Pressure is then read on the manometer dial. (Courtesy of
Drs. W. C. Waggoner and C. F. Cairy, Michigan State University, East Lansing, Mich.)

Cardiac Monitors

Since the importance of early recognition of cardiac arrest has
become apparent, apparatus for monitoring the heart have been
developed. These vary in size, cost, method of recording cardiac
function, and effectiveness. The smallest is the Veling monitor, a
model of which is marketed for veterinary use (Fig. 15–7). All
monitors act on the same principle used in electrocardiography.
Electrical waves, which are produced in the heart muscle and which
form the ECG complex, are picked up by leads attached to the body,
amplified, and fed to the output stage of the monitor. The Veling
monitor produces a sequence of "beeps" corresponding to the peaks

of the ECG complex. At its greatest amplitude three sounds may be heard corresponding with the peaks of the P, R, and T waves; hence, the sounds are a translation of the electrical activity of the heart. Irregularities of cardiac rhythm and changes in the frequency and amplitude of the ECG complex are said to be detected by changes in rate, tone, and number of sounds produced by the monitor. Booth (1962) has indicated that this instrument is not reliable for evaluating the functional competence of the heart in severe hypotension and barbiturate depression.

More expensive cardiac monitors have various refinements (Fig. 15–8). Some not only include audible indications of the electrocardiographic complex, but also produce a loud alarm at any predetermined interval after asystole. In some a coupled oscilloscope enables continuous observation of the electrocardiogram, the monitor converting the electrical activity of the heart into a light flash on the oscilloscope screen and also producing an audible sound.

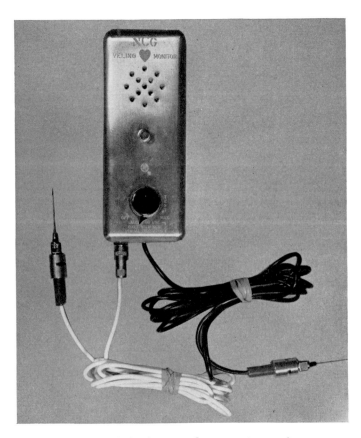

FIGURE 15–7. *(Continued on opposite page)*

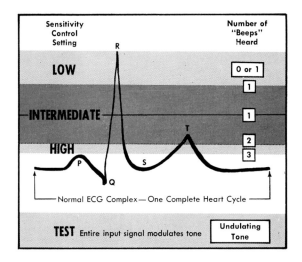

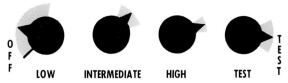

FIGURE 15–7. The Veling heart monitor. Wires connect the instrument to needle electrodes inserted in the patient. The principle of operation is illustrated. One, two or three sounds will be heard with each QRS complex depending upon the sensitivity setting. (Courtesy of National Cylinder Gas Division of Chemetron Corporation, Chicago, Ill.)

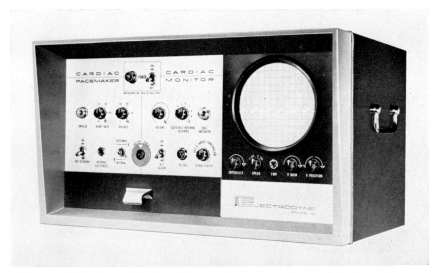

FIGURE 15–8. A combined cardiac monitor, pacemaker, and electrocardioscope. When connected to the patient by a 3-wire cable it provides a continuous visual display of the electrocardiogram. The QRS complex is also converted to a neon flash and a sharp audible note. An alarm sounds when cardiac arrest occurs. The pacemaker will automatically stimulate the arrested heart at a preset rate by means of externally located electrodes. (Courtesy of Electrodyne Company, Inc., Norwood, Mass.)

This sound may be adjusted in volume or eliminated completely
if desired. With some monitors, electrodes, which are placed on the
patient's chest, can be coupled so that at the onset of cardiac arrest
an artificial rhythmic systole is produced by electrical stimulation
(Nicholson *et al.*, 1959).

The value of cardiac monitors in small animal anesthesiology
remains to be seen. When an animal dies of respiratory arrest, the
heart may continue to send out electrical waves audible on the
monitor for many minutes, though no effective pulse is produced
and successful resuscitation is no longer possible. A blood pressure
recorder would indicate impending cardiovascular collapse long
before changes were detected in the ECG.

Because respiratory failure usually occurs before cardiac arrest,
a respiratory monitor is also a more valuable instrument.

Temperature

Determination of body temperature may be of interest in many
types of anesthesia and is absolutely essential in hypothermia.

For routine use a conventional rectal thermometer is quite

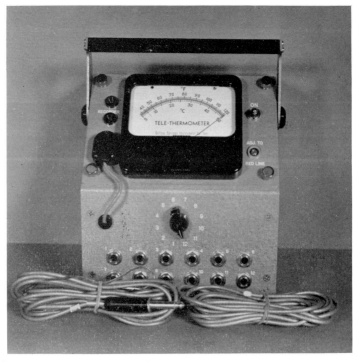

FIGURE 15–9. A multichannel thermistor thermometer. Two types of waterproof
probes are shown in the foreground.

adequate. It should be realized, however, that it has certain short-comings. The temperature of the liver and other deep organs is always 1° or 2° C. higher than the rectum. In addition, feces in the rectum will insulate the thermometer from rapid temperature changes. For these reasons when a hypothermia technique is being employed the thermometer is inserted in the thoracic esophagus.

Several types of thermistor thermometer are sold commercially (Fig. 15–9). These operate on the principle that electrical resistance of the thermistor changes with variation in temperature and this change is measured and recorded on a dial. Waterproof probes containing thermistors are available with cables of sufficient length that they can be inserted in the patient and monitored at some distance (Fig. 11–2, p. 207). Multichannel units are used when the temperature in more than one location is desired.

Electroencephalography

Caton (1875) first noted the occurrence of electrical potentials in the brains of animals. Other workers noted that anesthesia produced changes in these potentials but it was not until 1937 that Gibbs *et al.* published their work suggesting, "A practical application of these observations might be the use of the electroencephalogram as a measure of the depth of anesthesia during surgical operations. The anesthetist and surgeon could have before them on tape or screen a continuous record of the electrical activity of both heart and brain." Since then a number of investigators have reported the changes associated with various types of anesthesia.

The mechanism underlying normal cortical electrical activity is little understood but recent evidence suggests that the rhythms represent fluctuating potentials produced by dendrites. Sequential changes in the electroencephalographic pattern associated with anesthetic agents probably arise from chemical action primarily in this region of the neuron.

The useful effect of this phenomenon is that anesthetic agents tend to limit individual variation in wave patterns seen in the normal electroencephalogram, and a relatively characteristic series of changes is produced by any given agent. This "ironing out" of individual variation enables the practical use of electroencephalography for monitoring depth of anesthesia (Fig. 15–10).

With moderate to deep anesthesia there is a greater simplifying tendency which is apparent with the disappearance of local differences in cortical electrical activity. During the stage of "burst suppression" the entire brain may appear to discharge as a unit. This tends to indicate existence of a synchronizing system coordinating electrical activity in both cortical and subcortical regions. Such a network has been demonstrated by Swank (1949) and has been shown to be sensitive to blocking by anesthetic agents (French *et al.*, 1953).

The electroencephalographic pattern during light anesthesia is different from that seen during sleep. Therefore, it appears that anesthetic agents do not act by means of the same systems responsible for the sleep state.

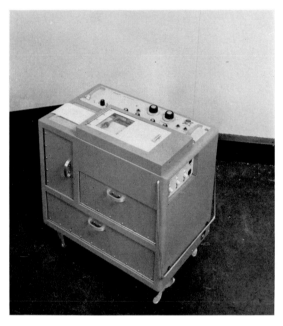

FIGURE 15–10.   A recording unit for continuous surveillance of the patient's electrocardiogram and electroencephalogram. (Courtesy of Epsco Medical, Cambridge, Mass.)

A basic pattern can be constructed which allows classification (Fig. 15–11). As induction of anesthesia is started, there is an increase in frequency to 20 to 30 cycles per second. The small rapid wave pattern is replaced, as consciousness is lost, by a large slow wave which increases in amplitude as it slows (50 to 300 microvolts, 1 to 5 cycles/second). As anesthesia deepens, the wave may become regular in form and repetition time, with secondary faster waves superimposed on it. Finally the amplitude begins to decrease with periods of relative cortical inactivity (burst suppression). These may continue until depression results in the entire loss of cortical activity with a flat tracing.

Courtin *et al.* (1950) first demonstrated the usefulness of electroencephalographic changes in clinical anesthesiology. They classified

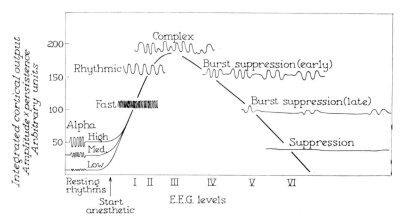

FIGURE 15–11.   Diagram of average changes in the electroencephalographic pattern during anesthesia. (From Martin, J. T., Faulconer, A., Jr., and Bickford, R. G.: Electroencephalography in Anesthesia. Anesthesiology, *20*, 359, 1959.)

ELECTROENCEPHALOGRAPHIC LEVELS OF ANESTHESIA

(Nitrous oxide – Oxygen – Ether)

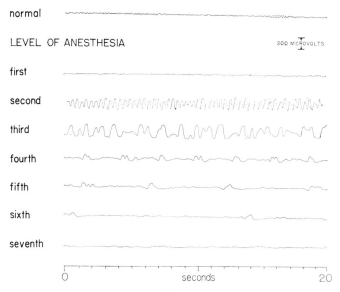

FIGURE 15–12.   Electroencephalographic patterns characteristic of successive electroencephalographic levels of anesthesia.   (From Courtin, R. F., Bickford, R. G., and Faulconer, A., Jr.:   Classification and Significance of Electroencephalographic Patterns Produced by Nitrous Oxide-Ether Anesthesia During Surgical Operations.   Proc. Staff Meet., Mayo Clin., *25*, 197, 1950.)

ether anesthesia into seven electroencephalographic levels which appeared to be relatively constant from one patient to another (Fig. 15–12). These levels taken with bipolar and fronto-occipital leads were as follows:

Level 1 (flat). The alpha waves disappear as consciousness is lost. Low amplitude (30 microvolts), fast discharges (20 to 30 cycles/second) may occasionally be seen. This stage with ether anesthesia lasts about the first 7 minutes of induction.

Level 2 (rhythmic). Slow waves (average 2 to 8 cycles/second) of high amplitude (200 to 300 microvolts) characterize this stage. There is definite rhythm with lack of interference. This level is of approximately 60 seconds' duration.

Level 3 (complex). The rhythmicity is abruptly lost and a series of slow waves are observed with faster waves superimposed. The wave amplitude is less than in Level 2. There is no suppression.

Level 4 (slight suppression). With deeper levels of anesthesia burst suppression occurs. At this level suppression does not last longer than 3 seconds with waves 2 to 4 cycles/second and an average amplitude of 150 microvolts. During the period of suppression activity is less than 20 microvolts in amplitude.

Level 5 (moderate suppression). Periods of suppression lasting 3 to 10 seconds are observed with intervening single waves of smaller amplitude than those of Level 4.

Level 6 (severe suppression). Activity does not occur more frequently than once every 10 seconds and regularity is absent. Amplitude is about 70 microvolts.

Level 7 (complete suppression). There are no measurable waves and activity does not exceed 20 microvolts.

During recovery the patterns closely mirror the tracings obtained during induction. As light anesthesia is reached the sleep rhythm may appear or low amplitude waves of 8 to 13 cycles/second may return prior to recovery.

Level 3 is required for incision of the skin without reflex movement. In Level 3 abdominal relaxation is poor, in 4 it is moderate, and in 5 it is excellent.

In man it has been shown that the mean concentration of ether in arterial blood at various encephalographic levels is almost in linear correlation with the levels outlined above. Thus the electroencephalogram can be used for quantitative assessment of this effect.

Considerable work has been done in both dogs and cats to determine the effects of preanesthetic and anesthetic agents, muscle relaxants, anoxia, carbon dioxide, and hypothermia on the electroencephalographic pattern. For a more complete review of this work the reader should consult Martin *et al.* (1959).

Servoanesthesia

Advantage has been taken of the fact that the electrical potential of the cortex decreases as anesthesia deepens, to produce a device which will automatically maintain anesthesia at any desired level. This apparatus stores energy to a set point at which it is then released, activating a mechanism which will deliver a calibrated dose of anesthetic to the patient. Energy storage then begins again until a sufficient amount accumulates to reactivate the dosimeter. In light stages of anesthesia, the cortex produces considerable electric energy and doses are administered frequently. As anesthesia deepens, the energy output slackens and administration becomes less frequent. It is thus possible to maintain any given level of electrical depression. This method of anesthesia has been termed *servoanesthesia*. At present the chief use for this apparatus is in the laboratory. Considerable refinement of the apparatus needs to be made before it can be placed in general use, since certain technical difficulties are attendant with it. A great amount of amplification is needed to make brain potentials large enough to be recorded. This in turn leads to development of artifacts. Interference in the operating room from other pieces of equipment commonly occurs. Also some variation will be encountered, depending upon placement of the electrodes.

Present Status and Uses for Electroencephalography

Electroencephalography has been shown to be useful in determining the degree of cortical electrical activity associated with various anesthetic drugs, hypoxia, hypothermia, and accumulation of carbon dioxide. However, Cullen (1961) has pointed out that the anesthetist cannot expect to manage anesthesia by substituting the electroencephalograph for clinical observation of traditional signs, unless he elects to be consistently behind in detecting serious change. Martin *et al.* (1959) believe that electroencephalography is still no more than a tool in the hands of the anesthesiologist. They list the following areas where it may make an important contribution to anesthesiology:

1. Maintenance of a steady state in laboratory investigations in which variations in depth of anesthesia are undesirable.
2. Early detection of inadequate cerebral perfusion, during whole-body perfusion with extracorporeal circulation.
3. Instruction in anesthesiology and clinical evaluation of new anesthetic agents.
4. Assessment of damage and recovery after severe hypoxic accidents during anesthesia or cardiac arrest.

5. Detection of critical changes in amplitude of cortical potentials during hypothermia.
6. Maintenance of a steady state of anesthesia in the operating room when all other signs of anesthesia are unavailable.

References

BOOTH, N. H.: Evaluation of a Cardiac Monitor. J.A.V.M.A., *140*, 664, 1962.

CATON, R.: Electric Currents of the Brain. Brit. Med., J. *2*, 278, 1875.

COURTIN, R. F., BICKFORD, R. G., and FAULCONER, A., JR.: Classification and Significance of Electroencephalographic Patterns Produced by Nitrous Oxide-Ether Anesthesia During Surgical Operations. Proc. Staff Meet., Mayo Clin., *25*, 197, 1950.

CULLEN, S. C.: Monitors and Clinical Judgment. Am. J. Surg., *102*, 300, 1961.

FRENCH, J. D., VERZEANO, M., and MAGOUN, H. W.: Neural Basis of Anesthetic State. A.M.A. Arch. Neurol. & Psychiat., *69*, 519, 1953.

GIBBS, F. A., GIBBS, E. L., and LENNOX, W. G.: Effect on Electroencephalogram of Certain Drugs which Influence Nervous Activity. Arch. Int. Med., *60*, 154, 1937.

MARTIN, J. T., FAULCONER, A., JR., and BICKFORD, R. G.: Electroencephalography in Anesthesiology. Anesthesiology, *20*, 359, 1959.

NICHOLSON, M. J., EVERSOLE, U. H., ORR, R. D., and CREHAN, J. T.: A Cardiac Monitor-Pacemaker: Use During and After Anesthesia. Anesthesiology, *38*, 335, 1959.

ROBINSON, R. E. and EASTWOOD, D. W.: Use of a Photo-Sphygmometer in Indirect Blood Pressure Measurements. Anesthesiology, *20*, 704, 1959.

SWANK, R. L.: Syncronization of Spontaneous Electrical Activity of Cerebrum by Barbiturate Narcosis. J. Neurophysiol., *12*, 161, 1949.

WEINREB, H. L., NAFTCHI, N., and MENDLOWITZ, M.: The Measurement of Digital Arterial Blood Pressure. A.M.A. Arch. Surg., *80*, 131, 1960.

DRUGS AND EQUIPMENT FOR ANESTHETIC EMERGENCIES

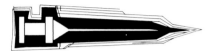

Chapter 16

Blood and Blood Substitutes
  Whole Blood
  Plasma
  Dextran (Expandex)
  Gelatin
Vasopressors
  Epinephrine Hydrochloride (Adrenalin)
  Levarterenol Bitartrate (Levophed)
  Methoxamine Hydrochloride (Vasoxyl)
  Phenylephrine Hydrochloride (Neo-synephrine)
  Mephentermine (Wyamine)
  Amphetamine Sulphate (Benzadrine Sulphate)
  Methamphetamine Hydrochloride (Desoxyephedrine)

Metaraminol Bitartrate (Aramine)
ACTH and the Adrenocortical Steroids
  Adrenocorticotrophic Hormone (ACTH)
  Adrenocortical Steroids
Cardiac Defibrillator and Arrest Kit
  Calcium Chloride
  Potassium Chloride
Analeptics
  Pentylenetetrazol (Metrazol)
  Methetharimide (Mikedimide, Megimide)
The Narcotic Antagonists
  Nalorphine Hydrochloride (Nalline)
  Levallorphan Tartrate (Lorfan)
Respirators

THE wide variety of drugs and equipment used in anesthetic emergencies warrants more detailed description than can be given in a chapter on management of emergencies. For this reason they are discussed first.

Blood and Blood Substitutes

Whole Blood

Use of whole blood in the prevention and treatment of shock has become commonplace in small animal practice. A canine donor is kept in many hospitals and blood withdrawn as needed. From the standpoint of availability in emergency situations, banking of whole blood is probably more desirable. In addition, plasma from blood which becomes outdated can be collected for storage and future use.

For optimum results, blood should be collected aseptically in sterile bottles containing a solution of citric acid, sodium citrate, and dextrose (ACD solution), which slows hemolysis and delays diffusion of potassium from red cells into the plasma. Stored blood should be maintained at a temperature of 38 to 42° F. If during storage the blood temperature rises to above 60° F., there is rapid destruction of blood cells even though the blood is subsequently cooled.

The length of time transfused red cells survive in the recipient is roughly in proportion to the duration of storage. Under optimum conditions more than 90% of the red cells will survive in the recipient when blood is stored for 1 to 10 days; from 10 to 21 days approximately 70% of the red cells will survive. Even when stored for 21 days, under optimum conditions 70 to 80% of transfused red blood cells survive in the recipient at least 5 days.

When time permits and when valuable animals are transfused, cross matching of donor and recipient is desirable. However, from a practical standpoint, this is seldom done since incompatabilities in small animals are rarely encountered.

Young *et al.* (1952) have demonstrated five different iso-antibodies in the serums of transfused dogs. These are designated anti-A, B, C, D, and E; anti-A is the only one causing severe hemolysis. Single random blood transfusions in dogs have been shown to be capable of stimulating production of anti-A iso-antibodies in approximately 23% of the recipients.

Hemolytic anemia in newborn puppies can be caused by previous transfusion of the dam with incompatible blood. This situation occurs when a type A-negative female is transfused with A-positive blood and develops anti-A iso-antibodies in her serum. If she subsequently whelps A-positive pups and nurses them, the antibodies are passed to the pups through the milk. Affected pups usually die within 2 or 3 days after whelping. If the puppies are prevented from nursing for the first 24 hours of life this difficulty can be avoided, since the antibodies cannot be absorbed through the intestinal mucosa after this period has elapsed.

Clark and Woodley (1959) found that average healthy dogs have a blood volume equal to 8.1% of their body weight. When they injected red blood cells by various routes into dogs they found that 81.7% of the red blood cells given intraperitoneally were absorbed intact, 48% being absorbed in the first 24 hours. Less than 3% of the red blood cells injected intramuscularly and subcutaneously were absorbed intact and over 97% were destroyed at the injection site. When intramedullary transfusions were given in the femur, red cells passed very rapidly into the circulation, 95.3% being absorbed intact.

Under most circumstances blood is administered intravenously, the rate of injection depending upon the degree of need and size of the animal. In the past, too rapid administration was thought to cause right heart embarrassment. However, Firt and Hejhal (1957) demonstrated rather conclusively in dogs that sodium citrate, rather than the rate of administration, is the cause of overloading and failure of the heart. Cardiac failure is produced by vasoconstriction of the pulmonary vascular bed and, in larger doses, depression of the myocardium. In shock, cardiac disease, severe anemia or liver damage, small intravenous doses of citrate, even the amount contained in a slow transfusion of a small quantity of blood, may be very dangerous. Heparinized blood, on the other hand, can be safely transfused at fast rates either intravenously or intra-arterially (over a pint a minute when given simultaneously in both jugular veins). The advantage of intra-arterial transfusion of citrated blood is thought to lie in the fact that citrate filters into the interstitial

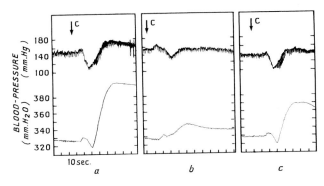

FIGURE 16–1.   The effect of calcium and procaine on pulmonary vasoconstriction and myocardial depression produced by injection of 1.5 ml./kg. of 3.8% citrate in a dog: (a) the effect of citrate alone; (b) the effect of citrate with 10% calcium gluconate 0.8 ml./kg. and 1% procaine 0.5 ml./kg.; (c) the effect of citrate with calcium alone (in the above dosage). Citrate and calcium injected at C. (From Firt, P. and Hejhal, L.: Treatment of Severe Haemorrhage. Lancet, *273*, 1132, 1957.)

fluid and a lower concentration reaches the myocardium and pulmonary vascular circuit.

The toxic effect of citrate during transfusion can be counteracted by simultaneous intravenous administration of calcium and procaine. Calcium cannot be given mixed with the transfusion blood, but should be given intravenously in a different vein than the one used for transfusion because of the danger of clotting.

Ten per cent calcium gluconate (0.7 ml./kg.) alone will reduce the effect of citrate 50 to 60%. For best results in dogs 10% calcium gluconate (0.6 ml./kg.) and 1% procaine hydrochloride (0.5 ml./kg.) are given intravenously, starting before and continuing during transfusion (Fig. 16–1).

The amount of whole blood needed will vary widely depending on the circumstances. The average intravenous dose is from 5 to 10 ml. per pound of body weight. In acute continuing hemorrhage, however, blood must be given until the hemorrhage stops. Occasionally, because of severe vascular collapse it is impossible to cannulate a vein for transfusion. In this situation a direct cut-down on a large vessel should be performed immediately. Hesitation may mean loss of a patient which otherwise could be saved.

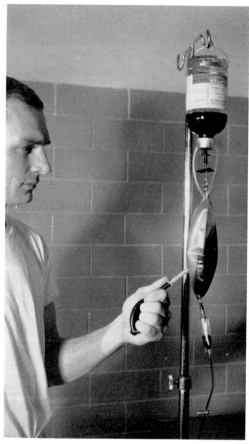

FIGURE 16-2.   Disposable equipment for administration of blood under pressure or by gravity flow. The plastic bag has two compartments, blood from the bottle flowing into one. When the second is inflated, by pumping the bulb syringe, pressure is exerted on the blood which is then forced into the patient. Because the two compartments do not communicate, danger of air embolism is eliminated.

In severe exsanguinating hemorrhage, intra-arterial administration of blood has been advocated. By so doing, it is possible to administer a large quantity of blood rapidly, thus maintaining the arterial pressure without the possibility of overburdening the heart. A simple pressurized transfusion set* has been developed which will

* See Appendix A, p. 404 for manufacturer.

allow administration of blood under pressure without fear of air embolism (Fig. 16–2).

Plasma

Plasma has all the properties of whole blood except its oxygen-carrying capacity. In shock not accompanied by loss of blood it is preferred to whole blood, since administration of the latter will produce a polycythemia with a disproportionate number of red blood cells in relation to the liquid portion of the circulating blood. On a volume for volume basis plasma contains almost twice as much protein as is found in whole blood, since 40 to 50% of whole blood is red blood corpuscles. Plasma contains 6 to 7% protein, 60% of which is albumin. However, because of its small molecular weight albumin exerts 80% of the colloidal osmotic pressure of the blood. One gram of albumin will retain 18 ml. of water within the circulation. In addition to their osmotic pressure effects the proteins of plasma can be metabolized by the body.

Plasma is usually obtained from banked whole blood which has become outdated. The supernatant plasma is siphoned into sterile containers and the cellular sediment discarded. Fifty per cent dextrose solution is added as a stabilizer to make a final concentration of 5% dextrose. Liquid plasma can be stored at room temperature for as long as 6 months without appreciable deterioration provided bacterial contamination has not occurred. If kept in a liquid state, however, it is more frequently stored under refrigeration at 38 to 40° F. Plasma stored in the liquid state should be filtered prior to use since flocculation rapidly occurs.

Frozen plasma may be kept indefinitely without flocculation or the danger of bacterial growth. When needed it should be quickly thawed at approximately 100° F. Filtration of frozen plasma generally is not necessary.

A working rule for plasma administration is to give 0.66 ml./lb. for each unit the hematocrit reading is over 45. The following is an example:

If the hematocrit is 60 in a 35 pound dog:

$$60-45 = 15$$
$$15 \times \tfrac{2}{3} \times 35 = 350 \text{ ml. of plasma}$$

Extra plasma is rapidly removed from the circulation and from a practical standpoint excessive amounts cannot be administered.

Dextran (Expandex)

Dextran is a water-soluble high molecular weight polysaccharide obtained by bacterial fermentation of sucrose. It is a polymer of glucose and has a molecular weight of approximately 75,000. Dextran exerts an "osmotic increment" effect on the circulating blood of about 100%. That is, it draws an equivalent amount of fluid from the tissues into the blood vessels to increase the circulating plasma volume. At 4 hours 80% of the dextran is still circulating in the blood; as much as 50% may be excreted in the urine within 24 hours. A small portion which is not excreted is oxidized over a period of weeks.

Dextran is antigenic and at any sign of reaction the infusion should be stopped. If a reaction is not experienced on the first njection, repeat infusions may usually be given without ill effect. Dextran is not stored in the body and has no harmful effect on renal, hepatic, or other body functions. Mild diuresis follows its injection. It has the advantage that it is not species specific as are blood and plasma.

The dose of dextran varies depending upon the need of the animal. A basic dose of 3 ml./lb. of body weight is suggested for both dogs and cats. There is little danger of toxic overdosage.

Because of the expense of dextran solution, its use in small animals has been quite limited. However, of the plasma expanders dextran comes closest to being ideal, and is the only expander being added to the national stockpile by the Federal Civil Defense Administration for use in event of national emergency.

In man, administration of more than 2,000 ml. of dextran intravenously may increase the bleeding time (Howard et al., 1959).

Gelatin

From the standpoint of expense, a sterile gelatin solution is the cheapest plasma expander made commercially. It has the advantage that it can be easily stored, is immediately available for use, and is not species specific. Commercial solutions contain 6 to 8% f gelatin, usually prepared from pigskin, in physiological saline solution. These preparations have an average molecular weight o approximately 33,000. The antigenic properties are destroyed by autoclaving, and there is no immediate toxic or antiphylactoid reaction following its use. Repeated injections at intervals will cause serious and sometimes fatal disturbances in dogs, chiefly by derangement of blood production. Intravenous injection of gelatin produces pseudoagglutination of erythrocytes, but the cells separate on passage through small vessels and there is no interference with blood flow.

About two-thirds of injected gelatin disappears from the circulation within 6 hours, 84% in 24 hours. It should not be used in the presence of renal disease because of the additional burden its excretion imposes on the kidneys.

The dose of gelatin depends upon the size and condition of the animal, ranging from 15 to 300 ml. in small animals; additional amounts may be administered periodically as deemed necessary. Gelatin should be given intravenously at a rate not to exceed 30 ml./minute.

VASOPRESSORS

Epinephrine Hydrochloride, U.S.P. (Adrenalin)

Epinephrine hydrochloride is a white crystalline odorless powder consisting of hormone formed by the adrenal medulla. It is produced commercially either by synthesis or extraction from the adrenal glands of animals. A 1:1000 aqueous solution of epinephrine is used clinically. It oxidizes upon exposure to air and light, first to a pink color and then to a reddish brown. For this reason, it is protected by packaging in brown bottles.

Epinephrine is ineffective when given orally. Solutions may be injected intramuscularly, subcutaneously and, in emergencies, intravenously or intracardially. Intravenous injections produce a rapid and marked effect. The intramuscular dose necessary to produce a comparable response is 25 to 50 times greater. For this reason, intravenous and intracardial epinephrine should be used with great caution. Epinephrine in the tissues is oxidized by amine and phenol oxidases and by the cytochrome system. The end products appear to be melanin pigments (Blaschko et al., 1937). A small amount of unoxidized epinephrine is conjugated with sulfuric acid and excreted in the urine.

Injection of epinephrine produces a quick rise in both systolic and diastolic blood pressure. This effect is due mainly to arteriolar constriction but is augmented by cardiac acceleration, increased myocardial contraction, and contraction of the spleen. The initial constrictor effect is due to epinephrine stimulating the myoneural junction of blood vessels. A second rise in blood pressure may occur due to stimulation of the vasoconstrictor center, thus on a recording two peaks or rises may be seen. After the rises, a fall below normal occurs followed by a return to the initial level. Subsequent intravenous injections of equal quantities of epinephrine cause progressively smaller pressor effects in the dog.

The vascular response to epinephrine varies depending upon the body location. Vessels of the abdominal viscera, including those of the kidneys, are constricted. On the other hand the arterioles of the skeletal muscles are usually dilated. This can be explained on the basis of Cannon's "Emergency Theory" which states that the effect of epinephrine is to supply blood to those organs most needed during an emergency.

Epinephrine is a powerful cardiac stimulant, producing increased force of contraction, shortening of systole, and increased output. It stimulates the cardiac accelerator nerve causing an increased heart rate. These effects produce stimulation of the carotico-aortic pressor receptive mechanism which, in turn, stimulates the vagus nerve to depress the heart. The heart rate is thus slowed even as the blood pressure reaches its maximum.

The stimulating action of epinephrine on the myocardium is used in combating cardiac arrest. In this situation 0.5 to 1.0 ml. of 1:10,000 epinephrine is injected directly into the left ventricle following which the heart is massaged to force epinephrine-containing blood into the coronary vessels.

Epinephrine may also be detrimental to the myocardium, a high concentration producing cardiac dilatation and ventricular fibrillation. Epinephrine-induced ventricular fibrillation is seen with chloroform and cyclopropane, these anesthetics sensitizing the myocardium to the stimulant action of the drug. Under these conditions, a dose of epinephrine which normally has no cardiac effect will induce fibrillation. Intravenous procaine has been shown to exert an inhibitory effect on epinephrine-induced fibrillation in dogs anesthetized with cyclopropane (Burstein and Marangoni, 1940).

Epinephrine is sometimes used for its direct effect upon the blood vessels. Mixed with local anesthetic agents, a solution of 1:100,000 produces local vasoconstriction, preventing toxic reactions and prolonging the action of the agent. A 1:10,000 or 1:20,000 solution is sometimes sprayed on mucous membranes or injected locally to prevent hemorrhage during surgical procedures. Systemic toxicity can result from extensive absorption of epinephrine when used for this purpose.

Epinephrine has no direct effect upon respiration and should not be used as a respiratory analeptic. If blood pressure response to epinephrine is appreciable, an inverse respiratory response occurs. Respirations are decreased during the period of increased blood pressure and then increased as the blood pressure falls. This response is probably due to blood pressure changes in the carotid sinus and aortic arch.

Epinephrine has little effect on other body organs or functions; the gastrointestinal tract is inhibited, the iris of the eye is dilated, and the basal metabolic rate is accelerated. Epinephrine causes glycogenolysis, hyperglycemia, and transient glycosuria; this action potentiates barbiturate anesthesia. In the cat, epinephrine stimulates salivary flow which is thick and viscid.

In excessive doses, epinephrine will cause tachycardia, palpitation, high blood pressure, dyspnea, pupillary dilatation, vertigo, rapid collapse, and death. The latter occurs from acute cardiac dilatation, pulmonary edema, and ventricular fibrillation. When injected subcutaneously or intramuscularly in dogs 0.5 to 1.0 ml. of 1:1,000 epinephrine may produce edematous swelling followed by necrosis at the site of injection.

Epinephrine should be used with caution or not at all. In debilitated or aged animals, particularly those with cardiac involvement, it is contraindicated for the treatment of vascular shock.

No treatment other than symptomatic is used in epinephrine poisoning. Because of its rapid metabolism by enzymes within the body the effects are very transient.

Levarterenol Bitartrate, U.S.P. (*l*-arterenol; *l*-norepinephrine; *l*-noradrenalin; Levophed)

Levarterenol is the principal pressor amine found in postganglionic adrenergic nerves. The bitartrate is a white water-soluble powder. On exposure to air and light it tends to darken and should be discarded. Levarterenol bitartrate is a water-soluble salt of the levorotatory isomer of arterenol. The latter is the unmethylated precursor of epinephrine.

Levarterenol has a marked vasopressor action, slowing the pulse rate and producing little effect on cardiac output. The vasopressor action is due to generalized vasoconstriction and this characteristic is used clinically in treatment of hypotension due to surgery, hemorrhage, anesthetic agents, or tranquilizers. It does not increase the circulating blood volume and therefore is not a substitute for administration of whole blood or plasma expanders. Rather, it is an adjunct to treatment of these conditions. Levarterenol should be used cautiously with cyclopropane, chloroform, or other anesthetic agents which sensitize the heart, because of the possibility of producing ventricular fibrillation.

The inactivation and excretion of levarterenol is similar to epinephrine. Very small quantities are excreted in the urine.

Because of its vasoconstrictor property, levarterenol when injected into tissues may produce necrosis and slough.

According to Jones (1957) an average dose of levarterenol bitartrate for dogs is 0.03 microgram of *levarterenol base*/lb./minute of intravenous infusion time. The duration of infusion is determined by return of blood pressure to a normal level. Patients should be "weaned" from levarterenol infusions since sudden withdrawal may cause hypotension. Withdrawal should take place over a period of several hours.

22

Dilution of levarterenol for infusion should be in 5% dextrose to protect against loss of potency by oxidation. The infusion fluid is prepared by diluting 4 ml. of 0.2% levarterenol bitartrate solution (equivalent to 0.1% of base) in 1,000 ml. of 5% dextrose. Saline should not be used for this purpose because oxidation occurs with saline solutions.

Methoxamine Hydrochloride, U.S.P. (Vasoxyl)

Methoxamine produces a marked vasopressor response which is due almost completely to increased peripheral resistance without direct myocardial stimulation. Compensatory bradycardia follows the rise in blood pressure. Following intravenous injection an immediate response occurs which persists for about 1 hour. On intramuscular injection response occurs within 15 minutes and lasts for approximately 90 minutes. Tachyphylaxis has been observed in experimental animals.

In dogs whose hearts were made susceptible to cardiac arrhythmias by the administration of cyclopropane, chloroform, the production of myocardial infarcts or diptheria toxin myocarditis, methoxamine failed to provoke arrhythmias. Moreover, it prevented epinephrine-cyclopropane or epinephrine-chloroform ventricular tachycardia and fibrillation. Slowing of the heart rate and, on overdose, sinus pauses and brief periods of A–V nodal rhythm are produced by methoxamine. With lethal doses, if death occurs from respiratory arrest, cardiac action continues for some time (Lahti et al., 1955).

De Beer et al. (1956) studied the effect of methoxamine and found it to be an effective agent for restoration of blood pressure in dogs in hypotensive states produced by hemorrhage, trauma, burns, tourniquet release, histamine, barbiturate overdose, and ganglionic blockade. It proved longer lasting than either ephedrine or d-desoxyephedrine in restoring and maintaining blood pressure. In normotensive dogs and cats 0.4 mg./kg. produced tachyphylaxis when given as a second dose following an initial dose of the same amount of drug. At 0.8 mg./kg., second doses actually produced a depressor effect. In hypotensive animals doses of 0.4 mg./kg. produced effective and prolonged response (Tables 16–1, 16–2).

Brill et al. (1959) have shown that methoxamine is capable of suppressing ventricular arrhythmias experimentally produced in dogs by several methods. The dose used was 0.5 to 1 mg./kg. of body weight. Arrhythmias were suppressed for periods of 30 to 60 minutes.

Methoxamine hydrochloride is marketed in 1 ml. ampules containing 20 mg. of the drug. Its chief advantage over other sym-

pathomimetic amines is its prolonged effect from a single intramuscular injection (Levarterenol, on the other hand, gives momen-
tary control of blood pressure through adjustment of the rate of
infusion since it is a very short-acting drug).

Methoxamine can be given either intramuscularly or intravenously. The former does not cause tissue necrosis.

Table 16–1.—Restorative Action of Methoxamine on Hemorrhagic
Hypotension in Dogs

Hemorrhage	Dose of Methoxamine	Number Animals	Arterial Pressure in mm. Hg.			
			Initial	Shock Level	Peak	Plateau
25 ml./kg.	0.4 mg./kg. i.v.	3	142 ± 13[1]	75 ± 24	154 ± 14	122 ± 26
	0.8 mg./kg. i.v.	38	135 ± 19	73 ± 24	167 ± 37	123 ± 31
26–35 ml./kg.	0.4 mg./kg. i.v.	9	135 ± 18	64 ± 21	150 ± 36	100 ± 32
	0.8 mg./kg. i.v.	21	146 ± 27	65 ± 20	169 ± 35	124 ± 26
36–45 ml./kg.	0.4 mg./kg. i.v.	4	153 ± 26	83 ± 17	155 ± 20	111 ± 39
	0.8 mg./kg. i.v.	7	143 ± 20	65 ± 28	135 ± 35	90 ± 26

[1] Mean ± standard deviation.

(DeBeer, E. J., Wnuck, A. L., Fanelli, R. V., Norton, S., and Ellis, C. H.: The
Restoration of Arterial Pressure from Various Hypotensive States by Methoxamine.
Arch. int. pharmacodyn., *104*, 487, 1956.)

Phenylephrine Hydrochloride, U.S.P. (Neosynephrine)

Phenylephrine is a synthetic sympathomimetic amine with action
essentially equal to levarterenol. It is less potent than the latter
and has a longer duration of action with minimal cardiac effect and
little central stimulation. Reflex bradycardia occurs following
injection. In cyclopropane-sensitized hearts ventricular tachycardia
or fibrillation are not produced. Phenylephrine hydrochloride is
available as a 1.0% sterile solution for injection. The intravenous
dose for dogs is 0.04 mg./lb., the subcutaneous or intramuscular
dose approximately 0.08 mg./lb.

Phenylephrine is sometimes added to solutions of local anesthetic
agents in a concentration of 1:2,500 to produce prolongation of
action of the local anesthetic and reduce its toxicity.

Mephentermine, U.S.P. (Wyamine)

Mephentermine produces peripheral vasoconstriction with little
change in cardiac output, heart rate, or the electrocardiogram.
Goldberg *et al.* (1953) in comparing sympathomimetic drugs found

Table 16–2.—Restorative Action of Methoxamine on Hypotension in Dogs Induced by Several Methods

Hypotensive Method	Dose of Methoxamine	Number of Animals	Arterial Pressure in mm. Hg.			
			Initial	Shock Level	Peak	Plateau
Trauma of leg	0.4	7	122(100–152)[1]	79(65–94)	160(124–208)	105(90–128)
	0.8	3				
Burn Shock	0.4	4	131(121–138)	73(45–94)	137(120–153)	112(99–120)
Tourniquet Shock	0.4	4	162(150–190)	60(26–90)	127(93–165)	94(62–138)
Histamine	0.4	2	143(143–143)	38(30–45)	110(98–122)	102(93–110)
	0.8	2	138(95–180)	70(55–85)	128(125–130)	162(120–204)
Anesthetic	0.4	7	139(110–184)	63(24–115)	127(70–184)	97(40–150)
	0.8	10	129(96–177)	58(28–85)	158(112–270)	87(38–124)
Ganglionic Blockade	0.4	2	124(122–125)	102(84–120)	204(160–248)	166(160–172)
	0.8	4	119(105–130)	88(82–100)	191(80–130)	125(78–170)

[1] Mean and range

(DeBeer, E. J., Fanelli, R. V., Wnuck, A. L., Norton, S. and Ellis, C. H.: The Restoration of Arterial Pressure from Various Hypotensive States by Methoxamine. Arch. int. pharmacodyn., 104, 487, 1956.)

that it had prominent inotropic and chronotropic actions on the dog heart.

Mephentermine when given intravenously produces a pressor effect for 30 to 50 minutes; on intramuscular injection it lasts up to 4 hours. Repeated intravenous injections in dogs will produce tachyphylaxis.

Mephentermine is marketed in sterile vials containing 1 or 10 ml. (15 mg./ml.) for parenteral administration. The intravenous dose for dogs is 0.3 mg./kg.

Amphetamine Sulfate, U.S.P. (Benzadrine Sulfate, N.N.R.)

Amphetamine is a racemic mixture of d, l, and dl-beta forms of the drug. The dextro-rotatory form is known as *Dextro-Amphetamine, U.S.P.* (Dexedrine Sulfate).

Amphetamine is classified both as a sympathomimetic amine and a respiratory analeptic. In the former capacity it produces an elevation of blood pressure due to peripheral vasoconstriction, stimulates the heart muscle, relaxes the bronchial and intestinal muscles and dilates the pupil. As a respiratory analeptic it stimulates the cerebrospinal axis, particularly the brain stem and cortex. It is a potent stimulant of the medullary respiratory center, thus relieving central depression caused by anesthetics. A marked increase in rate and depth of respiration results from its central stimulating action. Large doses of amphetamine have been shown to increase oxygen consumption markedly in experimental animals.

Some variation in cardiovascular response of animals occurs with amphetamine. Generally a rise in systolic and diastolic pressures results. This is accomplished through peripheral vasoconstriction and direct action on the myocardium. With repeated doses tachyphylaxis will occur.

Gunn (1939) showed that amphetamine produced uterine contraction in all animals examined, including non-pregnant cats. Mydriasis is also produced.

Amphetamine is destroyed in the body by deamination and excretion of the unchanged portion in the urine. Amine oxidase has little effect on this compound.

Amphetamine is available in 5.0% solution. Craige (1943) reports that 5 mg./kg. of amphetamine sulfate intravenously is the M.L.D. in normal unanesthetized dogs. The optimum dose for anesthetized, critically depressed dogs is 4.0 to 4.5 mg./kg. intravenously. Doses of less than 1 mg./kg. are ineffective in this situation, while larger doses are superfluous and may be fatal. Dogs dying from large doses have severe hemorrhagic gastroenteritis on necropsy.

When amphetamine was given to dogs anesthetized with pentobarbital sodium (28.5 mg./kg.), 1 of 10 dogs died following injection of 11 mg./kg. and the LD_{50} appeared to be in excess of 44 mg./kg.

Methamphetamine Hydrochloride, U.S.P. (Desoxyephedrine; Benzefet; Desoxyn; Methedrine)

Methamphetamine is closely related to amphetamine and ephedrine. The pharmacological actions are similar to those of amphetamine. The drug possesses a marked stimulant action on the central nervous system and produces a rise in blood pressure due to peripheral vasoconstriction and cardiac stimulation. Sinoauricular tachycardia is produced in dogs anesthetized with cyclopropane. Methamphetamine is a more potent central nervous stimulant than is amphetamine and produces slightly less effect on the cardiovascular system. If methamphetamine is used for its vasopressor effect, the central nervous and cardiac actions should be kept constantly in mind.

Methamphetamine is available as a sterile liquid containing 40 mg./ml. The dose for dogs is 0.1 to 0.5 ml./10 lb. of body weight given intravenously, intramuscularly or intraperitoneally.

Metaraminol Bitartrate (Aramine)

Metaraminol is a potent vasopressor with prolonged duration of action. It is available in solution containing 10 mg./ml. The dose for dogs is 0.05 to 0.20 mg./kg. intravenously or 0.5 to 1.0 mg./kg. intramuscularly.

Following injection in hypotensive dogs there is a rapid rise in blood pressure due to peripheral vasoconstriction. An increase in cardiac output and coronary blood flow also occurs due to amplified myocardial contractility (Sarnoff et al., 1954). In dogs with hemorrhagic hypotension a significant increase in survival has been noted by Sarnoff and Kaufman (1954).

The central nervous system is not stimulated as with some other sympathomimetic amines and there is a slight tendency to prolong barbiturate narcosis. Respiration is either unaffected or moderately slowed following injection.

There is little evidence of tachyphylaxis. Following administration of epinephrine and some other sympathomimetic amines, secondary vasodilation occurs. This is not observed with metaraminol.

Injection may be made intravenously, intramuscularly, or subcutaneously. The onset of action is approximately 1 minute, 10 minutes and 20 minutes respectively and lasts for 20 minutes to

1 hour. Metaraminol does not appear to cause cardiac arrhythmias but its use with cyclopropane and similar agents is not recommended.

ACTH AND THE ADRENOCORTICAL STEROIDS

Adrenocorticotropic Hormone (ACTH)

ACTH is formed by the basophilic cells of the anterior pituitary gland. It is a polypeptide of low molecular weight. Commercially, ACTH is extracted from the pituitary glands of cattle and swine and has a biological activity of about 400 I.U./mg. One U.S.P. unit equals one International Unit and represents the adrenocorticotropic activity of 1 mg. of the International Standard.

ACTH stimulates the adrenal cortex which in turn causes release of adrenocorticosteroid hormones into the blood stream. The function of ACTH is to enable the animal to withstand sudden stress by stimulating increased adrenocortical secretion. The stimulus for release of ACTH from the anterior pituitary is thought to be nerve impulses from the hypothalamus or a high blood level of epinephrine. When ACTH is injected intramuscularly a portion is destroyed by tissue enzymes but sufficient drug remains to produce a physiological response. A single intramuscular injection of ACTH produces a peak release of adrenocortical steroids at 3 hours and the action is finished by the sixth hour. When given intravenously or intramuscularly only small amounts of ACTH are found unchanged in the urine.

ACTH is prepared as *Corticotropin*, U.S.P., a lyophilized powdered tissue extract, which is dissolved in water for injection. *Corticotropin Injection*, U.S.P. is also available. The dose of these is 0.5 to 1 unit/lb./day given intramuscularly in four divided doses at 6-hour intervals. ACTH is also available in repository form containing 15% gelatin to delay absorption and prolong the action following intramuscular injection (*Repository Corticotropin Injection*, U.S.P.). The initial dose of ACTH gel is 0.5 to 1 unit/lb./day; this is gradually reduced as recovery becomes apparent.

Adrenocortical Steroids

Adrenocortical steroids assist in regulating the volume and composition of body fluids and support essential cellular metabolism, thus maintaining homeostasis in the body. They are of three types: (1) glucocorticoids which cause gluconeogenesis, eosinopenia, hyperglycemia, sodium retention, edema, and potassium loss (cortisone, hydrocortisone, and their derivatives); (2) mineralcorticoids which principally affect electrolyte and water metabolism (aldosterone, corticosterone, and desoxycorticosterone); (3) androgenic corticoids (adrenosterone).

Pharmacologically, cortisone, hydrocortisone, and their derivatives (Fig. 16–3) produce the same actions. These include gluconeogenesis, hyperglycemia, glycosuria, and a negative nitrogen balance. Sodium is retained by the kidneys and potassium is excreted. When large amounts of potassium are excreted diuresis occurs. Excessive therapy may produce sodium retention with edema, hypochloremia, hypocalcemia, hypopotassemia, and metabolic alkalosis. This can be corrected by concurrent administration of potassium. Prolonged therapy with corticosteroids should be

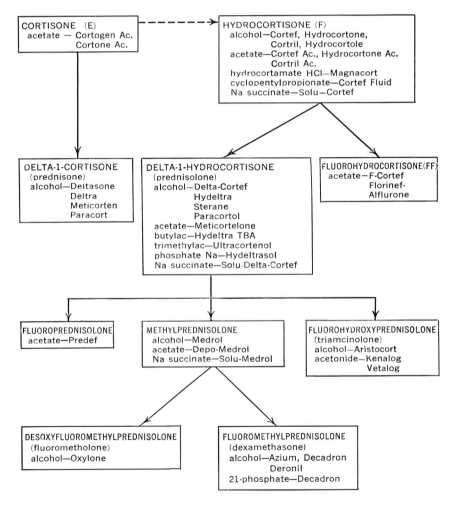

FIGURE 16–3. Corticosteroid derivations, their various forms, and their commercial availability. (Courtesy of Dr. K. B. Haas, The Upjohn Company, Kalamazoo, Michigan.)

avoided since this will produce atrophy of the adrenal cortex with elimination of calcium, phosphorus, and nitrogen, which in turn produces osteoporosis and occasional fractures.

These drugs reduce the inflammatory response to tissue insult. Vascularization and fibroblastic activity with formation of granulation tissue and intercellular ground substance are inhibited. This action slows wound healing and should be considered if these drugs are administered to surgical patients.

The glucocorticoids are absorbed readily from the gastrointestinal tract. For continuous therapy, however, they must be administered three or four times during a 24-hour period in order to obtain sustained hormonal effect.

Table 16–3.—Comparison of Various Corticoid Compounds

	Relative Glucocorticoid Activity	Relative Anti-inflammatory Activity
Cortisone	0.8	0.8
Hydrocortisone	1.0	1.0
Prednisone	4.0	2.5
Prednisolone	5.5	4.0
Methylprednisolone	10.5	5.0
Triamcinolone	—	5.0
Dexamethasone	—	9.4
Fluoroprednisolone	50.0	14.0

— Data not available.

(From data supplied by the Upjohn Company, Kalamazoo, Michigan.)

Metabolites of cortisone and hydrocortisone are eliminated through the kidneys in conjugation with glucuronic and sulfuric acids. These account for a small fraction of the total amount administered; the metabolism of the remainder is unknown.

Because less toxic derivatives with greater potency have been developed, little cortisone or hydrocortisone is used today; however, these drugs serve as criteria for comparison of newer drugs (Table 16–3).

Hydrocortisone is absorbed more slowly than cortisone following intramuscular injection. For most rapid effect hydrocortisone should be given by continuous intravenous infusion. Treatment by this method is highly effective but is not sustained once infusion is stopped. Therefore, it should be supplemented with intramuscular or repeated oral therapy if continued effect is desired.

For dogs Haas (1956) suggests 25 to 75 mg. of hydrocortisone in aqueous suspension every 24 hours until improvement occurs. The dose should then be reduced gradually to the smallest suitable maintenance level (usually 15 to 50 mg. or less, daily).

According to Davidson (1956) the dose of prednisolone (delta-hydrocortisone) is as follows:

5–15 pounds	1.25 mg. daily
15–40 pounds	1.25—5 mg. daily
40–80 pounds	2.5—12.5 mg. daily

The dose of prednisone (delta-cortisone) for dogs is 10 to 20 mg. daily for 3 days or less, then 2.5 to 5 mg. daily as required. The daily dose of either should be divided into 3 or 4 parts and given at regular intervals.

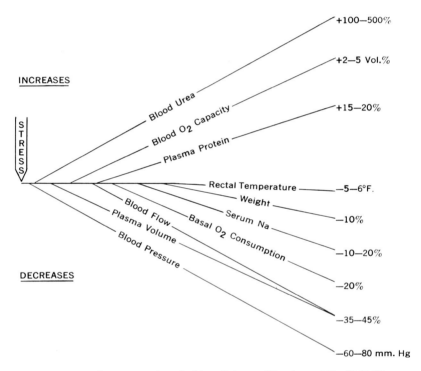

FIGURE 16–4. Symptoms of cortical insufficiency. (Courtesy of Dr. K. B. Haas, The Upjohn Company, Kalamazoo, Michigan.)

In periods of acute stress the normal output of cortical hormone may need to be multiplied as much as 10 times or even more. If the pituitary-adrenal axis is incapable of meeting this demand, falling blood pressure, increase in pulse rate, hemoconcentration, coma, and eventual death will occur (Fig. 16–4). Cortical hormone is involved in maintenance of capillary tone which in turn is important to homeostasis. In shock an intravenous preparation such as hydrocortisone sodium succinate or prednisolone sodium succinate will restore vascular sensitivity to vasopressors (Fig. 16–5). These drugs are indicated in poor surgical risks, shock from traumatic injury, overwhelming systemic infection, and emergency surgery. The dose of the former for small animals is 20 to 300 mg. depending upon the condition. In hypotensive shock an average of 200 mg. is required to elevate blood pressure to 90 mm. Hg.

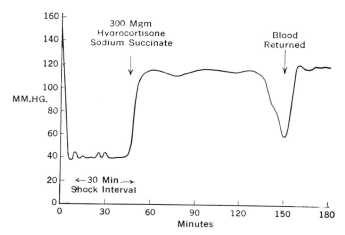

FIGURE 16–5. Effect of intravenous hydrocortisone sodium succinate on the blood pressure of a dog subjected to experimental hemorrhagic shock (From Connolly, J. E., Bruns, D. L. and Stofer, R. C.: The Use of Intravenous Hydrocortisone in Hemorrhagic Shock. Surgical Forum, 9, 17, 1958.)

The initial dose of prednisolone sodium succinate for small animals is 5 to 50 mg. For maintenance one-half the initial dose may be given at intervals of 1, 3, 6, and 10 hours afterward as deemed necessary. Repeated doses are important and are usually required in shock. Intramuscular injections of prednisolone can be given for prolonged therapy at the same time the first injection is made intravenously.

CARDIAC DEFIBRILLATOR AND ARREST KIT

Batelli introduced the electrical defibrillator in 1900. A number of models are available commercially, but expense has prevented their widespread use in veterinary practice.

Booth *et al.* (1958) have described a cardiac defibrillator which can be built for approximately 50 dollars (Fig. 16–6). The principal components are a variable transformer, an ammeter, and electrodes. The transformer has a range of 0 to 100 volts and the ammeter a range of 0 to 5 amperes. The electrodes are round brass plates, which in use are covered with saline-soaked gauze to prevent epicardial and myocardial burning.

To use the defibrillator the transformer is set between 70 and 90 volts. The operator grasps the insulated handles of the electrodes, places the electrodes on each side of the heart and the transformer switch is quickly turned on and off. This delivers a shock lasting only a fraction of a second and two or more amperes of current are allowed to flow through the myocardium. The operator should be prepared for the animal to have a tonic convulsion and be very

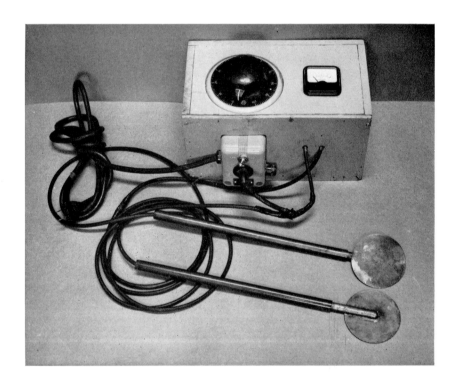

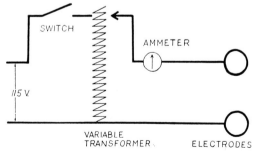

FIGURE 16-6. Cardiac defibrillator (top) showing inner and outer surfaces of electrodes. The electrical circuit is shown below.

careful that he does not contact the exposed electrodes, the animal, or the operating table.

In both experimental animals and clinic patients, this equipment combined with cardiac massage has proved highly effective in restoring normal cardiac rhythm. For a defibrillator to be of value it must be kept in a convenient location and saline for moistening the electrodes should be stored with it.

Since, in addition to the defibrillator, several drugs are necessary in treatment of cardiac arrest, an arrest kit containing all necessary supplies should be kept in readiness in the operating room. It should include:

> Instruments for thoracotomy
> Epinephrine hydrochloride, 1:10,000
> Calcium chloride or gluconate, 10%
> Potassium chloride, 5%
> Cardiac defibrillator and sterile saline

Calcium Chloride

The calcium ion increases contractility of the heart muscle and prolongs systole. When the heart is dilated and flaccid it enhances cardiac muscle tone and irritability.

Following massage, if the heart is flabby and ventricular standstill exists, 0.5 to 3 ml. of 10% calcium chloride or calcium gluconate should be injected directly into the left ventricle and massage continued.

Potassium Chloride

Ventricular fibrillation can be stopped by intraventricular injection of 50 mg./kg. of 5% potassium chloride. This effect is due to cardiac relaxation and inhibition produced by the potassium ion. In the absence of a defibrillator this technique coupled with massage may prove life-saving. However, it is not as effective as electrical defibrillation and should be used only as an adjunct.

ANALEPTICS

Drugs which stimulate the respiratory center and produce an increased respiratory exchange are termed *respiratory analeptics*. Those in common use include: pentylenetetrazol (Metrazol), methetharimide (Mikedimide), amphetamine (Benzedrine), and carbon dioxide. All but the latter produce an "arousal" effect characterized by a return toward consciousness of the patient. During the period of stimulation, which is short, animals may arouse enough to bump and bruise themselves severely or even have convulsions. In recent years, several investigators have stated that respiratory analeptics are contraindicated for respiratory depression produced by barbiturates. This is due to the fact that following stimulation for a brief period, the respiratory center becomes more depressed than it was prior to administration of the analeptic agent. Current belief is that artificial ventilation until the barbiturate is detoxified is the most effective means of management.

Pentylenetetrazol, U.S.P. (Metrazol, Leptazol)

Pentylenetetrazol is a white crystalline synthetic organic compound which is readily soluble in water. When administered intravenously it has a rapid effect upon the central nervous system. Small doses stimulate the medulla and midbrain while larger doses also excite the cerebral cortex and spinal cord. The effect appears to be direct and not reflex. Because of its action on the medulla, the drug is used for stimulation of the respiratory centers, both rate and depth of respiration being increased.

Pentylenetetrazol is not a cardiac stimulant and should not be used for this purpose. Any improvement in circulation which occurs following its administration is caused by more efficient and effective respiration.

Excessive doses of pentylenetetrazol will produce spinal convulsions. Since it excites the spinal cord, it should never be used in conjunction with morphine alone, morphine also being a spinal cord stimulant. This does not pertain if the animal is anesthetized, but only when the animal is under morphine narcosis.

Pentylenetetrazol is rapidly absorbed after intramuscular injection and this method of administration can be used in situations other than acute emergencies.

The liver inactivates most of the drug in dogs and cats, the kidney having little effect on detoxification. After large doses, only traces of drug can be found excreted unchanged in the urine of dogs. It has no particular tissue affinity, being distributed equally in the tissues. The rate of detoxification is proportional to the concentration of drug in the tissues (Tatum and Kozelka, 1941).

In anesthesia, pentylenetetrazol is used for respiratory failure from barbiturates and certain other central nervous system depressants. While it is available in tablet form, intravenous or intramuscular administration is recommended for emergencies. The dose of pentylenetetrazol in dogs is 3 to 5 mg./lb. of body weight repeated in 15 to 30 minutes as indicated. The tendency is to give too little for the desired effect. It has a relatively large margin of

safety though excessive doses will stimulate the spinal cord, producing convulsions and respiratory paralysis.

Methetharimide (Mikedimide, Megimide)

Methetharimide (3,3-methylethylglutarimide) is similar in chemical structure to the barbiturates and is antagonistic to them. The
drug is available as a 0.5% aqueous solution and a 3% solution in
propylene glycol. The aqueous solution is slightly less effective
(Cairy et al., 1961a). Both may be administered intravenously,
intramuscularly, intraperitoneally, subcutaneously, or intrathorac-

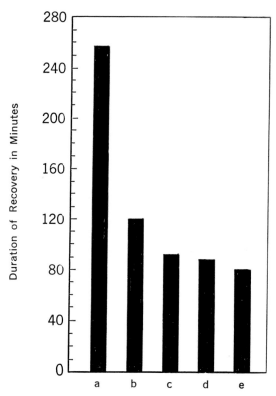

FIGURE 16-7. Average duration of recovery of cats from pentobarbital sodium
given intravenously, compared with intravenous pentobarbital sodium followed in 30
minutes with methetharimide by four routes of administration. Six operated cats were
used in each group.

  a—Pentobarbital sodium intravenously.
  b—Pentobarbital sodium followed by methetharimide intramuscularly.
  c—Pentobarbital sodium followed by methetharimide intraperitoneally.
  d—Pentobarbital sodium followed by methetharimide intrathoracically.
  e—Pentobarbital sodium followed by methetharimide intravenously.

(From Arañez, J. B. and Ramos, E. G.: 3,3-Methylethylglutarimide as an Analeptic
for Cats. Natural and Applied Sci. Bull., 17, 223, 1960.)

ically. However, in emergencies the intravenous route is recommended.

The antagonistic effect is evidenced by increased rate and depth of respiration, elevation of pulse rate and blood pressure, and return of reflexes. Overdosage can produce severe convulsions requiring administration of a thiobarbiturate for their control. For this reason slow intravenous administration "to effect" is most satisfactory. No attempt should be made to rouse depressed animals to the point that they are fully awake.

The dose of methetharimide is based on the amount of barbiturate administered and the depth of anesthesia. It is antagonistic to the barbiturate roughly on a milligram for milligram basis, 30 to 60 mg. (1–2 ml.)/5 lbs. of body weight usually being effective.

When given to dogs and cats the arousal time is shortened (Arañez and Paculdo, 1960; Arañez and Ramos, 1960) (Fig. 16–7). When combined with amphetamine, effectiveness in treatment of acute barbiturate depression is enhanced (Cairy et al., 1961b).

One drawback to methetharimide is a tendency for the animals to regress to their former anesthetized state unless repeated injections are made; therefore, treated animals should be watched closely during the recovery period.

Amphetamine and carbon dioxide are discussed elsewhere in the text.

THE NARCOTIC ANTAGONISTS

Nalorphine Hydrochloride (Nalline) and Levallorphan Tartrate (Lorfan)

Nalorphine and levallorphan are synthetic congeners of morphine which antagonize the respiratory depression caused by codeine, dihydrocodeine, morphine, meperidine, dihydromorphinone (Dilaudid), heroin, anileridine (Leritine), levorphan (Levo-dromoran), methadone, methyldihydromorphinone (Metopon), alphaprodine (Nisentil), and pantopon. They are specific antagonists for narcotics, and are not effective in respiratory depression due to barbiturates, anesthetics, or other agents. *They should not be used as general analeptics.*

When given intravenously to dogs deeply sedated with morphine the initial effects are observed within 15 seconds after injection (Aronson and Gans, 1959a). A deep inspiration is followed by change in the panting type respiration seen with morphine to breathing with a greater tidal volume and slower rate. After 90 seconds almost all signs of morphine hypnosis disappear. The same changes are seen with these drugs if given following other narcotics. When injected into pentobarbital-anesthetized dogs which have not received preanesthetic narcotic, a moderate depression of ventilation and a small but transient fall in blood pressure is observed.

When pentobarbital-anesthetized dogs are given morphine or meperidine intravenously followed by nalorphine, a rapid increase in ventilation, decrease in arterial carbon-dioxide content, and a return of blood pressure toward normal levels occurs without substantially altering the plane of anesthesia.

Nalorphine or levallorphan when given without prior administration of a narcotic will produce central nervous depression. The nature of the antagonism of these drugs for the narcotics has not been established, although many believe it to be a competitive inhibition.

One milligram of nalorphine is recommended for every 10 mg. of morphine or 20 mg. of meperidine used preanesthetically. One milligram of levallorphan is recommended for every 50 mg. of morphine or 100 mg. of meperidine. Since levallorphan and nalorphine are themselves depressant drugs, the total amount given in a 4-hour period should not exceed 5 mg. of levallorphan or 25 mg. of nalorphine for a 25 pound dog. In treating neonatal respiratory depression produced by narcotic analgesics, the dose of either drug should be approximately $\frac{1}{15}$ to $\frac{1}{20}$ of the adult dose. Good results have been reported by Kirk (1961), when narcotic depressed newborn pups were injected in the umbilical vessels with 0.1 ml. of nalorphine (0.5 mg.).

Aronson and Gans (1959b) have stated that administration of levallorphan or nalorphine in pentobarbital-anesthetized dogs depressed by narcotic analgesics permits resumption of adequate respiration without altering the level of anesthesia. In addition, narcotic analgesics may be given during prolonged surgery as supplemental anesthesia, respiratory depression being prevented or overcome by the use of these antagonists.

RESPIRATORS

These are discussed in Chapter 5, page 86.

References

Arañez, J. B. and Paculdo, D. J.: Barbiturate Antagonism. Vet. Med., *55*, 56, 1960.
Arañez, J. B. and Ramos, E. G.: 3,3-Methylethylglutarimide as an Analeptic for Cats. Nat. and Applied Sci. Bull., *17*, 223, 1960.
Aronson, A. L. and Gans, J. H.: The Narcotic Analgesics and Their Antagonists as Adjuncts to Barbiturate Anesthesia. I. Physiological and Pharmacological Considerations. Am. J. Vet. Res., *20*, 909, 1959.

ARONSON, A. L. and GANS, J. H.: The Narcotic Analgesics and Their Antagonists as Adjuncts to Barbiturate Anesthesia. II. Clinical Applications. J.A.V.M.A., *134*, 459, 1959.

BLASCHKO, H., RICHTER, D., and SCHLOSSMANN, H.: The Oxidation of Adrenaline and Other Amines. Biochem. J., *31*, 2187, 1937.

BOOTH, N. H., WILL, D. H., MOSS, L. C., and SWENSON, M. J.: An Electrical Apparatus and Its Application in Defibrillating the Heart of the Dog. J.A.V.M.A., *132*, 117, 1958.

BRILL, I. C., KRUEGER, J. D., and McCAWLEY, E. L.: Restoration of Sinus Rhythm in Experimental and Clinical Ventricular Arrhythmias by Methoxamine Hydrochloride. Am. J. Cardiology, *3*, 307, 1959.

BURSTEIN, C. L. and MARANGONI, B. A.: Protecting Action of Procaine against Ventricular Fibrillation Induced by Epinephrine During Cyclopropane Anesthesia. Proc. Soc. Exper. Biol. and Med., *43*, 210, 1940.

CAIRY, C. F., LEASH, A., and SISODIA, C. S.: Comparison of Several Drugs in Treating Acute Barbiturate Depression in the Dog. I. Single Drugs. J.A.V.M.A., *138*, 129, 1961.

CAIRY, C F., LEASH, A., and SISODIA, C. S.: Comparison of Several Drugs in Treating Acute Barbiturate Depression in the Dog. II. Pairs of Drugs. J.A.V.M.A., *138*, 132, 1961.

CLARK, C. H. and WOODLEY, C. H.: A Comparison of Blood Volumes as Measured by Rose Bengal, T-1824 (Evans Blue), Radiochromium-Tagged Erythrocytes, and a Combination of the Latter Two. Am. J. Vet. Res., *20*, 1067, 1959.

CRAIGE, A. H., JR.: Amphetamine in Veterinary Practice: Special Reference to Dosage. J.A.V.M.A., *103*, 28, 1943.

DAVIDSON, J. L.: Use of Newer Corticosteroids in Animals. Vet. Med., *51*, 222, 1956.

DE BEER, E. J., WNUCK, A. L., FANELLI, R. V., NORTON, S., and ELLIS, C. H.: The Restoration of Arterial Pressure from Various Hypotensive States by Methoxamine. Arch. internat. pharmacodyn., *104*, 487, 1956.

FIRT, P. and HEJHAL, L.: Treatment of Severe Haemorrhage. Lancet, *273*, 1132, 1957.

GOLDBERG, L. I., COTTEN, M. deV., DARBY, T. D., and HOWELL, E. V.: Comparative Heart Contractile Force Effects of Equipressor Doses of Several Sympathomimetic Amines. J. Pharm. & Exper. Therap., *108*, 177, 1953.

GUNN, J. A.: The Pharmacological Actions and Therapeutic Uses of Some Compounds Related to Adrenalin: Lecture I. Brit. Med. J., *2*, 155, 1939.: Lecture II, Ibid, *2*, 214, 1939.

HAAS, K. B.: Use of Newer Corticosteroids in Animals. N. Amer. Vet., *37*, 753, 1956.

HOWARD, J. M., EBERT, R. V., BLOOM, W. L., and SLOAN, M. H.: The Present Status of Dextran as a Plasma Expander. Am. J. Surg., *97*, 593, 1959.

JONES, L. M.: *Veterinary Pharmacology and Therapeutics.* 2nd ed. The Iowa State College Press, Ames, Iowa, 1957.

KIRK, R. W.: Personal Communication. Cornell University, Ithaca, New York, 1961.

LAHTI, R. E., BRILL, I. C., and McCAWLEY, E. L.: The Effect of Methoxamine Hydrochloride (Vasoxyl) on Cardiac Rhythm. J. Pharm. & Exper. Therap., *115*, 268, 1955.

SARNOFF, S. J., CASE, R. B., BERGLUND, E., and SARNOFF, L. C.: Ventricular Function. V. The Circulatory Effects of Aramine; Mechanism of Action of "Vasopressor" Drugs in Cardiogenic Shock. Circulation, *10*, 84, 1954.

SARNOFF, S. J. and KAUFMAN, H. E.: Effect of Aramine on the Survival of Dogs Subjected to Hemorrhagic Hypotension. Circulation Res., *2*, 420, 1954.

TATUM, H. J. and KOZELKA, F. L.: Distribution, Excretion and Rate and Site of Detoxification of Metrazol. J. Pharm. & Exper. Therap., *72*, 284, 1941.

YOUNG, L. E., O'BRIEN, W. A., SWISHER, S. N., MILLER, G. and YUILE, C. L.: Blood Groups in Dogs—Their Significance to the Veterinarian. Am. J. Vet. Res., *13*, 207, 1952.

ANESTHETIC EMERGENCIES

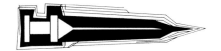

Chapter 17

DESPITE all precautionary measures anesthetic emergencies occasionally develop. It has been stated (————, 1950), "Although certain surgical procedures may be classified as 'minor operations' we need wider recognition of the fact that there is no such thing as a 'minor anesthetic'. . . . It is during . . . 'minor' procedures that the anesthetic accident often occurs." By scrupulous care many emergencies can be avoided; by prior preparation and training emergencies can usually be brought to a successful conclusion for the patient.

Classification of Anesthetic Emergencies

Anesthetic emergencies generally fall into one of the following categories.

- A. Respiratory System
  1. Hypopnea
  2. Apnea
  3. Hyperpnea
  4. Obstruction of airway
  5. Salivation and excessive mucus
  6. Laryngospasm and bronchospasm
- B. Cardiovascular System
  1. Hypotension and shock
  2. Cardiac arrest
- C. Regurgitation and Vomiting
- D. Convulsions
  1. From local anesthetics
  2. From hyperthermia

Hypoxia During Anesthesia

Hypoxia is probably the most common complication of anesthesia and may be due to many causes.

(355)

Hypopnea may occur even in lightly anesthetized animals due to depression of the respiratory centers by the anesthetic. Very shallow respirations and progressively developing cyanosis are the outward manifestations of this condition. Immediate corrective steps, such as endotracheal intubation and oxygen administration, should be taken since even mild hypoxia may eventually lead to respiratory or cardiac arrest.

Apnea usually results from an overdose of anesthetic. Thiobarbiturates commonly cause respiration to cease temporarily on induction. This is not a cause for alarm provided the animal does not become cyanotic, since ordinarily respirations resume as soon as carbon dioxide tension increases. However, in some animals this is not true and cyanosis develops followed by cardiac arrest. Because it is impossible to determine in which animals this will occur, stimulation of respiration by pressure on the chest reflex area, artificial respiration, and oxygen administration should be started early. In most situations oxygen given through a small gauge polyethylene endotracheal catheter is adequate, particularly if coupled with forcible compression of the rib cage to respirate the patient. In the event breathing does not resume and the mucous membranes remain cyanotic, a conventional endotracheal catheter should be inserted, the cuff inflated, and the catheter connected to a respirator if available. Since narcotics depress the respiratory center, a specific antagonist, such as nalorphine or levallorphan, should be administered to those animals which have received preanesthetic narcotics and are slow to respond to resuscitative measures.

Apnea also occurs with inhalation anesthetics and is a sign of dangerously deep anesthesia (Stage IV). Administration of anesthetic must be stopped immediately and the lungs flushed with air or oxygen to reduce the anesthetic concentration within the body.

Animals with diaphragmatic hernia will frequently evidence hyperpnea immediately following induction. The respiratory movements, though exaggerated, are ineffective and severe cyanosis develops followed by apnea and death. One should *always* intubate these patients as soon as anesthesia produces sufficient relaxation and immediately start artificial respiration. Hyperpnea may also develop when soda lime in a closed system becomes exhausted. The mucous membranes remain bright pink without evidence of cyanosis. Changing the soda lime will quickly correct the difficulty

Obstruction of the airway can occur from many causes. Unfavorable positioning of the patient during anesthesia may produce partial or complete block (Fig. 2-3). Care should be taken to see that draping material does not cover and occlude the mouth and nasal passages. If an endotracheal catheter is used, it must be remembered that it is the only opening through which the animal can breathe. For this reason it may present a hazard easily overlooked.

Occasionally the tongue may be swallowed occluding the pharynx. In brachycephalic dogs, elongation of the soft palate and eversion of the lateral ventricles may produce obstruction. When anesthetizing these breeds, one should *always* intubate the patient. Eversion of the lateral ventricles may pose a peculiar problem in that the laryngeal opening may not be large enough to admit a conventional endotracheal catheter. In this event a small gauge polyethylene catheter (.055″ I.D. × .075″ O.D.) should be inserted into the trachea to give oxygen.

Salivation and excessive mucus are common with thiobarbiturate anesthesia and with ether inhalation. Regardless of when they are encountered their formation should be treated by administration of atropine. Mucus and blood clots from surgery in the mouth or throat should be removed manually with sponges and with suction if available.

Laryngeal and bronchial spasms may develop in any species, but are seen most commonly in cats given ether or one of the thiobarbiturates. Spasms usually occur in lightly anesthetized animals from stimulation of the respiratory tract (intubation attempts, inhalation of concentrated anesthetic vapors). The result is coughing, and a high-pitched harsh inspiratory sound accompanied by some degree of cyanosis. Hall (1959) has suggested intravenous meperidine in this situation for its spasmolytic action. Preanesthetic atropine is preventive and can also be given intravenously as treatment. Oxygen should be administered intrapharyngeally until such time as the laryngospasms have relaxed and an endotracheal catheter can be inserted. Forcible intubation through a closed glottis may cause laryngeal edema and, therefore, should be done gently.

Treatment of Severe Hypoxia

Acute hypoxia produces damage in the brain. Intracellular edema occurring after a severe hypoxic episode is best treated by some form of dehydration therapy. Fifty per cent glucose or sucrose has been used; better results have been reported with concentrated plasma or serum given intravenously. The intravenous administration of urea solution* and/or carbonic anhydrase inhibiting diuretic agents is indicated. Li and Herring (1945) have shown that animals treated with corticosteroids or ACTH have an increased tolerance to low oxygen tension. Therefore, these drugs should also be given.

The thermoregulating center is sometimes affected by severe hypoxia, resulting in hyperthermia. In this case the patient should be cooled until consciousness returns. Hypothermia has been shown to be of value in protecting the brain from the after-effects of severe hypoxia by reducing the oxygen demand.

* Urevert. See Appendix A, p. 403 for manufacturer.

The heart is the only other organ which may be affected to any extent by a hypoxic episode. No strain should be placed on this organ and intravenous fluids should be kept to a minimum. The electrolyte balance should be watched to detect possible sodium retention.

Immediately following a severe hypoxic episode, if brain damage is suspected the following treatment is recommended:

1. Administration of 100% oxygen through an endotracheal or nasal catheter until the animal is fully capable of oxygenating himself.
2. Intravenous injection of a diuretic followed by additional injections at regular intervals. (The hematocrit is an indication of the effectiveness of this treatment.)
3. Injections of a corticosteroid for 3 days following which the dose is reduced gradually while ACTH is substituted.
4. Induction of hypothermia if possible. Antibiotics should be given to prevent pneumonia.

Shock

Shock is a general term implying the occurrence of prostration or stupor accompanied by decreased blood pressure. Shock is usually classified as primary or secondary, these differing not only in regard to cause, but also from the standpoint of prognosis and treatment. Primary shock is characterized by a sudden fall in blood pressure, due to vascular dilation, and is accompanied by warm extremities and a slow or normal pulse. Primary shock occurs immediately upon injury, is usually transient, and is thought to be a neurovascular reaction leading to capillary paralysis. It may be manifest as syncope from fear or excitement or may develop as a result of fall in blood pressure due to spinal anesthesia or spinal cord section. Primary shock, if due to nervous factors, may be transient and the patient recover rapidly. Conversely, the reaction may be deep and prolonged and merge into secondary shock without an intervening blood pressure rise, or it may even be fatal due to excessive neurovascular response or adrenal cortical deficiency. In primary shock there is only slight reduction in circulatory blood volume. This is shown in Table 17–1.

Dogs with primary shock have an almost normal bleeding volume, whereas those with secondary shock show marked reduction in volume. Hypotension which occurs with primary shock is usually corrected rapidly and spontaneously and will respond to adrenergic drugs.

Secondary shock is more severe and prolonged and may result from burns, trauma, manipulation of the abdominal viscera, perforation or strangulation of the bowel, peritonitis, or acute or sub-acute hemorrhage. Secondary shock is more delayed in onset, and does not occur immediately after injury, thus it is termed, "secondary". A humoral substance which causes damage to capillary walls is thought to be present. Regardless of cause, the common denominator in secondary shock is reduction in the effective circulating blood volume. This may be caused by external loss of blood or plasma, by internal hemorrhage into damaged organs, or by pooling of blood and leakage from dilated capillaries.

Table 17-1.—Bleeding Volume in Various Types of Shock

Series	Procedure	Number of cases	Average bleeding volume,* per cent of calculated blood volume	Average of group
1	Normal dogs	20	58.6	58.6 (normal)
2	Hyperventilation	5	56.2	
3	Anaphylaxis	5	51.0	
4	Histamine administration	6	50.5	49.9 (primary type of shock)
5	Spinal cord section	6	48.0	
6	Spinal anesthesia	6	44.0	
7	Trauma to an extremity	4	24.6	
8	Hemorrhage	7	24.9	21.8 (secondary type of shock)
9	Plasmapheresis	5	19.7	
10	Intestinal manipulation	6	18.0	

* The bleeding volume is the amount of blood that can be removed after maintaining the blood pressure at a low level by the procedure in question.

(From Drill, V. A.: *Pharmacology in Medicine.* McGraw-Hill Book Co., Inc., New York, 1954.)

Some physiological compensations take place to protect the animal. Among these are arterial and splenic constriction, increased cardiac rate, and selective distribution of the available blood supply. The vital organs are favored over the non-vital ones, causing superficial pallor, skin coldness, and weakened pulse. The most important organs are the central nervous system, heart, liver, and kidneys, the former being the most sensitive to decrease in blood flow. During shock the organism makes every effort to supply blood to the central nervous system and will survive as long as this is adequately maintained. On the other hand, if compensation is not adequate, shock will progress to the irreversible stage resulting in death of the patient. Stagnation of sludged blood in dilated capillaries reduces return flow to the heart. Decreased cardiac output further increases tissue hypoxia and permeability of capillaries. A point is reached at which hypoxic capillaries become permanently damaged and irreversibly permeable to plasma colloids. This state characterizes irreversible shock. When it is reached, the capillary bed will never again be able to retain blood or plasma transfused into the vascular system.

In shock, renal function is progressively diminished due to constriction of the renal vessels with decreased blood flow to the kidneys. A blood pressure of at least 70 mm. Hg is required for kidney function. The blood colloids have an osmotic pressure of 30 mm. Hg, and a pressure of 30 to 40 mm. Hg is required to overcome resistance of the kidney tubule and remainder of the urinary tract. Thus a prolonged fall in blood pressure will result in complete loss of kidney function.

Certain metabolic changes accompany the development of shock. Tissue hypoxia and circulatory stasis result in accumulation of metabolic products, such as carbon dioxide and lactic acid, which produce acidosis. As a consequence, the pH of the blood becomes progressively lower and, as the alkali reserve of the body is diminished, may fall below 7.0. Because of reduced kidney function, the non-protein nitrogen of the blood increases. There is loss of sodium and an increase in potassium of the blood. Coagulability of the blood is decreased. Hemoconcentration produces a rise in the hematocrit, which may serve as a rough measurement of the degree of shock since it is an indirect method of measuring capillary permeability.

Approximately 60% of the blood supply to the liver comes via the portal vein and 40% through the hepatic artery. Numerous workers have shown that interruption of the arterial blood supply to the liver will cause rapid death in dogs due to liver necrosis. If these dogs are treated with antibiotics just prior to ligation, most will survive. Death is due to inability of the liver, deprived of oxygen, to cope with normal clostridial saprophytes which are constantly present in this organ. Very little arterial blood is sufficient to prevent liver necrosis. Following hemorrhagic shock an increase in arterial blood flow to the liver will reduce mortality in dogs. Antibiotic therapy, to check bacterial proliferation, is also effective.

Clinically, shock is characterized by paleness of the skin and mucous membranes from diminished circulation to these organs. Decreased oxygenation due to reduced circulation results in cyanosis. In an effort to compensate for diminished cardiac output the heart rate increases. The pulse is fast and weak because of decreased circulating blood volume. If blood pressure determinations are made, the reading will be less than 90 mm. Hg. In the surgical field, lowered blood pressure and stagnation result in diminished bleeding, darkened blood, and cyanosis of the tissues. The blood viscosity is increased. As the heart becomes progressively more hypoxic, bradycardia will develop.

In an attempt to increase oxygenation of the blood, respirations are accelerated. Shallow respirations are an indication of pulmonary edema caused by increased capillary permeability. Restlessness, depression, weakness, and prostration become evident in unanesthetized animals. The body temperature falls and extremities become cold. There is increased thirst which may be accompanied by vomiting, dryness of the mucous membranes, and diarrhea. As functional activity gradually ebbs the animal will become comatose due to progressive uncompensated circulatory failure. This is an indication of the irreversibility of the shock mechanism. Terminally, the pupils become widely dilated.

In clinical practice, shock is occasionally seen on induction of anesthesia in animals which were normal, insofar as could be determined. This is primary shock due to the anesthetic agent, and is probably a combination of anesthetic toxicity, reduced respiratory exchange, and reduction in blood pressure due to loss of muscle tone with decreased venous return to the heart.

During surgery at least three factors may cause development of secondary shock. These include: (1) hemorrhage, (2) manipulation of the viscera or rough handling of tissues in general, and (3) cooling the abdominal cavity and its contents. According to Dukes (1947) a reduction of 40 to 50% in the blood volume of an unanesthetized dog will result in severe shock. Hay and Webb (1951) found that there is wide variation in the amount of blood loss necessary to produce irreversibility. Experimentally, it varied from 18 to 73% of the blood volume in dogs. Shock can be produced by trauma, such as compression or contusion of tissues, or manipulation of the intestine or other abdominal viscera. It has also been produced in dogs by cooling the abdominal cavity and its contents with water at 15°C. for 2 to 2½ hours. The effects of cooling should, for this reason, be considered in prolonged abdominal surgery.

Shock and the Pituitary-Adrenal System

Selye (1937; 1944) developed the concept of the general adaptation syndrome which explains body reactions occurring in response to systemic stress. In brief this concept consists of the following phases:

1. The alarm reaction.
   a. Shock phase.
   b. Counter-shock phase.
2. The stage of resistance.
3. The stage of exhaustion.

Noxious stimuli, chemical, physical, traumatic, or emotional, evoke non-specific phenomena in the body producing the alarm reaction. During the shock phase there is a fall in body temperature, lowered blood pressure, depression of the central nervous system, decreased muscle tone, excessive tissue breakdown, and anuria. Disturbance of cell membrane permeability results in hyperkalemia, hypochloremia, hemoconcentration, and sometimes acidosis. If death does not immediately intervene due to massive body damage, a phase of countershock follows, during which many of the changes seen in the shock phase are reversed. There is a rise in blood pressure and blood volume accompanied by increased blood chlorides and blood sugar. Pyrexia develops along with leukocytosis and marked eosinopenia. Alkalosis and diuresis may occur.

It should be emphasized that these changes are non-specific and that a wide variety of stressing agents will produce these results. In addition, superimposed on this picture is the direct effect of the stressing agent along with a wide variety of modifying factors which may be present.

If stress is maintained over a period of time, or is repetitive, the body adapts to the situation and is said to become resistant. The phase of resistance, therefore, is characterized by inability to produce the same degree of alarm reaction on repeated or continued application of the same stress.

If, however, the body is stressed repeatedly, or over a long period of time, resistance or adaptation may be overcome and the animal returns to the shock phase. In this so-called exhaustion phase, countershock does not occur and the animal dies.

Recovery from stress is dependent upon an adequate adrenal response or the administration of adrenocortical hormones. Corticotrophin (ACTH) from the anterior pituitary gland mediates activity of the adrenal gland. The release of corticotrophin may be produced by either nervous or humoral stimuli, adrenalin and reduced circulating corticosteroids being responsible for the latter. In stress situations, circulating corticoids are rapidly removed from the blood and metabolized in quantities which under normal circumstances would be toxic.

Unfortunately there is no simple reliable method for determining the adequacy of an animal's adrenal reserve or even its reaction during a stress situation. Eosinophil counts have been used, but this method is open to question. For this reason the decision to administer ACTH or corticosteroids must be based on clinical assessment of the animal's physical status combined with a knowledge of the proposed operative procedure. It is not suggested that corticoid therapy be undertaken as a routine procedure, but rather that it be given only to (1) those animals which are to undergo severe stress, (2) those that have undergone severe stress prior to operation, (3) those which clinically give evidence of deranged hormone balance, and (4) those which have received corticoid therapy within the past 6 months. In this regard, it is well to keep in mind the old adage, "An ounce of prevention is worth a pound of cure."

For best results corticoids should be administered *prior to anesthesia* rather than at the time shock develops. Demand for increased circulating corticoids will start when anesthesia is administered and will continue not only through the operative period, but also for 2 or 3 days immediately following the operation. This need then declines to the normal maintenance level at 8 to 10 days.

To produce and maintain a corticoid level it is necessary that administration be made parenterally and early, since oral medication is often not reliable and intramuscular injections are absorbed slowly. Intravenous corticoids can be given in saline or dextrose during the operative procedure. It is recommended that corticoid be given intramuscularly 24 hours prior to operation, again 12 hours prior to operation and every 12 hours thereafter for 48 to 72 hours. The dose should then be gradually reduced. Oral therapy can be substituted in the tapering off period. It is impossible, within reason, to administer too much corticoid during a stress period. Dangers of overdosage occur only with prolonged treatment.

Under certain circumstances corticoids may be contraindicated since the following may occur:

1. Controlled or inactive infections may spread during corticoid therapy.
2. Wound healing may be delayed resulting in dehiscence.
3. Diabetes mellitus may be aggravated by corticoid administration.
4. In congestive heart failure there will be increased water and salt retention with possible cardiac failure.
5. Administration of corticoids in early pregnancy may produce congenital abnormalities in the fetus.
6. Gastrointestinal ulcers may perforate.

Animals which have been on continuous corticoid therapy for some time must be continued on this treatment during the anesthetic period and throughout the period of recovery. Failure to do so will result in a depletion crisis at a time when there is a greatly increased demand for corticoid substances.

Treatment of Shock

Primary shock, as previously indicated, is often of short duration and can be successfully treated with adrenergic agents. The danger of primary shock lies in the fact that unless the situation is corrected, it may merge into secondary shock with eventual death of the patient. For this reason *immediate* corrective steps should be instituted. If improvement does not occur rapidly, more intensive measures should be undertaken as outlined under secondary shock.

The main treatment of secondary shock should be aimed at restoring the effective circulating blood volume to normal. Otherwise, the use of adrenergic drugs in treatment of secondary shock is valueless.

Under most circumstances whole blood is best for treatment of shock, since it has oxygen carrying ability which other agents do not. In shock without blood loss, such as occurs with burns, plasma is preferable since there is fluid loss without reduction in blood cellular elements. Plasma is also the preferred agent when whole blood is not available. In the absence of either whole blood or plasma, plasma expanders such as dextran or gelatin are indicated. Crystalloid solutions, such as isotonic or hypertonic sodium chloride or glucose, can be used, but do not have the osmotic effects of the foregoing and, therefore, are of only transitory effect. They are most valuable in conjunction with whole blood or plasma in the *prevention* of shock.

In man the results of shock therapy are judged by measuring the systolic blood pressure. Pressures below 90 mm. Hg call for rapid infusion of fluids and injection of vasoconstrictors; with pressures above 90 mm. the slow transfusion of fluids is indicated.

It has been previously stated that the use of vasoconstrictors alone in the treatment of secondary shock is not effective; however, their continuous infusion in conjunction with blood or blood substitutes will more quickly re-establish a normal blood pressure.

Because circulation is impaired, oxygen should be given to assure optimum oxygenation of the blood. Intravenous corticoids will improve the tone of the vascular system and make it responsive to vasoconstrictors. Antibiotic therapy should also be started to protect the animal against facultative pathogens and their toxins.

History of Cardiac Arrest and Resuscitation

In the 16th Century, Vesalius made three great discoveries which initiated the study of cardiac arrest and resuscitation. He developed a method for endotracheal intubation and artificial respiration, described ventricular fibrillation, and made the first attempt to resuscitate a non-beating heart. He also noticed that hypoxia predisposed to ventricular fibrillation.

William Harvey, in the 17th Century, was next to record attempts at cardiac resuscitation. His method differed from that of Vesalius in that he was the first to use manual manipulation as a resuscitative technique.

Moritz Schliff, a professor of physiology at Florence, Italy is credited with laying the basis for future work on cardiac arrest and resuscitation by his experimentation with dogs in the 1870's. He was able, by cardiac massage and endotracheal insufflation, to re-establish the heartbeat in dogs up to $11\frac{1}{2}$ minutes after it had stopped.

In 1900, J. Prus in Lemberg, Germany described studies in cardiac resuscitation of dogs. Artificial respiration and cardiac massage were used and in 16 of 21 killed with chloroform the heart action was restored.

Batelli introduced the electrical defibrillator in 1900, but it was not until 1947 that the first successful defibrillation of a human heart was reported.

Since 1900 many cases of human cardiac resuscitation have been recorded and there is a wealth of literature on this subject. A cardiac arrest registry has been established at the University of Missouri, School of Medicine, and physicians the world over are invited to cooperate in recording cases. Some interesting information has been compiled through this procedure. The incidence of cardiac arrest in man is approximately 1 in every 2,125 operations. The incidence in males is higher than females, the ratio being 1.5:1. Twenty-one per cent of arrests occur in persons in the age group from birth to 10 years of age. By far the greatest number happen in the operating room, 14.2% developing outside in a series of 1,710 cases. Of the 1,710 recorded cases only 11.3% evidenced ventricular fibrillation.

Causes of Cardiac Arrest

For many years hypoxia was thought to be the cause of cardiac arrest. However, in suffocation the heart does not stop in sudden arrest but increases in rate for a short time, following which it gradually slows and eventually stops completely. Hearts removed from animals may beat independently for as long as 10 to 15 minutes. Therefore, it seems that hypoxia *per se* does not cause sudden heart failure; however, it plays a predisposing part in the development of cardiac arrest.

It has been known for at least 50 years that irregularities in the heart beat are associated with the vagus nerve. The efferent vagus fibers are preganglionic and end in peripheral ganglia located in the auricle. Postganglionic fibers then innervate the SA node and the AV node along with the auricular muscle and AV bundle. A constant cardio-inhibitory tone is maintained by the vagus. Reflexes can travel to the heart from the respiratory and gastrointestinal tracts by three routes: (1) through the afferent vagal nerves to the vagal center, thence by an efferent branch to the heart, (2) by an axon reflex in the vagal system, from one branch to another thus bypassing the vagal center, and (3) by spread of vagal impulses to a ganglion, where they are transferred to a branch of the sympathetic system and then to the heart. Stimuli may originate anywhere that vagal nerve endings are present, such as in the pharynx, trachea, and bronchi, or in the large vessels close to the heart.

Young *et al.* (1951) showed that the effects of vagal stimulation on the heart were greatly increased by hypercapnia. As carbon dioxide increased and the blood pH fell, the degree and duration of cardiac asystole on vagal stimulation increased. Atropine sulfate abolished this effect.

In the dog, carbon dioxide accumulation (hypercapnia) and hyperpotassemia increase the cardio-inhibitory effect of vagal stimulation. Conditions which stimulate the vagus and tend to produce reflex inhibition of the heart include vagotomy, traction on the vagus nerve or the pulmonary hilus, endotracheal intubation, bronchoscopy, reflexes caused by aspiration of regurgitated gastric contents or vomition, swallowing of a large food bolus, or manipulation of various organs supplied by the vagus nerve. It has been shown experimentally that obstructive jaundice makes dogs more susceptible to reflex vagal cardiac irregularities, apparently due to increased vagal tone.

The *vago-vagal reflex* is a term used to describe heart block produced by vagal inhibition due to reflex stimuli from afferent vagal fibers. It is thought that the vago-vagal reflex will not produce cardiac arrest in a normal, healthy individual. Reid *et al.* (1952) have stated that three essential mechanisms are necessary for cardiac arrest to occur: (1) there must be disease of the ventricular conduction tissue, (2) there must be depression of the remaining ventricular conduction tissue by drugs or anesthetic agents, and (3) there must be suppression of stimulus formation in the auricles. Normally, regardless of periods of reflex inhibition of the atria, the ventricles can originate a spontaneous contraction. However, if vagal reflexes depress stimulus formation in the auricles and the conduction tissue of the ventricles is diseased, cardiac arrest may occur.

When long surgical procedures are undertaken with closed systems, blood carbon dioxide may accumulate regardless of the fact that the patient is well oxygenated. Under these circumstances the blood pH may fall to below 7.0. Low blood pH prolongs the conduction time of the heart and may lead indirectly to cardiac irregularities and arrest. Carbon dioxide delays conduction but does not suppress stimulus formation in the ventricle. This type of heart failure, which develops slowly, is due to inadequate oxygenation of the common myocardium.

Following prolonged exposure to high levels of carbon dioxide, the serum potassium rises. The source of this potassium is not definitely known but may be the liver, skeletal muscles, and bones. Serious changes in the electrocardiogram are noticed when the serum potassium reaches 8 mEq./liter and at 10 mEq. heart block usually occurs.

In 1913, Levy showed that ventricular fibrillation could be produced in cats under chloroform anesthesia by allowing the animals to struggle during induction, by intermittent administration of chloroform, or by increasing the chloroform concentration suddenly. A high incidence of cardiac arrhythmias occurs with cyclopropane anesthesia. For this reason it is contraindicated in cardiac surgery, in surgery of the great vessels, and in hyperthyroidism.

Curare and curare-like drugs produce a high incidence of anesthetic deaths due to cardiac arrest. Beecher and Todd (1954) have reported a series in which mortality was particularly high when curare and ether were combined.

Ethyl chloride has definite toxic effects on the heart as evidenced by cardiac arrhythmias and its use has been abandoned by most human anesthesiologists. In a series of 33 cats anesthetized with trichloroethylene, all had abnormal electrocardiograms (Johnson *et al.*, 1958). The most frequent abnormality was development of ectopic ventricular systoles and about two-thirds showed auricular fibrillation. They stated that trichloroethylene produced myocardial damage as evidenced by the electrocardiograms.

Surprisingly, the cat and species lower on the phylogenetic scale are capable of spontaneous ventricular defibrillation, whereas higher species including dogs, primates, and man are not.

Diagnosis of Cardiac Arrest

Frequently there is little indication that a patient is about to undergo cardiac arrest, although signs such as cyanosis, bradycardia, hypotension, changes in respiration, changes in the electrocardiogram (downward displacement of the pacemaker, repetitive ectopic beats, change in A-V or interventricular conduction), and unexplained changes in the level of anesthesia may serve as a warning. During open thoracic or abdominal procedures there is little problem since heart action and pulsation of the large vessels can be directly visualized. Palpation of large vessels, such as the femoral, is satisfactory to determine if there is cardiac output and a pulse. Examination of the fundus of the eye with an ophthalmoscope has been advocated, but it is highly unlikely that such an instrument will be available. Prolonged auscultation with a stethoscope is to be condemned. Swann and Brucer (1949) have pointed out that all heart sounds cease in dogs at a systolic pressure of 50 mm. Hg and, therefore, if no sounds are heard, circulation has probably failed. Electrocardiographic tracings will indicate cardiac standstill in most instances; however, an electrocardiograph is not often attached to the patient during an operation. The time necessary to attach one, allow it to warm up, and make a tracing is too long for successful resuscitation to follow. Cardiac monitors can be used on every patient undergoing general anesthesia; their worth, however, remains to be clearly proved.

Electroencephalographic tracings provide an excellent means of determining cessation of circulation. There will be an absence of alpha, beta, and gamma waves within about 20 seconds after total anoxia of the brain. Thus, cerebral anoxia may be noted before electrocardiographic tracings show cessation of electrical activity in the heart.

Respirations usually cease within a few seconds following cardiac arrest. Unfortunately, respiratory arrest is often the first sign noted though cardiac arrest has been present for some time. Cyanosis, on the other hand, is not necessarily a reliable sign of cardiac arrest.

It is now generally agreed that if there is a question of cardiac standstill, an open thoracotomy should be immediately performed. Johnson and Kirby (1954) state, "This may seem like an unnecessary, aggressive policy to those who are not familiar with this catastrophe because of the possibilities that the heart may be beating so feebly that signs of effective circulation are lacking. It is true that this possibility does exist, but we believe that this risk must be accepted."

Mistakes in diagnosis will inevitably occur; however, the fear of an occasional mistaken diagnosis should not deter immediate resuscitative measures. Mullens (1955), commenting on a case in which the heart was found to be beating with normal rhythm but very weakly, stated, "No surgeon should apologize for such an eventuality. The hesitant surgeon can convince himself of a distant beat in what is actually a silent chest. Thoracotomy is a much safer procedure than spending precious time at prolonged auscultation."

An alternative to direct cardiac massage is closed chest massage in which the heart is compressed by pressure on the chest wall. Swann and Brucer (1951) successfully resuscitated small dogs by closed chest cardiac massage and oxygen administration. Their technique was to place the dog on its side and, with a hand on either side of the chest, compress the chest over the heart 100 times a minute. A blood pressure of approximately 110/30 could be produced by this method.

Open and closed-chest massage have been compared in dogs by Redding and Cozine (1961). After producing ventricular fibrillation in pentobarbital-anesthetized dogs by electrical shock, closed-chest massage was begun by compressing the sternum against the vertebral column 100 times a minute (Fig. 17–1). Intermittent positive pressure breathing was also maintained. This combination was continued for 20 minutes following which an external defibrillator was applied to the chest and the heart defibrillated. In a like series of dogs, the chest was opened and the heart manually massaged following induction of fibrillation. Little difference was found in carotid blood pressures obtained with either method. With closed-chest massage, carotid blood flows averaged 12% of the control flow prior to ventricular fibrillation, while aortic blood pressure averaged 31% of the control. With open-chest massage, carotid flow was 19% and aortic blood pressure 37% of control values.

In pilot studies with the closed-chest technique, severe trauma resulted when maximal force was used to obtain the highest possible blood pressure. Mediastinal hemorrhage, fractured ribs, and lacerations of the liver were frequently produced. Survival depended upon the use of moderately forceful compression. Distortion of the chest contour was almost invariably produced, even in surviving animals, by fractures of the costal cartilages.

Fatigue of the operator produced by the two methods varied strikingly. With open-chest massage at least two operators were necessary, whereas one could effectively continue closed-chest massage for 20 minutes. With both methods circulation was effectively restored following defibrillation. It should be emphasized, however, that unless the animal is connected to an electrocardiograph, which is highly unlikely, there is no means of determining whether the heart is fibrillating unless the chest is opened.

Clinical attempts at cardiac resuscitation in small animals have been discouraging. While resuscitation can be performed almost routinely on dogs over-anesthetized with pentobarbital in the physiology laboratory, naturally occurring arrests do not respond as favorably. This is probably due to factors not found in normal dogs, since most patients are obviously not normal.

Hoerlein (1955) has reported one dog which survived but suffered permanent visual impairment. In several other animals he reports temporary cardiac recovery followed by fall in blood pressure and death. This has been the experience of many veterinarians, animals usually dying within 24 hours following arrest. An exception to this rule is arrest or fibrillation occurring during cardiac surgery. Here immediate steps can be taken and the success ratio is higher.

Cardiac arrest is essentially a 3-minute emergency and this must be kept constantly in mind. Delay in diagnosis and institution of resuscitation will invariably be fatal. Delay in diagnosis is responsible for approximately 85% of the failures to resuscitate successfully. The best rule of thumb is that if there is no palpable apex beat or evidence of pulse pressure, and both have disappeared suddenly, then cardiac arrest has occurred. Patients seldom survive a delay of more than 4 minutes before artificial circulation is maintained by massage. The greatest time lapse usually is between arrest and diagnosis. This period is often spent by the anesthetist in a futile search for a stethoscope, in injecting ineffective stimulants, in searching for an

24

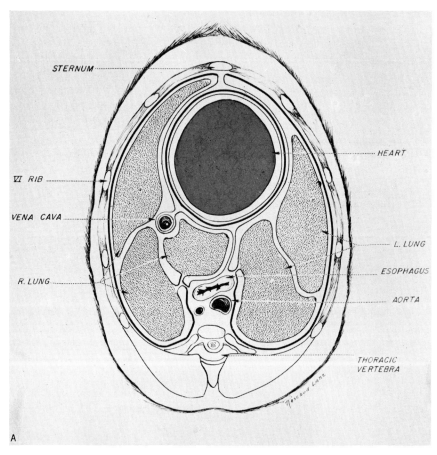

FIGURE 17–1A

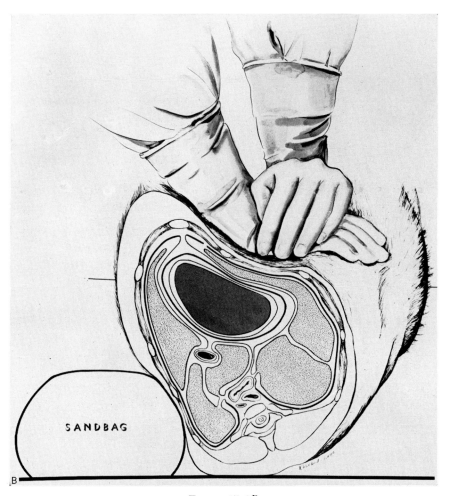

FIGURE 17–1B

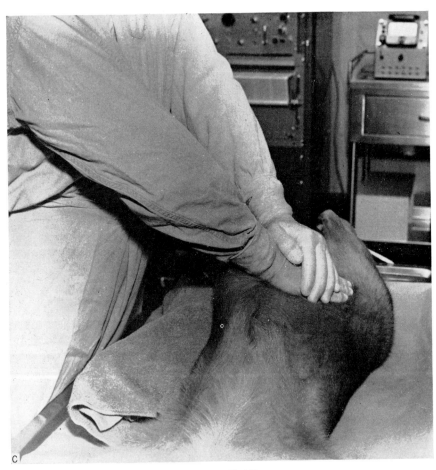

FIGURE 17–1C

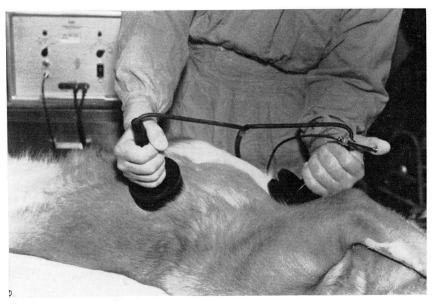

FIGURE 17–1D

FIGURE 17–1. Closed chest massage. Cross section of the canine thorax through sixth thoracic vertebra (A). External massage producing compression of heart (B). Position of hands; the heel of hand is placed slightly to left of the midsternum (C). Placement of external defibrillator electrodes over the manubrium and on the left precordial region. (From Ott, B. S.: Closed Chest Cardiac Resuscitation. Small Animal Clin., 2, 572, 1962.)

endotracheal catheter, in looking for the instruments necessary for thoracotomy, or in seeking a consultant.

Injection of epinephrine and other stimulants is to be at least partially condemned. It is unlikely that this procedure will revive arrested hearts, although this may occasionally occur. Analeptics increase the metabolic activity of the cortical cells and, if effective massage is instituted, will contribute to cortical hypoxia. A second disadvantage to injection of stimulants lies in the time lag involved in filling a syringe, making the injection, and waiting to see if the procedure is effective. This can easily prove fatal.

According to DeCamp (1953) the human heart stops in diastole 90% of the time and in ventricular fibrillation 10%. Booth *et al.* (1958) found 2 of 21 dogs' hearts developed fibrillation after a lethal dose of pentobarbital, the remaining 19 exhibiting complete arrest. Cessation in systole is extremely rare. The diagnosis of ventricular fibrillation sometimes presents a problem. Even with the chest open, it may be difficult to determine whether a heart is fibrillating, particularly when it is examined through the intact pericardial sac. Electrocution is probably the only situation in which ventricular fibrillation is a good possibility. Fibrillation can probably be diagnosed as well by palpation as by visualization. Many authors have described the "worm-like" nature of fibrillation. This is due to blocks of myocardial tissue contracting with different rates, rhythms, and degrees of strength.

Treatment of Cardiac Arrest

Cardiac arrest can be successfully corrected, provided it is recognized immediately and the appropriate steps speedily accomplished. Oxygenated blood must be pumped to the brain within 3 minutes after arrest occurs. The procedure is as follows:

1. An endotracheal catheter is inserted, the cuff inflated, and the catheter attached to a resuscitator, gas machine, or some other means of positive pressure ventilation. Rhythmic lung inflation ·is immediately commenced to assure adequate oxygenation of the blood.

2. Without any preparation, the chest is opened immediately through the sixth intercostal space on either side. A hand is inserted through the incision and the heart grasped between the thumb and forefingers. The heart is squeezed rhythmically at a rate of approximately 60 times a minute.

3. If an assistant is available the rib incision is enlarged and a rib retractor inserted in order to facilitate exposure of the heart. The assistant then starts an intravenous drip of dextran, gelatin, or other plasma substitute.

4. If the heart is flabby and without tone, continued massage may, by increasing the coronary circulation, initiate return of the beat. If the beat does not return, 1 to 5 ml. of 1% calcium chloride solution can be injected into the left ventricle. If the beat is still not produced, 1 to 3 ml. of 1:10,000 epinephrine hydrochloride may be injected into the left ventricle. Neither of these solutions should be repeated in less than 10 minutes.

5. If it is thought the heart is in ventricular fibrillation, the pericardium should be incised and the heart exposed. It will have a bluish tinge and contract like "a bundle of worms". Massage should be continued vigorously until cardiac tone and color improve. The electrodes of a defibrillator are then applied on either side of the heart and a shock administered. This procedure may need to be repeated several times in order to effect defibrillation. If not successful initially, 1 to 3 ml. of 1:10,000 epinephrine can be injected directly into the lumen of the left ventricle, followed by a short period of massage and then another shock with the defibrillator.

6. Following successful defibrillation the intravenous administration of plasma expander should be continued. A vasoconstrictor such as levarterenol can be added to this solution to maintain effective blood pressure. A corticosteroid should also be given, preferably by intravenous drip.

7. Following defibrillation the heart should be observed for at least 30 minutes prior to closure of the chest incision. Closure should not be done unless the heart is beating vigorously.

8. Further treatment should include administration of antibiotics to forestall infection and corticosteroid to combat stress. On theoretical grounds at least, once the shock state has passed a diuretic is indicated to prevent cerebral edema from the hypoxic episode.

Regurgitation and Vomiting

Regurgitation is the *passive* discharge of stomach contents into the pharynx. It may occur in dogs during anesthesia, despite adequate preanesthetic preparation, since relaxation of the cardia allows gastric contents to flow up the esophagus if the animal is positioned in dorsal recumbency. Often the flow of material from the mouth is the only evidence that this has occurred. Gastric juice is brown in color and contains dark flocculent material. While regurgitation under anesthesia is usually not as serious as vomition, immediate steps should be taken to remove regurgitated material as outlined below.

Occasionally it is necessary to anesthetize an animal without preanesthetic preparation and vomiting may occur on induction or during anesthesia. Usually vomition is preceded by several abortive retching movements which are easily recognized, having once been observed. *Immediate treatment is necessary* to prevent unfavorable sequelae and even fatality from this event. As soon as retching movements occur the following steps should be taken:

1. If anesthetic is being administered, it should be stopped immediately, the operating table tilted so that the patient is positioned with his head down, and oxygen given either through the mouth or with a nasal catheter.
2. The pharynx and larynx should be cleared of vomitus manually and with suction, if available.
3. The larynx and bronchial tree should be cleaned by direct laryngoscopy and bronchoscopy.
4. The bronchial tree should be lavaged with saline or mild sodium bicarbonate solution.
5. An endotracheal catheter should be inserted and the cuff inflated to prevent further aspiration in the event vomiting again occurs.

Specific drug therapy is indicated to prevent inflammation and infection in the respiratory tract. This should include:

1. A corticosteroid intravenously followed by intramuscular injections for the next 2 or 3 days.
2. ACTH gel, 5 to 15 units, daily for 4 days.
3. A broad spectrum antibiotic either intravenously or intramuscularly.
4. Continued administration of oxygen, either through a nasal catheter or in an oxygen chamber, if necessary to maintain adequate oxygenation.
5. Aminophylline (0.05 to 0.2 gm.) intravenously or in suppositories twice daily for 2 or 3 days for its bronchodilating effect.
6. Expectorant cough mixtures to produce thin bronchial secretions which may aid in removal of vomitus not removed by manual cleaning.
7. Inhalation of a detergent aerosol which may aid in prevention of atelectasis.

Convulsions

Convulsions during general anesthesia are quite rare and result most frequently from administration of ethyl or vinyl ether to a hyperthermic animal. Dehydration and acidosis are probably contributing factors. Convulsions usually occur at a rectal temperature between 41 and 42° C. Halothane has little tendency to produce this phenomenon, and therefore may be of particular value in anesthetizing febrile patients (Pittinger *et al.*, 1961). A thiobarbiturate should be injected intravenously to control convulsions, the inhalant anesthetic stopped, and the patient cooled by immersion in water.

Convulsions due to local anesthetics have been discussed in Chapter 13, p. 246.

References

BEECHER, H. K. and TODD, D. T.: A Study of the Deaths Associated with Anesthesia and Surgery. Ann. Surg., *140*, 2, 1954.

BOOTH, N. H., WILL, D. H., Moss, L. C., and SWENSON, M. J.: An Electrical Apparatus and Its Application in Defibrillating the Heart of the Dog. J.A.V.M.A., *132*, 117, 1958.

DeCAMP, P. T.: Nature and Management of Cardiac Arrest. J. Louisiana Med. Soc., *105*, 311, 1953.

DUKES, H. H.: *The Physiology of Domestic Animals.* 6th ed. Comstock Publishing Co., Inc., Ithaca, New York, 1947.

HALL, L. W.: Accidents and Emergencies in Anesthesia. Modern Vet. Practice, *40*, 28, 1959.

HAY, E. B. and WEBB, J. K.: The Effect of Increased Arterial Blood Flow to the Liver on the Mortality Rate Following Hemorrhagic Shock. Surgery, *29*, 826, 1951.

HOERLEIN, B. F.: Cardiac Resuscitation in a Dog with Cardiac Arrest. J.A.V.M.A., *127*, 210, 1955.

JOHNSON, J. and KIRBY, C. K.: Cardiac Standstill and Ventricular Fibrillation. Am. Pract. and Digest Treat., *5*, 264, 1954.

JOHNSON, V. L., KLAVANO, P. A., WRIGHT, R., and SACKS, D.: Some Effects of Trichlorethylene on the Electrocardiogram of the Cat. Vet. Med., *53*, 375, 1958.

LI, C. H. and HERRING, V. V.: Effect of Adrenocorticotropic Hormone on the Survival of Normal Rats During Anoxia. Am. J. Physiol., *143*, 548, 1945.

MULLENS, J. E.: Cardiac Arrest. Canad. M. A. J., *72*, 838, 1955.

PITTINGER, C., MITCHELL, C., ALEU, F., and PAGE, W.: Convulsive Phenomena in Hyperthermic Dogs During Anesthesia. Anesthesiology, *22*, 893, 1961.

PRUS, J.: Ueber Die Weiderbelebung in Todesfallen in Folge von Erstickung, Chloroformvergiftung und Elektrischem Schlage. 1. Weiderbelebung nach Erstickung; 2. Weiderbelebung nach Chloroformtod. Wein. klin. Wchnschr., *13*, 451, 1900.

REDDING, J. S. and COZINE, R. A.: A Comparison of Open-Chest and Closed-Chest Cardiac Massage in Dogs. Anesthesiology, *22*, 280, 1961.

REID, L. C., STEPHENSON, H. E., JR., and HINTON, J. W.: Cardiac Arrest. A.M.A. Arch. Surg., *64*, 409, 1952.

SELYE, H.: Studies on Adaptation. Endocrinology, *21*, 169, 1937.

SELYE, H.: General Adaptation Syndrome. Josiah Macy, Jr., Foundation Conference on Metabolic Aspects of Convalescence Including Bone and Wound Healing. 8th Meeting, New York City, October 1944.

SWANN, H. G. and BRUCER, M.: The Cardiorespiratory and Biochemical Events During Rapid Anoxic Death. I. Fulminating Anoxia. Texas Reports Biol. Med., *7*, 511, 1949.

SWANN, H. G. and BRUCER, M.: The Sequence of Circulatory, Respiratory and Cerebral Failure During the Process of Death; Its Relation to Resuscitability. Texas Reports Biol. Med., *9*, 180, 1951.

YOUNG, G. W., JR., SEALY, W. C., HARRIS, J., and BOTWIN, A.: The Effects of Hypercapnia and Hypoxia on the Response of the Heart to Vagal Stimulation. Surg. Gynec., & Obst., *93*, 51, 1951.

————: The Prevention of Anesthetic Accidents. Lederle Bulletin Newsletter, July, 1950.

AFTERCARE

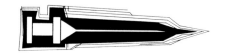

Chapter 18

WHILE in most instances recovery from anesthesia is uneventful, the patient should be kept under observation during the recovery period to prevent any untoward sequelae. In large hospitals it is wise to have a recovery room for this purpose, since all the necessary equipment, drugs, and materials can be kept in one place and there is less difficulty is watching several animals. In some instances the "prep" room may also serve as the recovery room.

Following removal from the operating room, the animal should be placed in its cage in lateral recumbency. A blanket, or even newspaper, should be placed under and over the patient to conserve body heat. The tongue should be pulled forward to preclude its blocking the pharynx. The water pan should always be removed from the cage to prevent accidental drowning in the event the semi-conscious patient should place his nose and mouth in the container. Under no circumstances should an anesthetized animal be placed in the same cage as a conscious one, since the former cannot protect itself. Cannibalism has been known to occur, particularly where the anesthetized patient had an open wound!

When preanesthetic sedation has not been used, animals may thrash and struggle, bruising themselves severely and even breaking teeth during the recovery period. Coursing breeds, such as greyhounds, Russian wolfhounds, and Afghans, are particularly prone to this phenomenon. Use of a narcotic, such as meperidine, in small doses will quiet animals in this condition. Plastic-covered sponge rubber mats in recovery cages will also afford protection.

Following pentobarbital an occasional animal will have an extremely prolonged recovery period. Cats are more prone to this than dogs, sometimes sleeping as long as 72 hours before arousing. Special attention must be given these animals to prevent hypostatic congestion and subsequent pneumonia. They should, of course, be kept warm and turned frequently. In addition, prophylactic antibiotic therapy should be given and a protective ophthalmic ointment instilled in the eyes to prevent corneal drying. Intravenous electrolyte solutions in moderate amounts will prevent dehydration. If barbiturates have been used, dextrose or lactate solutions should be avoided because of their re-anesthetizing potential.

Anesthetized animals should be kept warm but it must be remembered that they cannot escape from excessive heat. Occasionally they may be badly burned or even killed by injudicious use of heating pads or other warming devices (Fig. 18–1). Often during the recovery period, the temperature of cats will fall to as low as 94° F. without ill effect. It must be remembered that a low temperature *per se* is not a sign of impending catastrophe. Relatively safe methods for applying heat include infrared heat lamps, hot water bottles, and blankets.

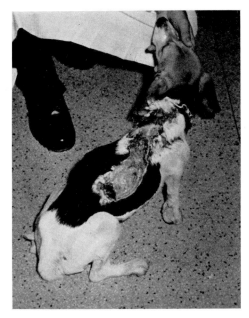

FIGURE 18–1.   Skin slough due to positioning animal during anesthesia on a heating pad which became excessively hot.

Proper ventilation of the area in which the animal is recovering must also be afforded. In hot humid climates animals may sometimes die from heat prostration caused by struggling during recovery.

Constrictive bandaging of the head or throat must be avoided because of the danger of asphyxiation. Occasionally cats which have been tightly bandaged around the abdomen will evidence posterior paralysis on recovery. This is apparently due to circulatory obstruction to the hindquarters and removal of the bandage quickly restores them to normal.

If an endotracheal catheter is left in position during the recovery period it must be removed as soon as the patient regains the swallowing reflex. Otherwise, it may be chewed and swallowed or aspirated.

As soon as the animal regains the righting reflex, the water pan should be returned to the cage and the animal encouraged to drink a small quantity. Food may be offered as soon as the patient can stand.

Further postanesthetic care will be dictated by the animal's condition and the procedure(s) for which anesthesia was administered.

It is unwise to send anesthetized animals home, since owners are generally unable to cope with any unusual situation which may arise. In addition, they may become alarmed by the signs of approaching consciousness and demand service unnecessarily during the night or other inconvenient hours.

STATISTICS
AND
RECORDS

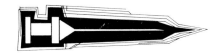

Chapter 19

Reasons for Keeping Records
Survey of Anesthetic Fatalities at the
  Angell Memorial Animal Hospital
Data Collection

Survey of Anesthetic Fatalities at Colorado
  State University
Non-Fatal Complications

Reasons for Keeping Records

Death of a patient from any cause is always unpleasant, but a fatality from anesthesia is even more so since it is obviously induced by the anesthetist. One will occasionally hear a veterinarian state that he has never lost an animal from anesthesia. This is conceivably true, though highly unlikely if a sizeable number of animals have been anesthetized. Obviously, the criteria for anesthetic mortality in this instance must be defined. It is human nature to forget the disagreeable and to excuse a fatality by blaming it onto something over which the anesthetist has no control.

As long as anesthetics are administered the hazard of death can never be eliminated completely; it can, however, be minimized, particularly if one is willing to investigate and learn from mistakes. Once an anesthetic fatality has occurred, a searching review should be made of events leading to it and a necropsy should be performed to piece together its pathogenesis and etiology. Armed with this information the anesthetist can then take steps to prevent a recurrence of this tragedy.

Unfortunately there is little recorded information concerning mortality in small animals anesthetized in clinical practice. This is due to the fact that (1) busy practitioners do not have time to collect the necessary data, (2) there is no economic gain to be derived from such collection, and (3) there is lack of interest on the part of individuals best able to obtain this data. Even clinics of veterinary schools in the United States have little valid information on this subject.

(381)

Survey of Anesthetic Fatalities at the Angell Memorial Animal Hospital

Albrecht and Blakely (1951) have presented a 5-year survey of anesthetic mortality at the Angell Memorial Animal Hospital, Boston, Massachusetts. The criterion they used for establishing death under anesthesia is one suggested by Waters and Gillespie (1944) which classifies any death occurring from the time of induction of anesthesia until the patient either returns to consciousness

Table 19–1.—Analysis of Anesthetic Deaths at the Angell Memorial Animal Hospital, 1946–1950

Anesthetic	Number Anesthetized	Number Died	Per Cent Mortality
Ether	577	3	0.519
Pentothal	3,828	6	0.156
Pentothal-ether	212	1	0.47
Pentobarbital-ether	233	4	1.71
Pentobarbital	16,747	50	0.29
Totala—all nesthetics	21,597	64	0.295

(From Albrecht, D. T. and Blakely, C. L.: Anesthetic Mortality: A Five-Year Survey of the Records of the Angell Memorial Animal Hospital. J.A.V.M.A., *119*, 429, 1951.)

Table 19–2.—Anesthetic Mortality According to Species (Angell Memorial Animal Hospital, 1946–1950)

Species of Animal	Number Anesthetized	Number of Fatalities	Per Cent Mortality	Ratio
Dogs	14,640	38	0.259	1:385
Cats	6,936	25	0.360	1:277
Misc.*	21	1	4.762	1:21

* Unspecified number of rabbits, monkeys, goats, 1 skunk, 1 raccoon.
(From Albrecht, D. T. and Blakely, C. L.: Anesthetic Mortality: A Five-Year Survey of the Records of the Angell Memorial Animal Hospital. J.A.V.M.A., *119*, 429, 1951.)

or to his original preoperative condition as an anesthetic death. Using this standard, deaths may be due to (1) the anesthetic (2) the surgical procedure (3) the condition of the patient or (4) any combination or all of the foregoing. In most cases the fatal outcome is the result of a combination of factors and it is difficult or impossible to assign the exact responsibility of each (Tables 19–1, 19–2).

It should be noted that these animals were all in-patients and these figures do not include animals anesthetized in the out-patient clinic. It is reasonable to assume that a somewhat higher mortality rate might result in out-patients since they are not anesthetized under such ideal conditions.

The average age of animals which died was 5 years, ranging from 12 weeks to 14 years. Little difference was noted between males and females, there being 29 males, 32 females, and 3 animals in which the

Table 19-3.—Summary of All Fatalities According to Diagnosis (Angell Memorial Animal Hospital, 1946–1950)

Diagnosis	Fatalities
Trauma	20
Spay for disease or pregnancy	9
Spay for sterilization	6
Abscess	6
Urethral calculi	5
Foreign body	4
Dentistry	4
Miscellaneous	10

(From Albrecht, D. T. and Blakely, C. L.: Anesthetic Mortality: A Five-Year Survey of the Records of the Angell Memorial Animal Hospital. J.A.V.M.A., *119*, 429, 1951.)

Table 19-4.—Breed Incidence of Fatalities, All Anesthetics (Angell Memorial Animal Hospital, 1946–1950)

Breed	Number
Fox Terrier	6
Boston Terrier	6
Terrier type	5
Cocker Spaniel	3
Boxer	2
Collie type	2
Irish Terrier	2
English Setter	1
Irish Setter	1
Chow	1
Scottish Terrier	1
Toy Collie	1
Spitz	1
Spitz-Pomeranian	1
Pug	1
Pekingese	1
Shepherd type	1
Beagle	1
Yorkshire Terrier	1
Total Dogs	38
Total Cats	25
Total Rabbits	1
TOTAL	64

(From Albrecht, D. T. and Blakely, C. L.: Anesthetic Mortality: A Five-Year Survey of the Records of the Angell Memorial Animal Hospital J.A.V.M.A., *119*, 429, 1951.)

sex was not recorded. Table 19–3 summarizes the fatalities according to clinical diagnosis prior to anesthesia. The breed incidence in dogs which died is listed in Table 19–4. The authors point out that 32% of the animals dying suffered from traumatic conditions and that the high incidence in fox terriers can probably be explained by the fact that five of six which died suffered from trauma. Also, 26.9% of the 37 dogs which died were brachycephalic breeds.

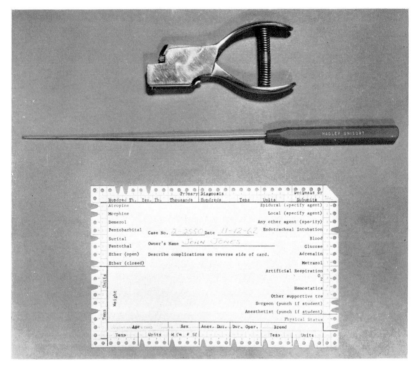

FIGURE 19–1.   A marginal punched card with punch and sorting needle. The card was made for a male cocker spaniel, 1 year of age, which weighed 25 pounds and was in physical status II. It was given preanesthetic morphine-atropine, anesthetized with Surital-ether, and a gastrotomy of 1-hour duration was performed. The anesthesia also lasted 1 hour.

Data Collection

To obtain meaningful data concerning anesthesia, certain information must be collected and definite criteria established. For those interested in keeping statistics the use of marginal punched cards (Fig. 19–1) is suggested. The holes along the margins are coded according to the information it is desired to record (Schwabe and Davis, 1954). The face of each card may have the code printed on it or a master code card may be used and the other cards punched using it as the key. A card is made for each animal anesthetized, with the owner's name and the case number written on it. The remainder of the data is punched around the margins. Additional information which cannot be recorded in code form may be written on the face and back of the card when necessary. Among the items which can be recorded are:

1. Species, breed, age, sex, weight, and physical status of the animal.
2. Surgical procedure or other reason for anesthesia.
3. Preanesthetic agents given.
4. Anesthetic agents used and method of administration.
5. Person administering anesthesia (veterinarian, student, lay personnel).
6. Duration of anesthesia.
7. Difficulties encountered and method of correction.

It can be seen that tabulation of this data will not only give extensive information on anesthesia but also the incidence of surgical diseases in various age groups and breeds.

Obviously, moribund patients are not good anesthetic risks, and if a single agent is used to anesthetize them the mortality rate for this agent may appear to be disproportionately high. In discussing anesthetic mortality, therefore, it is necessary to categorize the physical status of the patient (Table 2–1, p. 23).

It should be emphasized that physical status and anesthetic risk are entirely different. In determining anesthetic risk many factors must be considered including the degree of skill of the anesthetist, the anesthetic to be employed, and the physical status of the patient. In determining operative risk the foregoing must be appraised and, in addition, the operation to be performed and the skill of the surgeon must also be taken into consideration.

Survey of Anesthetic Fatalities at Colorado State University

During the years 1955 through 1957* records were kept of all small animal anesthesias at the Colorado State University Veterinary Hospital, using marginal punched cards as shown in Figure 19–1. Results of 2,912 anesthetic periods in dogs and cats, using a wide variety of preanesthetics and general anesthetics, are summarized in Tables 19–5 through 19–15.

An anesthetic death was defined as *any death occurring from the time of induction until the righting reflex returned, regardless of cause.* The mortality rate was considerably higher than that reported by Albrecht and Blakely (1951). Two reasons for this may be that (1) almost all animals at Colorado State University were anesthetized by students (92.54%), and (2) not all animals anesthetized at the Angell Memorial Animal Hospital were included in their survey.

* Except summer months.

Agent(s)	Species	Physical Status	Total	Died*	Per Cent Mortality†	Totals All Categories of Physical Status	
Pentobarbital	Canine	I	939	5	0.532		
		II	384	6	1.562	Total Anesthetized	1401
		III	62			Died	13
						Per Cent Mortality	0.928
		IV	16	2	12.50		
	Feline	I	234	3	1.282		
		II	37	1	2.702	Total Anesthetized	282
		III	10	1	10.00	Died	5
						Per Cent Mortality	1.773
		IV	1				
Thiamylal	Canine	I	118				
		II	361			Total Anesthetized	551
		III	64			Died	2
						Per Cent Mortality	0.363
		IV	8	2	25.00		
	Feline	I	114				
		II	44			Total Anesthetized	175
		III	15			Died	1
						Per Cent Mortality	0.571
		IV	2	1	50.00		
Thiopental	Canine	I					
		II	1			Total Anesthetized	1
		III				Died	
						Per Cent Mortality	0.0
		IV					
	Feline	I	1				
		II				Total Anesthetized	1
		III				Died	
						Per Cent Mortality	0.0
		IV			·		
Combuthal	Canine	I	3				
		II	5			Total Anesthetized	9
		III	1	1	100.00	Died	1
						Per Cent Mortality	11.111
		IV					

Agent(s)	Species	Physical Status	Total	Died*	Per Cent Mortality†	Totals All Categories of Physical Status
Combuthal	Feline	I	2			
		II	1			Total Anesthetized 3
		III				Died
		IV				Per Cent Mortality 0.0
Pentobarbital-Thiamylal	Canine	I	11			
		II	14			Total Anesthetized 28
		III	1			Died 1
		IV	2	1	50.00	Per Cent Mortality 3.571
	Feline	I	2			
		II	1			Total Anesthetized 4
		III	1			Died
		IV				Per Cent Mortality 0.0
Ether (S)‡	Canine	I				
		II	1			Total Anesthetized 1
		III				Died
		IV				Per Cent Mortality 0.0
Ether (C)§	Canine	I	1			
		II	4			Total Anesthetized 6
		III	1			Died
		IV				Per Cent Mortality 0.0
	Feline	I				
		II				Total Anesthetized 6
		III	2			Died 1
		IV	4	1	25.00	Per Cent Mortality 16.667
Ether (S & C)	Canine	I				
		II				Total Anesthetized 2
		III	1			Died 1
		IV	1	1	100.00	Per Cent Mortality 50.00

Table 19-5.—Physical Status and Per Cent Mortality of 2912 Dogs and Cats Anesthetized with Various Agents (Colorado State University, 1955-1957) (Continued)

Agent(s)	Species	Physical Status	Total	Died*	Per Cent Mortality†	Totals All Categories of Physical Status
Pentobarbital-Ether (S)		I	9			
		II	3			Total Anesthetized 13
	Canine					Died
		III	1			Per Cent Mortality 0.0
		IV				
		I	5	1	20.00	
		II	1			Total Anesthetized 6
	Feline					Died 1
		III				Per Cent Mortality 16.667
		IV				
Pentobarbital-Ether (C)		I	4			
		II	9			Total Anesthetized 16
	Canine					Died
		III	1			Per Cent Mortality 0.0
		IV	2			
		I	1			
		II				Total Anesthetized 1
	Feline					Died
		III				Per Cent Mortality 0.0
		IV				
Thiamylal-Ether (C)		I	55	1	1.818	
		II	113	1	0.885	Total Anesthetized 232
	Canine					Died 8
		III	40	1	2.50	Per Cent Mortality 3.448
		IV	24	5	20.833	
		I				
		II				Total Anesthetized 1
	Feline					Died 1
		III				Per Cent Mortality 100.0
		IV	1	1	100.00	
Thiamylal-Ether (S)		I				
		II	1			Total Anesthetized 1
	Feline					Died
		III				Per Cent Mortality 0.0
		IV				

Agent(s)	Species	Physical Status	Total	Died*	Per Cent Mortality†	Totals All Categories of Physical Status	
Combuthal-Ether (C)	Canine	I	1				
		II				Total Anesthetized	1
		III				Died	
		IV				Per Cent Mortality	0.0
Thiopental-Ether (C)	Canine	I					
		II	2			Total Anesthetized	2
		III				Died	
		IV				Per Cent Mortality	0.0
Pentobarbital-Thiamylal-Ether (C)	Canine	I	1				
		II				Total Anesthetized	1
		III				Died	
		IV				Per Cent Mortality	0.0
Halothane (C)	Canine	I					
		II				Total Anesthetized	1
		III	1			Died	
		IV				Per Cent Mortality	0.0
Pentobarbital-Halothane (C)	Canine	I	1				
		II	2			Total Anesthetized	4
		III				Died	
		IV	1			Per Cent Mortality	0.0
Thiamylal-Halothane (C)	Canine	I	39	1	2.564		
		II	65			Total Anesthetized	134
		III	24			Died	1
		IV	6			Per Cent Mortality	0.746
Thiopental-Halothane (C)	Canine	I					
		II				Total Anesthetized	1
		III	1			Died	
		IV				Per Cent Mortality	0.0

Table 19–5.—Physical Status and Per Cent Mortality of 2912 Dogs and Cats Anesthetized with Various Agents (Colorado State University, 1955–1957) (Continued)

Agent(s)	Species	Physical Status	Total	Died*	Per Cent Mortality†	Totals All Categories of Physical Status
Combuthal-Halothane (C)	Canine	I	2			
		II				Total Anesthetized 2
		III				Died
		IV				Per Cent Mortality 0.0
Thiamylal-Cyclopropane (C)	Feline	I				
		II				Total Anesthetized 1
		III				Died
		IV	1			Per Cent Mortality 0.0
Ethyl Chloride (S)	Feline	I	1			
		II				Total Anesthetized 3
		III	2			Died
		IV				Per Cent Mortality 0.0
Trichloro-ethylene (S)	Feline	I	17			
		II	5			Total Anesthetized 22
		III				Died
		IV				Per Cent Mortality 0.0
All agents—both species			2912	36	1.236	

* Includes all animals dying for any reason between induction of anesthesia and return of righting reflex.

† Per cent mortality $= \dfrac{\text{Number dead}}{\text{Number anesthetized}}$

‡ S = Administered by semi-open drop method.

§ C = Administered in a closed system with carbon dioxide absorption by soda lime.

Table 19–6.—Mean Age and Sex of Dogs and Cats Anesthetized at Colorado State University, 1955–1957

			Sex			
Species	Total Anesthetized	Mean Age*	M	CM†	F	SF‡
Canine	2406	2.798	967	38	1103	298
Feline	506	1.818	201	33	250	22
Canine and Feline	2912	2.308	1168	71	1353	320

* Of animals with known age. Animals less than 1 year figured as 7 months.
† CM = Castrated male
‡ SF = Spayed female

Table 19–7.—Age of Animals Dying under Anesthesia (Colorado State University, 1955–1957)

Canine		Feline	
Age in Years	Number	Age in Years	Number
<1	1	<1	2
1	6	1	1
2	5	2	1
3	2	3	2
4	2	9	1
5	1	Unknown	2
6	2		
7	3		
Unknown	5		
Mean Age* 3.122 Years		Mean Age* 2.738 Years	

* Of animals with known age. Animals less than 1 year figured as 7 months.

Table 19–8.—Sex of Animals Dying Under Anesthesia Compared to Total Anesthetized (Colorado State University, 1955–1957)

	Sex	Deaths	Total Anesthetized	Per Cent Mortality	Ratio
Canine	Male	11	967	1.137	1:87.9
	Castrated Male	0	38	—	—
	Female	11	1103	0.997	1:100
	Spayed Female	5	298	1.678	1:59.6
Feline	Male	2	201	0.995	1:100
	Castrated Male	0	33	—	—
	Female	5	250	2.00	1:50
	Spayed Female	2	22	9.09	1:11

The mean age of both dogs and cats dying under anesthesia was slightly higher than the mean age for each species (Tables 19–6, 19–7). Mortality in spayed females of both species was higher than in intact animals of either sex (Table 19–8). This suggests that body changes produced by spaying may have an adverse affect on the animal's ability to withstand the stress of anesthesia and surgery. On the other hand, the mean age of all spayed animals (4.465 years) was considerably higher than the mean age of the group.

Breed-wise, the highest mortality was in the cocker spaniel, which at this time was probably the most common purebred seen at the clinic (Table 19–9). Only two brachycephalic dogs died, a bulldog and a pekingese.

Table 19–9.—Breed of Animals Dying Under Anesthesia (Colorado State University, 1955–1957)

Dogs			Cats	
Breed	*Number*		*Breed*	*Number*
Mixed breed	13		Domestic	9
Cocker Spaniel	4			
Chihuahua	2			
Dachshund	2			
Bulldog	1			
Chesapeake Retriever	1			
English Cocker Spaniel	1			
Greyhound	1			
Labrador Retriever	1			
Pekingese	1			

Table 19–10 lists the relationship of physical status to deaths. As expected, the mortality rate increased sharply as physical status deteriorated. There were a wide variety of reasons for poor physical status (Table 19–11). In some instances anesthesia was administered and surgery performed as a last resort on animals which otherwise would have died within hours. The per cent mortality in all categories of physical status was higher in cats than dogs indicating a species intolerance to the anesthetics used.

A high mortality in healthy animals was associated with ovariohysterectomy. Four cats and four dogs died during or following this operation. All eight were anesthetized and operated upon by students. Three of these animals died of hemoperitoneum with associated cardiovascular collapse.

Some deaths occurred from poor judgment on the part of the anesthetist. Examples include administration of morphine, pentobarbital, or pentobarbital-thiamylal to animals in physical status IV (Table 19–12). A more serious error was injection of a gross overdose of pentobarbital. Six animals received glucose which may have deepened barbiturate anesthesia in the presence of shock. One death occurred because of ineptitude in placement of an endotracheal catheter.

Cardiac massage was performed in four dogs. Two of these resumed function only to stop after 8 and 14 hours respectively.

Approximately two-thirds of the fatalities occurred after surgery was completed and the animal was presumably recovering (Table 19–13). Of the 36 animals which died, seven were found dead without previous knowledge of complication. Continuous surveillance of

Table 19–10.—Relationship of Physical Status to Anesthetic Deaths (Colorado State University, 1955–1957)

	Physical Status	Deaths	Total Anesthetized	Per Cent Mortality	Ratio
Canine	I	7	1184	0.591	1:169
	II	7	964	0.726	1:138
	III	2	198	1.010	1:99
	IV	11	60	18.333	1:5.4
Feline	I	4	377	1.061	1:94
	II	1	90	1.111	1:90
	III	1	30	3.333	1:30
	IV	3	9	33.333	1:3

these animals was not maintained. Closer postoperative observation would probably have saved some of these.

Two cats given pentobarbital remained anesthetized 24 and 36 hours and succumbed despite resuscitative measures.

Non-Fatal Complications

Complications requiring some type of corrective measure arose in 5.46% of animals anesthetized with a general anesthetic. Hypopnea and respiratory arrest were most common and occurred with a variety of anesthetic agents (Table 19–14). Shock and hemorrhage were encountered less frequently, occurring in 18 dogs and 3 cats.

A number of animals remained anesthetized for prolonged periods and eventually aroused (Table 19–15). The susceptibility of cats to pentobarbital, and even thiamylal, was very evident; 4.6% of all cats receiving pentobarbital were anesthetized 14 hours or more, whereas only 0.57% of the dogs were so affected. When thiamylal was used in cats, 1.14% were anesthetized 15 hours or longer.

Table 19–11.—Analysis of Anesthetic Deaths in 36 Dogs and Cats (Colorado State University, 1955–1957)

A. Canine

Anesthetic Agent	P.S.*	Sex	Age	Breed	Reason for Anesthesia	Reason for Physical Status	Reason for Death, if Known
Pentobarbital	I	♀	2 yr.	Lab. Ret.	Ovariohysterectomy	Healthy	Hemoperitoneum
		♀	Unknown	Mixed	Ovariohysterectomy	Healthy	Hemoperitoneum
		♀	1 yr.	Mixed	Ovariohysterectomy	Healthy	Respiratory failure followed by cardiac failure. Cardiac massage unsuccessful.
		♀	7 yr.	C. Spaniel	Ovariohysterectomy	Healthy	Gross overdose of anesthetic
		♂	Unknown	Mixed	Liver biopsy	Healthy	Undetermined. Died during night.
	II	Sp ♀	2 yr.	Mixed	Excision of nasal tumor	Nasal tumor	Died on induction. Thoracotomy and cardiac massage, died 14 hours later.
		Sp ♀	2 yr.	Chihuahua	Umbilical herniorraphy	Umbilical hernia	Undetermined. Found dead 13 hours postinduction.
		♂	Unknown	Bulldog	Entropion operation	Entropion	Died before surgery. Endotracheal catheter in esophagus. Cardiac massage unsuccessful.
		♂	2 yr.	Mixed	To perform cerebral angiogram	Anesthetized previous day with pentobarbital and not fully recovered	Died after both carotid arteries injected with diodrast

* P.S. = Physical Status

(394)

Agent	Class	Sex	Age	Breed	Operation	Condition	Outcome
		♂	1 yr.	Mixed	Prostatectomy	Suppurating wound on thorax	Respiratory arrest during operation
	IV	♂	Unknown	Mixed	Castration	Distemper, without systemic symptoms	Undetermined. Died during night.
		♀	4 yr.	Pekingese	Lumbar myelogram	Ruptured intervertebral disc with systemic infection, urinary retention	Died 3 hours following myelogram
		♀	<1 yr.	Mixed	To control convulsions	Distemper with encephalitis	Died 1 hour postinduction
Thiamylal	IV	♀	3 yr.	Cocker Spaniel	Debridement and suturing of severe skin laceration	Severe skin laceration with hemorrhage, shock, internal injuries	Respiratory failure during operation, shock, internal hemorrhage
		♀	1 yr.	Mixed	Ligation of hepatic artery	Systolic murmur, ascites	Cardiac failure
Thiamylal-Ether (Closed system)	I	♂	7 yr.	Mixed	Esophagogastrectomy	Healthy	Surgical shock
	II	Sp ♀	1 yr.	Mixed	Diaphragmatic herniorrhaphy	Had recent surgery	Hemothorax and shock
	III	♀	1 yr.	Chihuahua	Cesarean section	Dystocia, dehydrated, thin	Shock from intrauterine hemorrhage
	IV	♂	2 yr.	C. Spaniel	Diaphragmatic herniorrhaphy	Diaphragmatic hernia with severe dyspnea	Died from shock during surgery
		♂	6 yr.	English C. Spaniel	Herniorrhaphy and partial splenectomy	Traumatic ventral hernia	Shock
		♂	7 yr.	C. Spaniel	Thoracotomy	Debilitated, weak, temperature 104° F.	Undetermined. Died during night

Table 19-11.—Analysis of Anesthetic Deaths in 36 Dogs and Cats (Colorado State University, 1955–1957) (Continued)

Anesthetic Agent	P.S.	Sex	Age	Breed	Reason for Anesthesia	Reason for Physical Status	Reason for Death, if Known
		Sp ♀	7 yr.	Dachshund	Exploratory celiotomy	Nephritis	Died on induction. Toxemia and shock.
		Sp ♀	4 yr.	Mixed	Intestinal anastomosis	Peritonitis from perforated intestine. Vomiting, dehydrated. Temperature 100.4° F.	Shock, toxemia
Thiamylal-Halothane (Closed system)	I	♀	1 yr.	Mixed	Ovariohysterectomy	Healthy	Died during induction of halothane. Probably gross overdose. Cardiac massage, died 8 hours later.
Combuthal	III	♂	5 yr.	Dachshund	Excision of intervertebral disc.	Ruptured intervertebral disc	Respiratory arrest
Pentobarbital-Thiamylal	IV	♂	6 yr.	Chesapeake	Liver biopsy	Generalized neoplastic disease	Undetermined. Died during night.
Ether (Open and closed system)	IV	♀	3 yr.	Greyhound	Ovariohysterectomy	Dystocia with metritis, toxemia, temperature 106° F. Macerated foetuses.	Toxemia. Died on induction.

B. Feline

Anesthetic Agent	P.S.	Sex	Age	Breed	Reason for Anesthesia	Reason for Physical Status	Reason for Death, if Known
Pentobarbital	I	Sp ♀	7 yr.	Domestic	Splenectomy	Healthy	Found dead following morning
		♀	1 yr.	Domestic	Ovariohysterectomy	Healthy	Hemoperitoneum

(396)

							Undetermined. Found dead 9 hours postoperatively.
	II	♀	<1 yr.	Domestic	Overiohysterectomy	Healthy	Died 36 hours following induction without arousing
	III	♀	3 yr.	Domestic	Ovariohysterectomy	Thin but otherwise asymptomatic	Died 24 hours following induction without arousing
Pentobarbital-Ether (Open)	I	Sp ♀	7 yr.	Domestic	Splenectomy	Off feed, dehydrated, infected skin wound, temperature 101.8° F.	Pentobarbital anesthesia lightened so ether administered by cone. Respirations and heartbeat ceased.
Ether (Closed system)	IV	♀	2 yr.	Domestic	Ovariohysterectomy	Healthy	Surgical shock. Common bile duct occluded at duodenum.
Thiamylal	IV	♂	9 yr.	Domestic	Excision of ampulla of Vater, with reimplantation into duodenum	Cachetic, jaundiced, dyspnea	Respiratory arrest. Bladder ruptured on induction.
Thiamylal-Ether (Closed system)	IV	♂	<1 yr.	Domestic	Catheterization of urethra	Urinary retention, uremia, depression	Airway occluded by pus from abscess
		♀	3 yr.	Domestic	Pulmonary lobectomy	Emaciated, dehydrated, temperature 102.8° F. Pulmonary abscess diagnosed radiographically	

Table 19–12.—*Preanesthetic and Anesthetic Agents Used in Fatalities (Colorado State University, 1955–1957)*

A. Canine

Preanesthetic(s)	Anesthetic(s)	P.S.	Fatalities
Atropine	Thiamylal-Ether (C)	I	1
		III	1
		IV	2
	Ether (O and C)	IV	1
Morphine-Atropine	Pentobarbital	I	5
		II	6
		IV	2
	Pentobarbital-Thiamylal	IV	1
	Combuthal	III	1
	Thiamylal-Ether	II	1
		IV	2
	Thiamylal	I	1
		IV	1
None	Thiamylal	IV	1
	Thiamylal-Ether	IV	1

B. Feline

Preanesthetic(s)	Anesthetic(s)	P.S.	Fatalities
Atropine	Pentobarbital	I	1
	Thiamylal-Ether (C)	IV	1
None	Pentobarbital	I	2
		II	1
		III	1
	Pentobarbital-Ether	I	1
	Ether	IV	1
	Thiamylal	IV	1

P.S. = Physical Status
O = Semi-open
C = Closed system with carbon dioxide absorption by soda lime.

Table 19–13.—Time of Death
(Colorado State University, 1955–1957)

Species	Before Surgery	During Surgery	After Surgery
Canine (27 deaths)	6	6	15
Feline (9 deaths)	0	2	7

Table 19–14.—Hypopnea and Respiratory Arrest
(Colorado State University, 1955–1957)

Agent	Hypopnea		Respiratory Arrest	
	Canine	Feline	Canine	Feline
Pentobarbital	32	1	22	1
Thiamylal	2	2	8	—
Thiamylal-Ether	—	—	3	—
Thiamylal-Halothane	—	—	5	—

Table 19–15.—Prolonged Anesthesia
(Colorado State University, 1955–1957)

Duration of Anesthesia in Hours	Pentobarbital		Thiamylal	Thiamylal-Pentobarbital
	Canine	Feline	Feline	Canine
14	3	2	—	—
15	—	—	1	—
16	1	2	—	—
17	—	4	—	—
18	1	2	1	—
19	2	—	—	—
22	—	1	—	—
24	—	1	—	—
30	1	—	—	—
31	—	—	—	1
72	—	1	—	—
Totals	8	13	2	1

Violent excitement on recovery was seen in eight dogs, four greyhounds and four of mixed breeding. These quieted on administration of meperidine.

Other miscellaneous complications included one case of hyperpnea, due to exhaustion of soda-lime during thiamylal-ether anesthesia, and one instance of mechanical failure of a gas machine.

Reflex contraction of the diaphragm synchronous with the heartbeat developed in a dog following a hypoxic episode (Brown and

Lumb, 1958). This was successfully treated by intravenous administration of 1 ml. of 50% calcium gluconate.

Cardiac arrest occurred in one dog and cat. Direct cardiac massage was successful in the dog but it was blind and ataxic thereafter. The cat was treated with external massage and intracardial ephinephrine and made a complete recovery.

References

ALBRECHT, D. T. and BLAKELY, C. L.: Anesthetic Mortality: A 5-Year Survey of the Records of the Angell Memorial Animal Hospital. J.A.V.M.A., *119*, 429, 1951.

BROWN, J. D. and LUMB, W. V.: Tracheal Obstruction in a Dog. J.A.V.M.A., *132*, 521, 1958.

SCHWABE, C. W. and DAVIS, L. R.: Marginal Punched Cards in Veterinary Research. Am. J. Vet. Res., *15*, 634, 1954.

WATERS, R. M. and GILLESPIE, N. A.: Deaths in the Operating Room. Anesthesiology, *5*, 1113, 1944.

APPENDIX A

Sources for Drugs and Equipment
Described in the Text

1. Drugs

Generic Name	Trade Name	Manufacturers
Adrenocorticotropic Hormone	Acthar	5
Amobarbital Sodium	Amytal	33
Amphetamine Sulfate	Amfetasul	44
Anileridine	Leritine	36
Apomorphine Hydrochloride		33
Atropine Sulfate		37
Barbital Sodium		36
Benzoquinonium Chloride	Mytolon	58
Butacaine Sulfate	Butyn Sulfate	1
Calcium Chloride Solution		54
Chloral Hydrate		
(See also Pentobarbital Sodium)		36
Chloralose, Alpha		47
Chlorobutanol	Chloretone	43
Chloroform		36
Chloroprocaine Hydrochloride	Nesacaine	55
Chlorpromazine Hydrochloride	Thorazine	44
Chondodendron tomentosum		
Extract, Purified	Intocostrin	52
Cocaine Hydrochloride		36
Cyclopropane		40
d-Tubocurarine Chloride		54
Decamethonium Bromide	Syncurine	10
Dextran	Expandex	13
Dibucaine Hydrochloride	Nupercaine	11
Dimethyl Tubocurarine	Metubine	33
	Mecostrin	52
Dyclonine Hydrochloride	Dyclone	44
Edrophonium Chloride	Tensilon	26
Epinephrine Hydrochloride	Adrenalin	43
Ether		52
Ethyl Chloride		23
Ethyl Isobutrazine	Diquel	28
Ethylene		40
Gallamine Triethiodide	Flaxedil	2
Gelatin Solution	Intragel	21
Halothane	Fluothane	7
Heparin Sodium		54

(401)

Generic Name	Trade Name	Manufacturers
Hexabiscarbacholine	Imbretil	10
Hexadimethrine Bromide	Polybrene	1
Hexamethonium Bromide	Bistrum Bromide	52
Hexobarbital Sodium	Evipal	58
Hexylcaine Hydrochloride	Cyclaine	36
Hyaluronidase	Wydase	59
Hydroxydione Sodium	Viadril	45
Levallorphan Tartrate	Lorfan	26
Levarterenol Bitartrate	Levophed	58
Lidocaine Hydrochloride	Xylocaine	6
Mepazine	Paxital	56
Meperidine Hydrochloride	Demerol	58
Mephenesin	Myanesin	9
	Tolserol	52
Mephentermine Sulfate	Wyamine Sulfate	59
Mephobarbital Sodium	Mebaral	58
Meprobamate	Equanil	59
Metaraminol Bitartrate	Aramine	36
Methadone Hydrochloride		1
Methamphetamine Hydrochloride	Desoxyn	1
Methetharimide	Mikedimide	42
Methitural Sodium	Neraval	50
Methohexital Sodium	Brevane	14
Methoxamine Hydrochloride	Vasoxyl	10
Methoxyflurane	Penthrane	1
Morphine Sulfate		33
Nalorphine Hydrochloride	Nalline	36
Neostigmine Methylsulfate	Prostigmine	26
Nicotine, Alkaloidal		41
Nitrous Oxide		40
Paraldehyde		36
Pentobarbital Sodium	Nembutal	1
	Toxital (For bears)	28
	Bulk Powder (For euthanasia solution)	22
Pentobarbital Sodium, Chloral Hydrate, and Magnesium Sulfate	Equithesin (For birds)	28
	Sedax (For birds)	15
Pentobarbital Sodium and Thiopental Sodium	Combuthal	16
	Pento-Short	25
Pentylenetetrazol	Metrazol	30
Perphenazine	Trilafon	50
Phenobarbital Sodium		37
Phenylephrine Hydrochloride	Neosynephrine	58
Piperocaine Hydrochloride	Metycaine	33
Potassium Chloride Solution		53
Prednisolone Sodium Succinate	Solu-Delta-Cortef	54
Procaine Hydrochloride	Novocaine	58
Promazine Hydrochloride	Sparine	59
Propiopromazine Hydrochloride	Tranvet	16
Protamine Sulfate		54

Generic Name	Trade Name	Manufacturers
Reserpine	Serpasil	11
Scopolamine Hydrobromide		24
Secobarbital Sodium	Seconal	33
Secobarbital Sodium and		
Mephenesin	Myothesia	35
Succinylcholine Chloride	Anectine	10
	Sucostrin	52
Tetracaine Hydrochloride	Pontocaine	58
Tetraethylammonium Chloride	Etamon	43
Thialbarbitone Sodium	Kemithal	21
Thiamylal Sodium	Surital	43
Thiopental Sodium	Pentothal	1
Tribromoethanol Solution	Avertin	58
Tricaine Methanesulfonate	M. S. 222	48
Trichloroethylene	Trimar	40
Triflupromazine Hydrochloride	Vetame	52
Trimethaphan	Arfonad	26
Urethane		36
Urea and Invert Sugar Solution	Urevert	53
Vinyl Ether	Vinethene	36

2. Equipment

Description or Trade Name	Manufacturers
Air Injector Valve	39
Ambu Resuscitator	19
AVR Unit	46
Blood Pressure Recorder	8
Cap-Chur Gun	41
Cardiac Monitors	
Veling	38
Electrodyne PMS-5	17
Electroencephalograph	18
Endotracheal Catheters	40, 20, 46, 38
Esophageal Stethoscope	40
Ethaire Unit	19
Gas Analyzer	8
Halsan Apparatus	21
Handy Resuscitator	38
Knowles Diffusion Respirator	46
Lewis-Leigh Valve	20
Metal Trough	32, 51
Oximeter	57
Oxygen Chambers and Cages	29, 46
Oxygen Control Unit (electronic)	39
Oxygenator (plastic, disposable, for heart-lung bypass)	53
PR-3 Resuscitator	46
Pumps (for heart-lung bypass)	49, 34, 27
PVS Fluothane Anesthesia Apparatus	46
Reelite(for electric clippers)	4

Description or Trade Name	*Manufacturers*
Soda Lime	40, 38
Stephen-Slater Valve	20
Thermometer (thermistor)	60
Transfusion Equipment (pressurized)	3
Trimar Inhaler	40
Ventimeter	40

Manufacturers

1. Abbott Laboratories
   North Chicago, Illinois
2. American Cyanamid Co.
   Surgical Products Division
   Dansbury, Connecticut
3. Amsco Laboratories
   Erie, Pennsylvania
4. Appleton Electric Co.
   Chicago, Illinois
5. Armour Pharmaceutical Co.
   Kankakee, Illinois
6. Astra Pharmaceutical Products
   Worcester 6, Massachusetts
7. Ayerst Laboratories
   685 3rd Ave.
   New York 17, New York
8. Beckman Instruments Co.
   Palo Alto, California
9. Biorganic Laboratories
   East Patterson, New Jersey
10. Burroughs Wellcome and Co., Inc.
    Tuckahoe, New York
11. Ciba Pharmaceutical Co.
    Summitt, New Jersey
12. City Chemical Corp.
    132 W. 22nd St.
    New York 11, New York
13. Commercial Solvents Corp.
    260 Madison Ave.
    New York 16, New York
14. Corn States Laboratories, Inc.
    Omaha, Nebraska
15. Detroit Veterinary Supply
    Detroit, Michigan
16. Diamond Laboratories, Inc.
    Des Moines, Iowa
17. Electrodyne Co., Inc.
    Norwood, Massachusetts
18. Epsco Medical
    Cambridge, Massachusetts
19. Ethical Veterinary Supply Co.
    34 31st St.
    Long Island City, 6, New York

Manufacturers

20. Foregger Co., Inc. (The)
    Roslyn Heights,
    Long Island, New York
21. Fort Dodge Laboratories
    Fort Dodge, Iowa
22. Ganes Chemical Works
    535 5th Ave.
    New York 17, New York
23. Gebauer Chemical Co.
    Cleveland, Ohio
24. Gotham Pharmaceutical Co., Inc.
    Brooklyn, New York
25. Haver-Lockhart Laboratories
    Kansas City, Missouri
26. Hoffman-LaRoche, Inc.
    Nutley 10, New Jersey
27. International Medical Instrument
    Corp.
    Stoneham, Massachusetts
28. Jensen-Salsbery Laboratories, Inc.
    Kansas City, Missouri
29. Kirschner Manufacturing Co.
    Vashon, Washington
30. Knoll Pharmaceutical Co.
    Orange, New Jersey
31. Lederle Laboratories
    Division of American Cyanamid Co.
    Pearl River, New York
32. Leighton, R. L. (Dr.)
    150 Thornbury Rd.
    Scarsdale, New York
33. Lilly, Eli and Company
    Indianapolis, Indiana
34. Mark Company (The)
    Randolph, Massachusetts
35. Massengill, S. E., Co.
    Bristol, Tennessee
36. Merck, Sharpe & Dohme
    Philadelphia 1, Pennsylvania
37. Moore Kirk Laboratories, Inc.
    Worcester 1, Massachusetts

Manufacturers

38. National Cylinder Gas, Division of Chemetron Corp.
840 N. Michigan Ave.
Chicago 11, Illinois
39. O. E. M. Division
Shampaine Industries, Inc.
1115 Lousons Rd.
Union, New Jersey
40. Ohio Chemical and Surgical Equipment Co.
1400 E. Washington Ave.
Madison 10, Wisconsin
41. Palmer Chemical and Equipment Co., Inc.
Atlanta 9, Georgia
42. Panray/Parlam Corp.
Englewood, New Jersey
43. Parke, Davis & Company
Joseph Campau Ave. at the River
Detroit 32, Michigan
44. Pitman-Moore Company
Indianapolis 6, Indiana
45. Pfizer, Charles & Co., Inc.
New York 17, New York
46. Professional Veterinary Services, Inc.
2855 E. 11th Ave.
Hialeah, Florida
47. Prolabo
12 Rue Pelee,
Paris 11, France

Manufacturers

48. Sandoz Pharmaceuticals
Hanover, New Jersey
49. Sarns, Inc.
Ann Arbor, Michigan
50. Schering Corp.
Bloomfield, New Jersey
51. Schroer Manufacturing Co.
2217 Campbell St.
Kansas City 8, Missouri
52. Squibb, E. R., & Sons
745 5th Ave.
New York 22, New York
53. Travenol Laboratories, Inc.
Morton Grove, Illinois
54. Upjohn Co. (The)
301 Henrietta St.
Kalamazoo 99, Michigan
55. Wallace Laboratories
Half Acre Rd.
Cranbury, New Jersey
56. Warner-Chilcott
Morris Plains, New Jersey
57. Waters Corp. (The)
Rochester, Minnesota
58. Winthrop Laboratories
1450 Broadway
New York 18, New York
59. Wyeth Laboratories
Box 8299, Philadelphia 1,
Pennsylvania
60. Yellow Springs Instrument Co., Inc.
Yellow Springs, Ohio

APPENDIX B

Standard Values and Equivalents

METRIC WEIGHTS

1 gram (1 gm.)	=	Weight of 1 cc. water at 4° C.
1000 gm.	=	1 kilogram (kg.)
0.1 gm.	=	1 decigram (dg.)
0.01 gm.	=	1 centigram (cg.)
0.001 gm.	=	1 milligram (mg.)
0.001 mg.	=	1 microgram (ug.)

METRIC VOLUMES

1 liter (L.)	=	1 cubic decimeter or 1000 cubic centimeters (cc.)
0.001 liter	=	1 milliliter (ml.)

SOLUTION EQUIVALENTS

1 part in 10	=	10.00 % (1 ml. contains 100 mg.)
1 part in 50	=	2.00 % (1 ml. contains 20 mg.)
1 part in 100	=	1.00 % (1 ml. contains 10 mg.)
1 part in 200	=	0.50 % (1 ml. contains 5 mg.)
1 part in 500	=	0.20 % (1 ml. contains 2 mg.)
1 part in 1,000	=	0.10 % (1 ml. contains 1 mg.)
1 part in 1,500	=	0.066% (1 ml. contains 0.66 mg.)
1 part in 2,600	=	0.038% (1 ml. contains 0.38 mg.)
1 part in 5,000	=	0.02 % (1 ml. contains 0.20 mg.)
1 part in 50,000	=	0.002% (1 ml. contains 0.02 mg.)

The number of milligrams in 1 milliliter of any solution of known percentage strength is obtained by moving the decimal one place to the right.

APOTHECARIES' OR TROY WEIGHT

(Used in Prescriptions)

1 pound (lb.)	= 12 ounces	= 5,760 grains
1 ounce (℥)	= 8 drams	= 480 grains
1 dram (ʒ)	= 60 grains	

Apothecaries' Volume

1 pint (O)	= 16 fluid ounces	
1 fluid ounce (fl. ℥)	= 8 fluid dram	= 480 minims (min.)
1 fluid dram (fl. ʒ)	= 60 minims	

AVOIRDUPOIS OR IMPERIAL WEIGHT

(Used in Commerce in the United States and in the British Pharmacopeia)

Grain	= same as Troy grain.	
Ounce (oz.)	=	$437\frac{1}{2}$ grains.
Pound (lb.)	= 16 oz.	= 7000 grains.
Ton	= 2000 lb.	

IMPERIAL VOLUME

		Apothecaries' System
Minims (min.)	=	0.96 ℳ
Fluidrachm (fl. dr.)	= 60 min.	= 0.96 fl.ℨ
Fluidounce (fl. oz.)	= 8 drachms	= 0.96 fl.ℨ
Pint (O)	= 20 fluidounces	= 1.2 O
Gallon (C)	= 8 pints	= 1.2 C

APPROXIMATE EQUIVALENT WEIGHTS

1 kilogram	=	2.2 Avoirdupois or Imperial pounds
1 kilogram	=	2.6 Apothecary or Troy pounds
1 gram	=	15 (15.4) grains
1 milligram	=	1/60 (1/64) grain
1 ounce	=	30 grams
(Avoirdupois or Imperial	=	28.350 grams)
(Apothecary or Troy	=	31.1035 grams)
1 dram	=	4 grams
1 grain	=	60 milligrams

VOLUMES

1 liter	=	1 quart
1 milliliter or cubic centimeter	=	15 minims
1 pint	=	500 cubic centimeters
1 fluid ounce	=	30 cubic centimeters
(Imperial	=	28.412 cubic centimeters)
(Apothecary	=	29.574 cubic centimeters)
1 fluid dram	=	4 cubic centimeters

Appendix B

EQUIVALENTS OF CENTIGRADE AND FAHRENHEIT THERMOMETRIC SCALES

Centigrade Degree	Fahrenheit Degree	Centigrade Degree	Fahrenheit Degree
—17	+ 1.4	14	57.2
—16	3.2	15	59.0
—15	5.0	16	60.8
—14	6.8	17	62.6
—13	8.6	18	64.4
—12	10.4	19	66.2
—11	12.2	20	68.0
—10	14.0	21	69.8
— 9	15.8	22	71.6
— 8	17.6	23	73.4
— 7	19.4	24	75.2
— 6	21.2	25	77.0
— 5	23.0	26	78.8
— 4	24.8	27	80.6
— 3	26.6	28	82.4
— 2	28.4	29	84.2
— 1	30.2	30	86.0
0	32.0	31	87.8
+ 1	33.8	32	89.6
2	35.6	33	91.4
3	37.4	34	93.2
4	39.2	35	95.0
5	41.0	36	96.8
6	42.8	37	98.6
7	44.6	38	100.4
8	46.4	39	102.2
9	48.2	40	104.0
10	50.0	41	105.8
11	51.8	42	107.6
12	53.6	43	109.4
13	55.4	44	111.2
		45	113.0

GAS DENSITIES

(Wt. of Unit Vol.)

22.4 liters of any gas is equal to its molecular weight in grams at a pressure of 760 mm. of mercury and 0° C.

MOLECULAR WEIGHTS

Ethylene	=	28 gm.
Air	=	29 gm.
Oxygen	=	32 gm.
Cyclopropane	=	42 gm.
Nitrous oxide	=	44 gm.
Carbon dioxide	=	44 gm.
Ether	=	74 gm.
Chloroform	=	119 gm.

(From A.M.A. *Fundamentals of Anesthesia*. 3d ed. W. B. Saunders Co., 1954.)

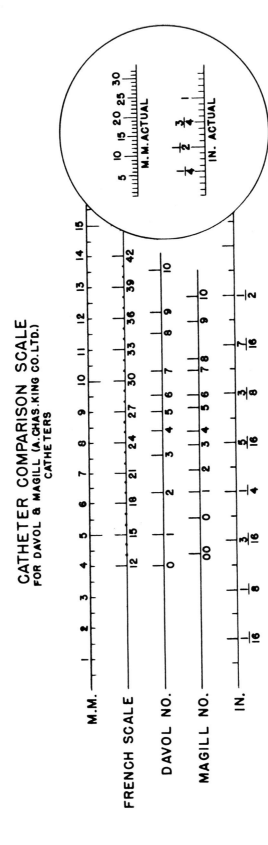

To compare catheter sizes place a rule on one of the calibrations and check along the edge for the corresponding figures. The scale is enlarged eight times for easy reading. An actual size scale is shown in the circle if measurements are required. (Courtesy of The British Oxygen Co. Ltd., London)

APPENDIX C

Euthanasia Solution

Pentobarbital sodium, powder	259.2 gm.
Ethyl alcohol, 95%	400.0 ml.
Sodium hydroxide solution, 10%	80.0 ml.
Hot water q.s.	2000.0 ml.

Give 1 ml./5 lb. intravenously, more if necessary.

INDEX

A

A.C.E. MIXTURE, 11, 125
Acid-Base balance, 29, 51–52
Acidosis, 51–52
ACTH (See *Adrenocorticotrophic hormone*)
Adrenalin (See *Epinephrine hydrochloride*)
Adrenocortical steroids, 29, 343–347, 357, 402
    in cardiac arrest, 375
    in shock, 362–364
Adrenocorticotrophic hormone, 343, 357, 362, 401
Aftercare, 378–380
Air, injector valve, 70, 403
    pendulum, 62
Alcohol, 10, 251–252
    in frogs, 273
Alkalosis, 51–52
Ambu resuscitator, 85, 146, 403
Amidone (See *Methadone hydrochloride*)
Amobarbital sodium, 177, 401
    effect of sex, 20
    in baboons, 294
    in fish, 269–270
    in rats, 20
Amphetamine sulfate, 341–342, 401
Amphibians, 180, 220, 273–274
Amytal (See *Amobarbital sodium*)
Analeptics, 349–352
    amphetamine sulfate, 341–342
Analgesia, 9
Anectine (See *Succinylcholine*)
Anemia, 29, 125, 330. (Also see *Blood*)
Anesthesia (Also see *General anesthesia*)
    definition, 9
    emergencies during, 355–377
    epidural (See *Epidural anesthesia*)
    facilities and equipment, 32–36 (Also see *Equipment*)
    factors altering, 18–22
    fatalities from, 382–393
    general (See *General anesthesia*)
    history of small animal, 10–12
    indications and contraindications, 26–27
    inhalation, 16 (Also see *Inhalation anesthetics*)
    monitoring, 311–328
    nerve block (See *Nerve block anesthesia*)
    non-fatal complications, 393–400
    personnel for, 36
    positioning of patient, 29–31
    prolonged, 378, 393

Anesthesia, reasons for administration, 15
    risk of, 385
    selection of, 23–28
    spinal (See *Spinal anesthesia*)
    theories of, 12–15
    types, 16–17
Anileridine, 109–110, 401
Animals, laboratory and zoo, 269–310
    (Also see respective species)
Anoxia, 52 (Also see *Hypoxia*)
Antelope, 292, 302–304
Antibiotics, effect on anesthesia, 22
    in patient preparation, 28
    in shock, 28, 364
    procaine penicillin toxicity in parakeets, 277
Anticholinergics, 93–95. (Also see Specific drugs)
Anticurariform agents, 232 (Also see *Benzoquinonium chloride, Neostigmine methylsulfate*)
Apnea, 355–356
    carotid body, 44
    definition, 37
Apomorphine hydrochloride, 106, 401
Aramine (See *Metaraminol bitartrate*)
Arfonad (See *Trimethaphan*)
Ascites, 29
Ascorbic acid, deficiency, 13, 21
    effect on brain metabolism, 14
Asphyxia, 10
Atropine sulfate, 93–94, 401
    for laryngospasm, 357
    for salivation and mucus, 357
    in birds, 275
    in deer, 297
    in goats, 296
    in guinea pigs, 283
    in sheep, 296
    in swine, 294
Avertin (See *Tribromoethanol solution*)
AVR unit, 91, 148–152, 403

B

BABOONS (See *Primates*)
Barbital sodium, 172–176, 401
Barbitone (See *Barbital sodium*)
Barbiturates, 170–195
    addiction, 172
    administration, intramuscular, 193
        intraperitoneal, 179, 193

(411)